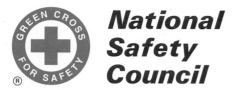

National Safety Council

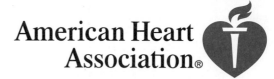

American Heart Association®

Fighting Heart Disease and Stroke

HEARTSAVER FACTS™

FIRST AID   AED   CPR   TRAINING   SYSTEM

JONES AND BARTLETT PUBLISHERS

Sudbury, Massachusetts

BOSTON   TORONTO   LONDON   SINGAPORE

American Heart Association
National Center
7272 Greenville Avenue
Dallas, Texas 75231-4596
800-242-8721
www.americanheart.org

Care has been taken to confirm the accuracy of the information presented and to describe generally accepted practices. However, the authors, editors, and publisher are not responsible for errors or omissions or for any consequences from application of the information in this publication, and make no warranty, express or implied, with respect to the contents of this publication.

World Headquarters
Jones and Bartlett Publishers
40 Tall Pine Drive
Sudbury, MA 01776
978-443-5000
info@jbpub.com
www.jbpub.com/FACTS

Jones and Bartlett Publishers
Canada
2406 Nikanna Road
Mississauga, ON L5C 2W6
CANADA

Jones and Bartlett Publishers
International
Barb House, Barb Mews
London W6 7PA
UK

Library of Congress Cataloging-in-Publication Data

Heartsaver facts : first aid, AED, CPR training system / National
     Safety Council, American Heart Association.
          p.   cm.
     Includes index.
     ISBN 07637-0954-9 (soft/perfect bound)
     1. First aid in illness and injury. 2. CPR (First aid)
3. Defibrillators.   I. National Safety Council.   II. American Heart
Association.
     RC86.7.H387   1998
     616.02   52—dc21   98-43210
                                                       CIP

Printed in the United States of America

02   10 9 8 7 6 5 4 3

Photo credits:
     Bruce Argyle, M.D.
     H.B. Bectal, M.D.
     Michael D. Ellis
     Murray P. Hamlet, D.V.M.
     Axel W. Hoke, M.D.
     Sherman A. Minton, M.D.
     Eugene Roberston, M.D.
     Richard C. Ruffalo, D.M.D.
     Jeffrey Saffle, M.D.
     Clifford C. Snyder, M.D.
     Charles E. Stewart, M.D.

The American Heart Association and the National Safety Council gratefully acknowledge the many individuals, agencies, and organizations who contributed to the development of the HEARTSAVER *FACTS*™ program.

Contributors to the American Heart Association CPR and AED section of this text:

Editors
     Tom P. Aufderheide, MD
     Edward R. Stapleton, EMT-P
     Mary Fran Hazinski, RN, MSN

Senior Science Editor
     Richard O. Cummins, MD, MPH, MSc

Subcommittee on Basic Life Support, 1997–1998
     Tom P. Aufderheide, MD, Chair
     Lance B. Becker, MD, Immediate Past Chair
     Thomas A. Barnes, EdD, RRT
     Robert A. Berg, MD
     Nisha Chandra, MD
     Ahamed H. Idris, MD
     L. Murray Lorance, EMT-D
     Keith Lurie, MD
     Graham Nichol, MD, MPH
     James W. Parham, Jr, MA, RN
     Paul E. Pepe, MD, MPH
     Edward R. Stapleton, EMT-P
     Wanchun Tang, MD
     Terence D. Valenzuela, MD

Special Contributors

Alidene M. Doherty, RN
Anita Bailey, NREMT-P
Terence D. Valenzuela, MD
Stacey Baker
L. Murray Lorance, EMT-D
Jim Scappini, EMT-D
Ronald W. Quinsey
William H. Montgomery, MD
AHA volunteers of Florida and Texas who participated in pilot evaluations of the Heartsaver AED course
AHA ECC Subcommittees on Advanced Cardiac Life Support, Pediatric Resuscitation, and Program Administration 1997–1998

Reviewers

Donald Gordon, PhD, MD
Jo Haag, RN
Joanne L. Hirsch
Peter Kudenchuk, MD
Mary E. Mancini, RN, MSN
Eric Niegelberg, EMT-P
Greg Wayrich, EMT-P
John L. Zirkle

Contributors to the National Safety Council first aid section of this text:

Editors

Alton L. Thygerson, EdD
Tom Lachaas

Reviewers/Special Contributors

American Academy of Ophthalmology
American Academy of Orthopaedic Surgeons
American Academy of Safety Education
American Alliance for Health, Physical Education, Recreation, and Dance
American Burn Association
American Camping Association
American Civil Defense Association
American College of Surgeons
American Dental Association
American Diabetes Association
American Equine Association
American Medical Association
American Trauma Association
Aquatic Exercise Association
Association for the Advancement of Automotive Medicine
Boy Scouts of America
Canadian Association of Fire Chiefs
Ellis & Associates
Emergency Nurses Association
Emergency Response Institute
Epilepsy Foundation
Girl Scouts, USA

International Association of Fire Fighters
International Society of Fire Service Instructors
Medic Alert Foundation
Mine Safety and Health Administration
National Academy of Emergency Medical Dispatch
National Association of EMS Physicians
National Athletic Trainers Association
National Center on Child Abuse and Neglect
National Cotton Ginners' Association
National Emergency Number Association
National Highway Traffic Safety Administration
National Institute of Burn Medicine
National Oceanic and Atmospheric Administration
National Recreation and Park Association
National Registry of Emergency Medical Technicians
National Rescue Consultants
National Ski Patrol
Occupational Safety and Health Administration
Prevent Blindness America
U.S. Air Force
U.S. Army
U.S. Centers for Disease Control and Prevention
U.S. Coast Guard
U.S. Consumer Product Safety Commission
U.S. Department of Health and Human Services
U.S. Public Health Service
Wilderness Medical Society
Young Men's Christian Association

Training organizations who pilot tested the first aid materials:

Arizona Chapter National Safety Council
Phoenix, AZ

Safety Center, Inc.
Sacramento, CA

Central Florida Chapter,
National Safety Council
Orlando, FL

Safety & Health Council of Western Missouri and Kansas
Kansas City, MO

Massachusetts Safety Council, Inc.
Braintree, MA

Safety Council of Greater St. Louis
St. Louis, MO

Northeastern New York Safety and Health Council
Albany, NY

Greater Los Angeles Chapter
National Safety Council
Los Angeles, CA

Colorado Safety Association
  Denver, CO

Hoosier Safety Council
  Indianapolis, IN

Safety Council of Maryland
  Baltimore, MD

Minnesota Safety Council, Inc.
  St. Paul, MN

New Jersey State Safety Council
  Cranford, NJ

Safety Council of Northeastern Ohio
  Youngstown, OH

Safety and Health Council of North Carolina
  Charlotte, NC

Western Pennsylvania Safety Council
  Monroeville, PA

The Palmetto Chapter
  National Safety Council
  Irmo, SC

Texas Safety Association, Inc.
  Pflugerville, TX

Utah Safety Council
  Salt Lake City, UT

Evergreen Safety Council
  Seattle, WA

Lehigh Valley Chapter
  National Safety Council
  Bethlehem, PA

ABOUT THIS COURSE

You can save the life of a loved one, friend, coworker, or a citizen in your community with the skills you learn in the HEARTSAVER *FACTS*™ course. This course was developed through a partnership between the American Heart Association and the National Safety Council. Some of you will be taking this course for general information, while others will be taking it because of an expectation to respond to an emergency at home or work.

What makes this course unique is that it combines the strengths of two of the best-respected national organizations to provide you with the knowledge and skills necessary to give appropriate care for both the most serious situations that you might encounter and those most likely to occur.

Part One of the HEARTSAVER *FACTS* course teaches the basic techniques of adult CPR and the use of an AED. You will also learn about using barrier devices in CPR and giving care for someone who is choking. This section follows the AHA guidelines for performing CPR and using an AED. These are integrated skills that you can learn best in a minimum 3½-hour course. The course instructor may adjust some details of CPR and AED operation to fit your particular setting and the brand of AED you are using.

The first half of this course was developed by the American Heart Association to support the growing movement toward public access defibrillation. In public access defibrillation, or "witness defibrillation," the person who recognizes someone in cardiac arrest gives the victim defibrillation shocks. The "witness" is often a lay rescuer, perhaps the victim's friend or coworker. The automated external defibrillator (AED) is a new and important device used in emergency cardiovascular care. AEDs are accurate, easy to operate, and have saved many lives. They can be used effectively by laypeople with minimal training.

You may work in a place where someone has decided to start a public access defibrillation program. More and more people like you who are trained in cardiopulmonary resuscitation (CPR) also need to learn how to use AEDs. In many communities AEDs are in use by firefighters, police, security guards, commercial airline crews, trained laypersons, and family members of cardiac patients who are at high risk for cardiac arrest. Both early CPR and early defibrillation—two links in the Chain of Survival—save lives. Getting the defibrillator—and someone to operate it—to a collapsed person in the first few minutes is the first step in achieving early defibrillation and saving a life.

Public access defibrillation using AEDs is a new and dynamic field. In most states, public access defibrillation is so new that legislators must revise state laws and regulations to allow defibrillation by nonprofessionals or "Good Samaritans." The information in this course will change over time. The AHA will continue to reevaluate the guidelines for CPR and AED use and revise them when necessary. You can stay informed about any changes through the AHA's newsletter *Currents in Emergency Care*.

Part Two of the **HEARTSAVER *FACTS*** course teaches first aid procedures for injuries, including bleeding control; bone, joint, and muscle injuries; burns; and specific injuries to the head, chest, abdomen, pelvis, and spine. It also addresses sudden illnesses, including seizures, diabetic emergencies, poisoning, bites and stings, and heat and cold emergencies. These are integrated skills that you can learn in a minimum 4-hour course. The course instructor may adjust some details of the course to fit your particular setting and expectation to respond to emergencies.

The second half of this course was developed by the National Safety Council to teach basic level first aid procedures. Most people will eventually find themselves in a situation requiring first aid, either for themselves or for others. Throughout the world, injuries are the leading cause of death through middle age. This does not even consider the millions more who suffer less severe injuries or illnesses requiring medical care each year. Properly applied, first aid can mean the difference between life and death, rapid recovery and long hospitalization, or temporary versus permanent disability.

This book contains several features designed to help you learn the essential skills of CPR, AED operation, and first aid. These features include learning objectives, review questions, and skill review sheets. These help make learning easier and more complete. Read the chapter objectives to help you understand essential information in the chapter. When you finish reading the chapter, answer the questions at the end of each chapter.

The skill sheets and flowcharts found throughout this text will help you to successfully perform the critical skills in the course and apply your knowledge to action steps.

The major knowledge objectives of the **HEARTSAVER *FACTS*** course are:

1. Describe the links in the AHA Chain of Survival

2. Describe how to activate the local emergency medical services (EMS) system

3. Recognize the signs and symptoms of 4 major emergencies:
   a. Heart attack
   b. Cardiac arrest
   c. Stroke
   d. Foreign-body airway obstruction

4. Recognize the signs and symptoms of the following sudden illnesses and injuries:
   a. Poisoning
   b. Allergic reaction
   c. Seizures
   d. Serious bone, joint, or muscle injuries

5. Describe how to provide care for wounds, burns, and bone and muscle injuries

6. Describe how to provide care for sudden illnesses

The major skills objectives of the **HEARTSAVER *FACTS*** course are:

1. Demonstrate the following skills using an adult manikin, AED (or suitable trainer model), pocket mask, and telephone:
   a. Calling 911 and getting the AED
   b. Rescue breathing using mouth-to-mouth and mouth-to-face mask techniques
   c. One-rescuer adult CPR
   d. Relief of adult foreign-body airway obstruction
   e. Safe defibrillation with an AED within less than 90 seconds of AED placement at the training manikin's side (less than 90 seconds is the maximum acceptable time)

2. Demonstrate how to troubleshoot the most common problems you might encounter while using an AED

3. Using first aid supplies and equipment, demonstrate how to:
   a. Assess an injured or suddenly ill victim
   b. Control bleeding
   c. Immobilize a serious bone, joint, or muscle injury

We wish you success as you learn the skills of **HEARTSAVER *FACTS***. When you complete the course, you will be better prepared to face future emergencies with powerful tools and effective skills.

CONTENTS

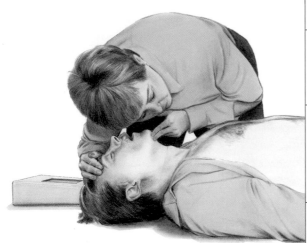

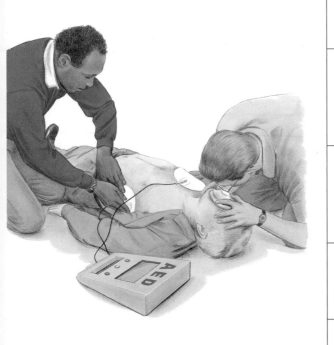

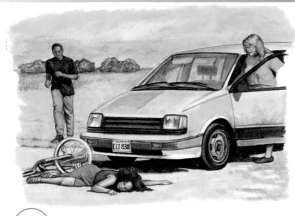

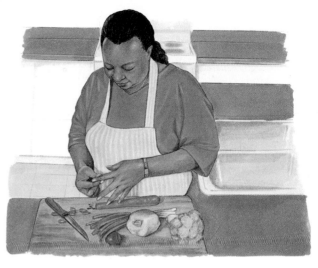

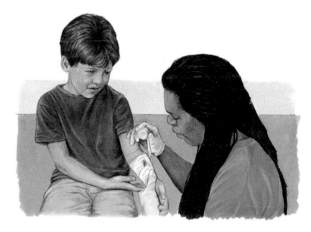

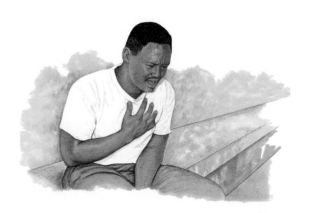

On August 15, 2000, the AHA released the new *Guidelines 2000 for Cardiopulmonary Resuscitation and Emergency Cardiovascular Care: International Consensus on Science.* These evidence-based science guidelines recommended several changes in the teaching and practice of BLS for lay rescuers to simplify the steps and increase the effectiveness of CPR. This page and the next summarize those changes.

When the AHA revises the Heartsaver AED Course materials in 2001, all new science changes will be incorporated into all the course materials. Until the release of the revised materials the instructor should reproduce these 2 pages, and participants should insert them into their course manuals and use these pages to correct their manual. General changes in science are provided below, followed by a list of the pages in the student manual where changes should be made to reflect the new recommendations.

MAJOR CHANGES IN CPR RECOMMENDATIONS

- **For the adult victim the lay rescuer should provide rescue breaths over 2 seconds rather than over 1½ to 2 seconds.** This slower delivery of rescue breaths should ensure that the breaths enter the victim's lungs rather than the stomach.

- **The lay rescuer no longer checks for a pulse to determine if chest compressions and use of an AED are required.** New science has documented that the pulse check is a very unreliable indicator of the presence or absence of cardiac arrest and that rescuer attempts to locate a pulse may delay the performance of chest compressions. **The rescuer should look for "signs of circulation" rather than a pulse to determine if chest compressions and use of an AED are required.** The absence of signs of circulation is one

of the signs of cardiac arrest, and the rescuer should perform chest compressions and attach an AED when signs of circulation are absent. When reviewing the student manual or observing videos, participants should replace **check for a pulse** with **check for signs of circulation** in every instance.

Signs of circulation include a check for **normal breathing, coughing, or movement.** To check for signs of circulation you should place your ear next to the victim's mouth and nose and look, listen, and feel for normal breathing or coughing. Then quickly scan the victim to check for movement. If the victim is not breathing normally, not coughing, and not moving, you should perform chest compressions or use the AED as instructed in the manual or video.

- **The new rate for chest compressions should be approximately 100 compressions per minute rather than 80 to 100 compressions per minute.** New science supports a faster compression rate to achieve optimal circulation during the performance of CPR.

- **The new ratio for chest compressions during 2-rescuer CPR should be 15 compressions to 2 breaths for 1 or 2 rescuers.** New science supports longer series of compressions to achieve optimal circulation during the performance of CPR.

- **New science supports simplification of the approach to lay rescuer management of foreign-body airway obstruction in the unresponsive victim.** If the lay rescuer encounters a responsive victim of FBAO who becomes unresponsive or if the rescuer suspects an airway obstruction in an unresponsive victim, the lay rescuer should perform CPR. Each time the airway is opened, the rescuer looks for an obstructing object in the back of the throat. If the rescuer sees an object, she or he should remove it. This simplification should improve the learning and retention of core CPR skills.

PAGES IN PARTICIPANT MANUAL ON WHICH TO MAKE SCIENCE CHANGES

Participants may wish to make corrections in this manual to reflect the 2000 science changes.

Science Changes	Manual Page	Suggested Revision
Simplification of procedure for managing an unconscious victim of foreign-body airway obstruction	13, 26-28	**Replace the complete procedure for the unresponsive/unconscious FBAO victim with the following:** If a responsive/conscious victim of FBAO becomes unresponsive/unconscious or if you encounter an unsuspected airway obstruction in an unresponsive victim, perform CPR. After attempting and reattempting ventilation during the performance of CPR, continue the sequence of chest compressions and ventilations. Each time the airway is opened, look for an obstructing object in the back of the throat. If you see an object, remove it.
Increased time for delivery of rescue breaths for adult victims	21 (box), 91, 94-95	**Replace rescue breaths taking 1½ to 2 seconds with breaths that take longer:** Give 2 slow breaths (take 2 seconds for each breath).
Signs of cardiac arrest in adults: Unresponsiveness and breathlessness are still valid signs of cardiac arrest. However, "pulse" is replaced with "signs of circulation."	10-11, 20* (*change occurs several times), 21, 22*, 29*, 30*, 37, 41*, 42, 45*, 46*, 52*, 53*, 54*, 57*, 62*, 63*, 79, 80*, 83, 91*, 337, 93*, 94, 98, 101, 102*, 104*, 105*	Replace "no pulse" with "no signs of circulation (no normal breathing, coughing, or movement in response to the 2 rescue breaths)." Replace "pulse" or "pulse present" with "signs of circulation" or "signs of circulation present."
All references to checking for a pulse (for adult and pediatric victims) should be changed to checking for signs of circulation (normal breathing, coughing, or movement)	18, 20*, 21*, 22*, 30*, 33, 40*, 41*, 43, 48, 52*, 53*, 57, 91, 101, 102*, 103, 104*, 105*	Whenever the text instructs rescuers to "check for a pulse," lay rescuers should substitute "check for signs of circulation (normal breathing, coughing, or movement)."
Increased rate of chest compression for adult victims	22	Replace compress "at a rate of 80 to 100" with "at a rate of approximately 100 per minute."
Compression-ventilation ratio for 2-rescuer CPR	24	The ratio for 2-rescuer CPR is 15 compressions to 2 ventilations (same as 1-rescuer CPR).
Skills performance sheet	91	In HS-AED skills performance sheet, substitute "check for signs of circulation (normal breathing, coughing, movement)" for "check for pulse" and "check for carotid pulse" as an indication to begin chest compressions and attach the AED for performance criteria and critical actions.

Part

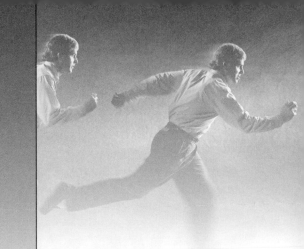

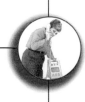

EARLY ACTION SAVES LIVES

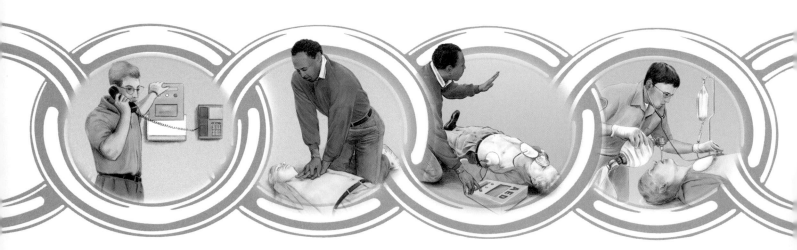

CONTENTS

1

Every year

250,000

adult

Americans

die from

cardiac arrest.

LEARNING OBJECTIVES

After reading this chapter, you should be able to

1. Name the links in the AHA adult Chain of Survival and discuss the role you play in the chain.
2. List the signs of these 4 major emergencies:
   a. Heart attack
   b. Cardiac arrest
   c. Stroke
   d. Airway obstruction by a foreign body (conscious choking)

STUDY QUESTIONS

As you read this chapter, try to answer these questions:

Chain of Survival

1. There are 4 links in the AHA Chain of Survival. What are they?
2. In the Heartsaver AED Course you are learning to perform the critical actions that compose 3 of the 4 links in the Chain of Survival. What are they?
3. Why is it important that *you* defibrillate with an AED rather than wait for emergency rescuers who are better trained than you are?

Heart Attack

1. How do people who are having a heart attack usually describe the pain?
2. Where is this pain usually located?
3. How long does the pain of a heart attack usually last?

Cardiac Arrest

1. There are 3 major signs of a cardiac arrest. What are they?

Stroke

1. How is the headache caused by a stroke often described?
2. What abnormalities may you see in facial muscles, arm movement, and speech in a person with stroke?
3. When should you activate the EMS system if you think someone has had a stroke?

Foreign-Body Airway Obstruction (Conscious Choking)

1. What is the universal sign that a person who cannot speak may use to indicate that he or she is choking?
2. A choking person says, "Help me! I'm choking!" How do you help him or her?
3. A person who is choking falls to the floor unconscious. How do you treat this person?

Cardiovascular disease is the single greatest cause of death in the United States. Every year more than 480,000 adult Americans die of a **heart attack** or its complications. About half (250,000) of these deaths result from **sudden cardiac arrest,** a complication of heart attack. A cardiac arrest can occur within seconds of the heart attack, before the victim arrives at the hospital. It will result in death unless immediate emergency treatment is provided.

The victim of an emergency such as a heart attack, cardiac arrest, stroke, or foreign-body airway obstruction can be saved if people at the scene act quickly to start the **Chain of Survival.** In this chapter you will learn the critical actions that compose the 4 links in the AHA Chain of Survival. You will learn how to recognize the symptoms of a heart attack, cardiac arrest, stroke, and foreign-body airway obstruction (choking) and when to call 911.

Onc link in the Chain of Survival is **cardiopulmonary resuscitation, or CPR.** With CPR you provide oxygen-rich blood to the brain and heart until defibrillation and more advanced care can be given.

Another link in the Chain of Survival is **defibrillation.** Defibrillation delivers an electric current ("shock") to the heart to stop abnormal electric activity. This allows the heart to resume normal function. You will learn to provide defibrillation using an **automated external defibrillator (AED).** An AED is a device that evaluates the victim's heart rhythm, generates and delivers an electric charge, and reevaluates the heart rhythm. All AEDs provide both voice and visual prompts to lead you through important rescue steps.

When you recognize an emergency, the first three links in the Chain of Survival are in **your** *hands.* **You** *call 911.* **You** *begin CPR.* **You** *use the AED.*

THE AHA CHAIN OF SURVIVAL SYMBOL

The AHA Chain of Survival symbol (**FIGURE 1**) depicts the critical actions required to treat any life-threatening emergency, including heart attack, cardiac arrest, stroke, and airway obstruction by a foreign body.

Once you recognize an emergency, you should *immediately*

- **Call 911** to activate the emergency medical services (EMS) system and send someone to get the AED.
- **Begin CPR.**
- **Use the AED.**
- **Transfer to advanced care** (when skilled EMS rescuers arrive).

You must know when to activate the Chain of Survival. You must recognize that an emergency exists. When you recognize the emergency, the first 3 links — call 911, begin CPR, and use the AED — are in your hands. *You* perform these actions. *You* connect the links that increase a person's chance of survival. Skilled emergency professionals will respond to the 911 call. You can then transfer the person to them for advanced care.

To save people with heart attack, cardiac arrest, or stroke, *each set of actions or link in the Chain of Survival must be performed as soon as possible*. If any link in the chain is weak, delayed, or missing, the chances of survival are lessened.

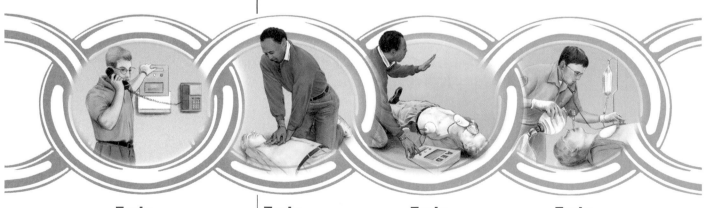

| Early Access | Early CPR | Early Defibrillation | Early Advanced Care |

FIGURE 1
The AHA Chain of Survival. The 4 links or actions in the chain are (1) call 911 and get the AED, (2) begin CPR, (3) use the AED, and (4) transfer to advanced care.

THE LINKS IN THE CHAIN OF SURVIVAL

Recognize an Emergency

First, you or other witnesses must recognize the emergency. You must recognize the warning signs of a heart attack, cardiac arrest, stroke, or choking. *Anyone* who is *unresponsive* should receive emergency care. Heart attack, cardiac arrest, stroke, and foreign-body airway obstruction can each cause unresponsiveness. Although many conditions — not just cardiac arrest — can cause unresponsiveness, *all* unresponsive victims will benefit from activation of the Chain of Survival.

Call 911 (or the EMS System in Your Area) and Get the AED

As soon as an emergency is recognized, call 911. Keep the AED near the telephone in the home, worksite, or public building. The person who calls 911 can return with the AED.

When you or another rescuer calls 911, let the emergency medical dispatcher ask you questions. While the dispatcher interviews you, he or she will enter the data on a computer. The information you give will be relayed to a response team. Answer in short, specific replies, giving only the requested information. The dispatcher will probably ask

- **"What is your emergency?"** You might answer, *"A customer had sudden chest pain and has now collapsed."*
- **"What's happening now?"** *"My friend is giving CPR! We have an AED."*
- **"Where is the victim located?"** *"We are at the Evergreen Company, here at 1234 Fifth Avenue NE, in the back hall."*
- **"What number are you calling from?"** *"The number is 555-1313."*

At this point the dispatcher may give you directions such as, **"Stay on the line until I tell you to hang up. Rescuers are being sent to your location. Please meet them and direct them to the scene."**

Dispatcher-Assisted CPR and Defibrillation and Enhanced 911

In many areas of the country emergency medical dispatchers are taught how to help callers give emergency care. With help from the dispatcher, callers can give CPR and use an AED. The instructions are basic and simple, but they will help the victim until EMS personnel arrive. Remember, early CPR and early defibrillation are critical links in the Chain of Survival and need to be started immediately.

Unresponsiveness is a red flag for an emergency — you need to act immediately!

PUBLIC ACCESS DEFIBRILLATION

The AHA promotes the most rapid possible defibrillation of victims of cardiac arrest. To do this the AHA wants to place AEDs in the hands of trained, nontraditional rescuers. These include police, security guards, and family members of patients at high risk for cardiac arrest.

Public access defibrillation (PAD) programs place AEDs in homes, police cars, worksites, and public gathering places, under the supervision of licensed physicians. PAD rescuers must be trained in CPR and use of an AED. When AEDs are readily available, rescuers can provide defibrillation within the first few minutes of out-of-hospital cardiac arrest. This dramatically increases the victim's chances of survival.

The Heartsaver FACTS Course has been developed to support the PAD movement and specific PAD programs. The course is designed to help you learn how to give CPR and use an AED. These skills are essential in caring for the victim of cardiac arrest.

fyi

Using a prepared list of instructions, the emergency medical dispatcher can coach you through the basic steps of CPR and in the use of your AED. At a worksite you will usually have help. Use this approach:

- Repeat the dispatcher's instructions loudly to the other rescuers and confirm that they are following that step.
- If the victim vomits or other complications arise, tell the dispatcher. Do not expect that you will perform perfectly in such a crisis.
- Be sure that rescuers follow each instruction, even if it takes extra seconds.
- Ensure rescuer safety at all times.
- When EMS personnel arrive at the victim's side, the dispatcher will tell you that he or she is hanging up.
- You hang up last.

Public access defibrillation programs and AED manufacturers should work with local EMS systems. Program authorities or manufacturers should notify EMS directors of AEDs placed in homes, businesses, or other public areas.

Find out if your community has *enhanced 911*. In enhanced 911 a computer automatically confirms the caller's address. Also ask if your 911 dispatchers are trained to offer prearrival instructions to rescuers. This means that they can give instructions for immediate care based on the clinical *criteria* of the emergency. If not, become a vocal advocate for such services in your community. Enhanced 911 can save precious seconds, minutes, and even lives.

Begin Cardiopulmonary Resuscitation

CPR is the critical link that buys time between the first link (call 911) and the third link (use the AED). The earlier you give CPR to a person in cardiac or respiratory arrest, the greater his or her chance of survival. CPR keeps oxygenated blood flowing to the brain and heart until defibrillation or other advanced care can restore normal heart action.

Use the Automated External Defibrillator to Treat Ventricular Fibrillation

Most sudden cardiac arrest victims are in **ventricular fibrillation (VF)**. VF is an abnormal, chaotic heart rhythm that prevents the heart from pumping blood. VF causes more cardiac arrests than any other rhythm.

You must defibrillate a victim immediately to stop VF and allow a normal heart rhythm to resume. The sooner you provide defibrillation with the AED, the better the victim's chances of survival. If you provide defibrillation within the first 5 minutes of a cardiac arrest, the odds are about 50% that you can save the victim's life. But with each passing minute during a cardiac arrest, the chance of successful resuscitation is reduced by 7% to 10%. After 10 minutes there is very little chance of successful rescue.

Transfer to Advanced Care

The fourth link in the Chain of Survival is advanced care. This link is provided by highly trained EMS personnel called "paramedics." Paramedics give CPR and defibrillation as well as more advanced care. They can give cardiac drugs and insert endotracheal breathing tubes. These advanced actions (1) help the heart in VF respond to defibrillation or (2) maintain a normal rhythm after successful defibrillation.

HOW TO RECOGNIZE MAJOR EMERGENCIES: HEART ATTACK, CARDIAC ARREST, STROKE, AND FOREIGN-BODY AIRWAY OBSTRUCTION (CHOKING)

How to Recognize a Heart Attack

A heart attack means some heart muscle has suddenly started to die. The muscle is dying because one of the heart's major blood vessels (a coronary artery) has become blocked. The artery can be blocked by buildup of cholesterol deposits or by a blood clot. *Acute myocardial infarction* is the medical term for heart attack.

A person having a heart attack is usually awake and can talk to you but feels severe pain. The most critical time for treatment of heart attack is the first 30 minutes after symptoms begin. If you suspect someone is having a heart attack, activate the EMS system immediately. These minutes count! Know the symptoms!

The most important and most common symptom of a heart attack is chest pain or pressure in the center of the chest, behind the breastbone (sternum). The pain lasts more than 3 to 5 minutes. Consider **chest pain** *a* **red flag.** *The flag says* **Warning! You should think of a heart attack.**

You can ask these questions:

- *"What is the pain like?"* People describe the pain of a heart attack in many ways: a "pressure," "fullness," "squeezing," or "heaviness."

- *"Where is the pain located?"* Usually people feel the pain right behind the breastbone, deep in the center of the chest **(FIGURE 2)**. After a few moments the pain may seem to spread to the shoulder, the neck, the lower jaw, or down the

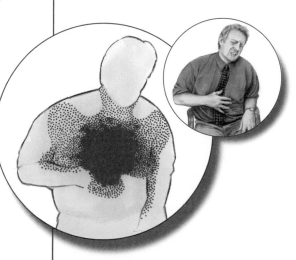

FIGURE 2
Typical locations of chest pain in persons having a heart attack.

Not *all* warning symptoms occur in *every* heart attack. If any occur, don't wait. Get help immediately. Call 911. Delay can be deadly! People who are having a heart attack may complain of signs or symptoms other than chest pain. These additional *red flags,* or warning symptoms, of a heart attack include

- *Lightheadedness,* "feeling dizzy" during the pain
- *Fainting,* completely losing consciousness, especially when the pain starts
- *Sweating,* breaking out in a "cold sweat all over" but without a fever
- *Nausea,* usually without vomiting — "I feel sick"
- *Shortness of breath,* especially worrisome if the victim is short of breath during pain, while lying still or resting, or when moving only a little

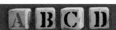

arm. The pain may be on the left side or the right side or on both sides. Sometimes the pain or discomfort may even be felt in the back, between the shoulder blades.

- *"How long* does the pain last?"* The discomfort of a heart attack usually lasts more than a few minutes. Sharp, stabbing, knifelike pain that lasts only a second and then disappears is almost never heart attack pain. Heart attack chest pain sometimes "stutters." This means the pain may stop completely but returns a short time later.

Many people will not admit that their symptoms may indicate a heart attack. People react with a variety of statements or excuses. They may say "I'm too healthy" or "I don't want to bother the doctor" or "I don't want to frighten my wife" or "I'll feel ridiculous if it isn't a heart attack" or "I hate red lights and sirens."

When a person with symptoms of a heart attack tries to downplay what he or she is feeling, **you** must take responsibility and act at once. Tell the victim to sit quietly. Tell the nearest person to call 911 and get the AED. Be prepared to perform CPR if necessary.

After you or someone else calls 911, have the person rest quietly and calmly. Help the person into a position that is the most comfortable and that allows the easiest breathing.

How to Recognize a Cardiac Arrest

When blocked arteries deprive the heart muscle of oxygen during a heart attack, the heart may actually stop beating. This produces a **cardiac arrest:** no blood flow and no pulse. Without blood flow to the brain, the person becomes unconscious, collapses, and stops breathing normally. Often VF stops the rhythmic contractions of the heart. VF leads to chaotic, quivering, and uncoordinated spasms of the heart muscle.

VF starts in the same damaged areas of the heart muscle that produce the severe chest pain of a heart attack. VF can begin in mildly damaged areas of the heart, even in men or women without chest pain. Sudden VF and cardiac arrest may be the only sign of a heart attack in some victims. The only treatment for VF is electrical shocks from a defibrillator.

*It is critical for you to recognize that an unresponsive person may be in cardiac arrest. Unresponsiveness is a **red flag** for an emergency — you need to act immediately!*

1. *Unresponsiveness:* The person is unconscious and does not respond when you call their name or touch them. At this point tell someone to activate the EMS system and get the AED.

2. *Breathlessness:* The person does not take a normal breath when you check for several seconds. You discover that the person is breathless only after you begin the sequence of CPR: open the airway and look, listen, and feel for respirations.

3. *Pulselessness:* You feel no pulse in the person's neck. You confirm that the person is pulseless only after you have delivered 2 breaths to the breathless victim.

How to Recognize a Stroke

Stroke happens fast. Stroke is the rapid onset of neurological problems like weakness, paralysis in one or more limbs (particularly the hand), difficulties with speaking, visual problems, intense dizziness, facial weakness, altered consciousness, or severe headache. Stroke occurs when one of two events happen in the brain: (1) a blood vessel is blocked by a blood clot so that an area of the brain receives no blood flow and no oxygen or (2) a blood vessel breaks open and blood pours out into or over the brain. Strokes are common, serious, and often sudden. *Stroke is a leading cause of death and serious disability among Americans.*

Strokes sometimes cause such severe brain damage that the victim stops breathing or develops a blocked airway. You may need to perform some or all of the steps of CPR: rescue breathing, chest compressions, or both. Although most strokes occur in older people, *strokes can happen in persons of all ages.*

You should know the **red flags** or **signs of stroke** so that you can activate the EMS system. Signs of stroke range from very mild signs to loss of consciousness and coma. The most common complaints include the following:

- Severe headache (often described as "the worst headache of my life")
- Visual disturbances such as blurring or double vision
- Slurring, or loss of speech, or incoherent speech
- Loss of movement, weakness, unsteadiness, or falls
- Dizziness or nausea

Unfortunately, many of the signs of stroke can be vague or ignored by the victim. If you are concerned that someone has had a stroke, look closely for one of the following 3 signs:

CRITICAL CONCEPTS: REMEMBER THE *CRITICAL ACTIONS* TO DO AS SOON AS YOU FIND SOMEONE WHO IS *UNRESPONSIVE:*

- Call 911 and send someone to get the AED.
- Begin the steps of CPR and provide as much support as needed.

FOUNDATION FACTS: DO STROKE VICTIMS EVER NEED CPR?

- Acute stroke victims may become confused or may almost become unconscious. This can reduce breathing or cause airway obstruction or choking. You must provide CPR for these victims. CPR can be lifesaving simply by
  — Placing the unconscious but breathing person in the "recovery position" (see Chapter 2, Figure 9)
  — Opening the airway if airway obstruction is present
  — Performing rescue breathing if the victim is unconscious and not breathing
- Note that chest compressions are rarely needed during the first minutes after a stroke.

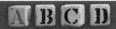

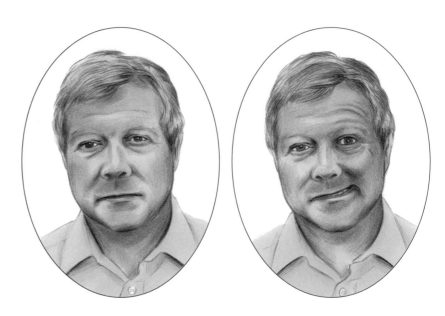

FIGURE 3
Stroke victim with facial droop (right side of the victim's face). Left, Victim in repose. Right, After the command, "Look up and smile showing all your teeth."

1. **Facial droop:** This is most obvious if the victim smiles or grimaces. If one side of the face droops or the face does not move **(FIGURE 3)**, a stroke may have occurred.

2. **Arm weakness:** This is most obvious if the victim extends his or her arms with eyes closed. If one arm drifts downward or the arms can't move, this may indicate a stroke.

3. **Speech difficulties:** This is most obvious if the victim is unable to speak or slurs words. Ask the victim to repeat a sentence such as "You can't teach an old dog new tricks." If the victim cannot repeat the phrase or sentence accurately and clearly, a stroke may have occurred.

Whenever you see signs of stroke, call 911. EMS personnel will examine the person and transport him or her to a hospital for evaluation and treatment. Wonderful new treatments for stroke are now available. These include "clot busters" for the brain (thrombolytic agents), which may reduce or eliminate brain damage from a stroke. These treatments, however, must be given within minutes of the onset of stroke. To help treat a stroke victim, bystanders and lay rescuers must

- Recognize the signs of stroke.

- Call 911.

- Provide CPR if needed.

- Transfer the victim to trained EMS personnel for rapid transport to the emergency department.

Do not make the mistake of thinking that a stroke victim's symptoms are caused by alcohol or drug intoxication or medical conditions such as low blood sugar. If you suspect that a person is having a stroke, call 911 at once.

How to Recognize Airway Obstruction by a Foreign Body (Choking)

Every year airway obstruction by foreign bodies or choking causes about 3185 deaths. Foreign-body obstruction of the airway in the adult usually occurs during eating. Meat is the most frequent cause of choking in adults, but a variety of foods and foreign bodies have caused airway obstruction in children and some adults.

To treat airway obstruction successfully, **you must recognize it.** For all choking victims, if a foreign body is obstructing the airway it must be removed. Otherwise breathing or rescue breathing won't work. For conscious choking victims you help clear the airway. For unconscious choking victims you open the airway and forcefully remove the blocking object either by the Heimlich maneuver or by using your fingers.

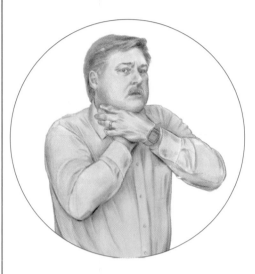

FIGURE 4
Universal choking signal.

CRITICAL CONCEPTS:
RED-FLAG SIGNS OF SEVERE FOREIGN-BODY AIRWAY OBSTRUCTION

- The *"universal choking signal"* (clutching the neck with one or both hands) (**FIGURE 4**)
- Poor, ineffective coughs
- Inability to speak
- High-pitched sounds while inhaling
- Increased difficulty breathing
- Blue lips or skin (cyanosis)
- Loss of consciousness and responsiveness

CHAPTER 1

SUMMARY

To rescue someone, you must first recognize that the person is having an emergency. The Chain of Survival for heart attack, cardiac arrest, stroke, and foreign-body airway obstruction starts with an alert fellow citizen who recognizes the emergency and takes action. This is an important step and one that will be practiced over and over again in this course.

This course encourages each participant to become a part of the community's Chain of Survival:

- Learn to recognize 4 conditions that are major killers in the United States: heart attack, cardiac arrest, stroke, and foreign-body airway obstruction.
- Know to call 911 and activate the EMS system for these emergencies.
- Know how to open or clear an obstructed airway.
- Know how to perform CPR.
- Know how to use an AED.

With this knowledge and these skills, you can become an effective and vital link in the community's Chain of Survival.

REVIEW QUESTIONS

1. When you find an unresponsive victim, which link in the Chain of Survival should be accomplished first?

    a. call 911

    b. begin CPR

    c. use the AED

    d. transfer to advanced care

2. Which of the following is a *red-flag* symptom of a heart attack?

    a. squeezing or crushing chest pain behind the breastbone that lasts more than a few minutes

    b. sharp, stabbing chest pain that lasts only a few seconds

    c. shortness of breath

    d. "the worst headache of my life"

3. Which of the following groups of signs or symptoms are the *red-flag* signs of cardiac arrest?

    a. facial droop, arm weakness, speech difficulties

    b. chest pain, lightheadedness, sweating, and nausea

    c. unresponsiveness, breathlessness, and pulselessness

    d. unresponsiveness, spontaneous breathing, and chest pain

4. Which of the following are *red-flag* signs and symptoms of a stroke?

    a. sudden loss of consciousness and cardiac arrest

    b. facial droop, arm weakness, and speech difficulties

    c. unresponsiveness, breathlessness, and pulselessness

    d. crushing chest pain that lasts a few minutes, nausea, and sweating

5. What are the *red-flag* signs of severe airway obstruction that require your intervention?

    a. wheezing between coughs and hoarse speech

    b. severe, forceful coughing

    c. inability to speak, breathe, or cough and blue skin or lips

    d. unresponsiveness, breathlessness, and pulselessness

HOW DID YOU DO?

1. a; **2.** a; **3.** c; **4.** b; **5.** c

THE ABCs: TECHNIQUES OF ADULT CPR

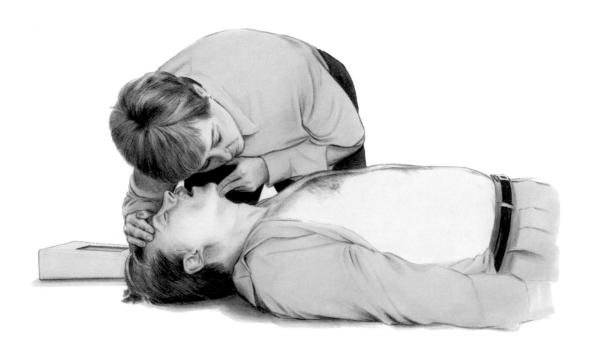

CONTENTS

2

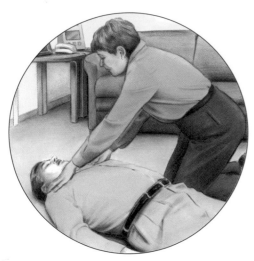

FIGURE 1
Unresponsive.

**CRITICAL CONCEPTS:
UNRESPONSIVE —
911 — AED**

To help you remember these first actions, think of this short phrase: Unresponsive — 911 — AED. These are critical steps you must do before the ABCs. Whether you are responding in a crowded worksite with many helpers or you are alone — what we call "the Lone Rescuer" — you still have to make sure that either you or another person takes these actions.

LEARNING OBJECTIVES

After reading this chapter you should be able to

1. Describe and demonstrate one-rescuer CPR

2. Describe and demonstrate how to use pocket face masks during CPR

3. Recognize when someone is choking due to a foreign-body airway obstruction

4. Describe and demonstrate how to clear the airway of a conscious or unconscious person who has a foreign body blocking the airway

CPR: THE SECOND LINK IN THE CHAIN OF SURVIVAL

CPR skills include a combination of rescue breathing (blowing) and chest compressions (pumping). If you find an *unresponsive* person, send someone to *call 911* and *get the AED. Then you start CPR.* CPR is the second link in the Chain of Survival. Continue CPR until additional treatment (for example, defibrillation with an AED) restores normal heart action.

CPR helps the heart respond better to defibrillation shocks. For this reason it is critical to begin CPR at once. Do not wait for the AED to arrive. You will also give CPR *between* AED shocks (usually after every 3 shocks). You do this to provide oxygen to the heart and to increase the chances that defibrillation will succeed.

Check the victim: If the victim is *unresponsive*, *call 911* and *get the AED.*

NOTE: In Chapters 3 and 4 you will learn how to combine CPR and defibrillation. Defibrillation provides a step "D" to go with the ABCs of CPR. Always begin with the ABCs when you find an unconscious victim. Go to step D if the victim does not have a pulse. The AED appears in the figures for this chapter but is not taught until Chapters 3 and 4.

When you encounter an emergency — at home, at work, or in the community — quickly determine unresponsiveness to decide whether to call 911. Then get the AED from its location near the telephone:

1. **First, check to see if the victim is unresponsive** by gently shaking the victim and shouting, "Are you OK?" **(FIGURE 1).**

   - **If the victim does not respond,** send someone to **call 911 and get the AED!** This activates the EMS system, ensures that professional help is on the way, and brings the AED to your side in a few moments.

- **If you are alone** and find an unresponsive victim, you will have to leave the victim to call 911 and get the AED. As standard practice the AED should be stored next to a telephone. You should be able to call 911 while reaching for the AED in its carrying case **(FIGURE 2)**.

- When you have sent someone to call 911 and get the AED, kneel at the victim's side near his or her head to start CPR. The victim should be on his or her back. If not, carefully turn the victim onto his or her back.

2. **Airway: open the airway with the head tilt–chin lift maneuver (FIGURE 3).**

   - Tilt the head back by lifting the chin gently with one hand while pushing down on the forehead with the other hand.

3. **Breathing: head tilt–chin lift; look, listen, and feel; 2 slow breaths:**

   To check for breathing, _look, listen, and feel:_

   a. Place your ear next to the victim's mouth and nose **(FIGURE 3)** and listen for breathing, turning your head to observe the chest.

   b. Look for the chest to rise. Listen and feel for air movement on your cheek.

   If not breathing, give 2 slow rescue breaths (FIGURE 4). To perform rescue breathing in the home:

   a. Place your mouth around the victim's mouth and pinch the nose closed.

   b. Continue to tilt the head and lift the chin.

   c. Give **2 slow breaths.**

   d. Be sure the victim's chest rises each time you give a rescue breath.

   To perform rescue breathing in the workplace or in a public setting:

   a. Quickly assemble the pocket face mask (available in the AED case).

   b. Place the mask over the victim's nose and mouth.

   c. Continue to tilt the head and lift the chin.

   d. Provide **2 slow breaths** into the opening of the pocket face mask.

   e. Adjust the mask as needed to ensure a tight seal. Be sure the victim's chest rises each time you blow into the mask.

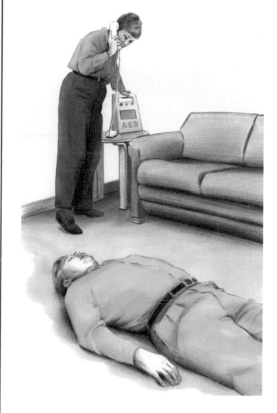

FIGURE 2
Call 911 — get the AED.

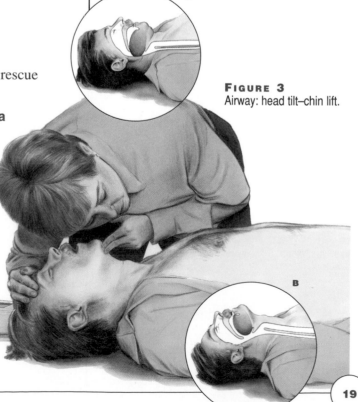

FIGURE 3
Airway: head tilt–chin lift.

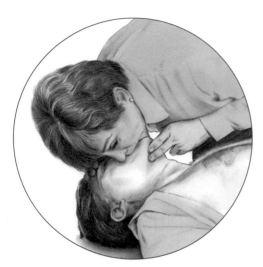

FIGURE 4
Breathing: give 2 slow breaths.

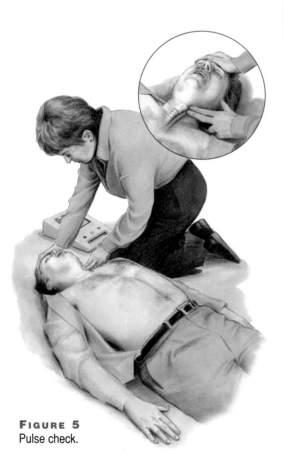

FIGURE 5
Pulse check.

4. **Circulation: check for a pulse. If no pulse, start chest compressions.** If the victim has a pulse but is not breathing, give rescue breaths (1 breath every 5 seconds).

   Ensure that someone has called *911* and is getting the *AED*.

   a. Maintain head tilt.

   b. Place 2 or 3 fingers on the Adam's apple (voice box). Slide the fingers into the groove between the Adam's apple and the muscle **(FIGURE 5)**.

   c. Feel for the pulse with your fingers for 10 seconds.

CRITICAL CONCEPTS: AIRWAY

In CPR your first action focuses on the **Airway.** You *must* open the airway. Remember, the **tongue** is the **most common cause** of a blocked airway in the unconscious victim. When a victim is unconscious, the muscles of the jaw and neck relax, allowing the tongue to fall back against the throat and block the airway **(FIGURE 3A).**

The tongue is attached to the lower jaw, so tilting the head and lifting the chin pulls the tongue away from the back of the throat and opens the airway. Open the airway by tilting the head back and lifting the chin. This is called the *head tilt–chin lift* maneuver.

If the victim has been injured with possible head and neck trauma, open the airway with a *jaw thrust*. Grasp the angles of the victim's jaw and lift it upward without tilting the head. This method of opening the airway, the *jaw-thrust maneuver,* will also pull the tongue away from the back of the throat **(FIGURE 6).** The jaw thrust causes less neck movement but is a bit more difficult to perform, so it should be saved for victims with possible head or neck injuries.

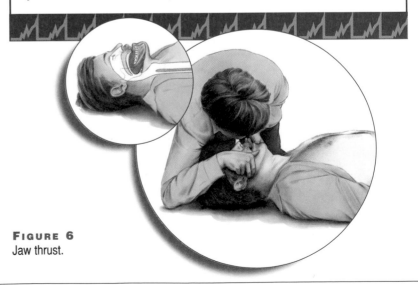

FIGURE 6
Jaw thrust.

FOUNDATION FACTS: WHY BREATHING?

When breathing stops, oxygen delivery to the heart and brain stops. If oxygen delivery is not restored immediately, the heart and brain may be damaged. The longer the victim is deprived of oxygen, the smaller the chance that he or she will respond to CPR. Mouth-to-mouth or mouth-to-mask breathing is the quickest way to deliver oxygen to the victim's lungs and blood.

When providing rescue breathing, check to see that the victim's chest rises with each breath you give. This is critical because it is the only way you can tell that you are giving good rescue breaths.

Breaths must be delivered slowly. Take 1 1/2 to 2 seconds to deliver each breath. You do not want to give rapid, forceful breaths, which can blow air into the esophagus and stomach instead of the lungs. Air in the stomach can cause vomiting, which complicates CPR in many ways.

If a victim has dentures, leave them in place. Dentures help provide a good mouth-to-mouth or mouth-to-mask seal. An exception to this rule occurs when the dentures are extremely loose. Loose dentures should be removed so that they do not fall back into the throat and obstruct the airway.

When you *look, listen, and feel* for breathing and find that the victim *is breathing,* you don't need to provide the 2 rescue breaths. Watch the victim to be sure that breathing continues. If the breathing is adequate, you may place the victim on his or her side in the recovery position to keep the airway open.

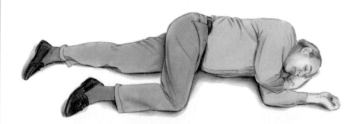

CRITICAL CONCEPTS: CHECK FOR THE CAROTID PULSE

Blood must circulate to deliver oxygen to the brain, heart, and other vital organs. If you can feel the pulse in the neck (the carotid artery), the victim's heart is beating adequately, and chest compressions are unnecessary. If you *cannot* feel the victim's carotid pulse within 10 seconds, then *both* chest compressions and attachment of the AED are needed.

FOUNDATION FACTS: AGONAL BREATHING

People in cardiac arrest soon stop breathing because oxygen is no longer delivered to the brain. Some victims, however, may display irregular, infrequent, gasping breaths called "agonal breaths." Agonal breaths may fool some rescuers into thinking that the victim is still alive, still responsive, and not in need of CPR or defibrillation. This could cause a missed opportunity to save a person's life.

If the victim is unconscious and pulseless, start CPR and attach the AED — even if you observe sporadic, gasping breaths. The AED can still identify the presence or absence of VF and clarify the victim's status.

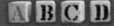

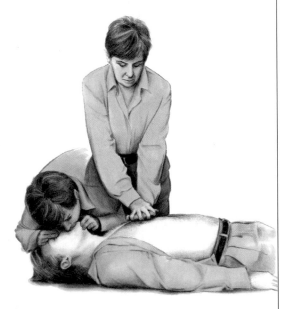

FIGURE 7
Position for chest compressions, on the lower half of the sternum.

d. If no pulse, start chest compressions. Find a position on the lower half of the sternum, right between the nipples (**FIGURE 7**).

e. Place the heel of one hand on the *center* of the breastbone right between the nipples.

f. Place the heel of the second hand on top of the first hand.

g. Position your body directly over your hands. Your shoulders should be above your hands, and you should look down on your hands.

h. Provide 15 compressions at a rate of 80 to 100 compressions per minute (slightly faster than 1 compression per second). Your instructor will give you suggestions about ways to maintain the correct speed.

5. **"Pump and blow":* Cycles: 15 chest compressions, 2 rescue breaths.**

   a. Continue one-rescuer CPR with **15** chest compressions ("pump") and 2 slow breaths ("blow") (**FIGURE 8**).

   b. After 1 minute of CPR (4 cycles of 15 compressions and 2 breaths), check the pulse to see if circulation has been restored. *Check the pulse* every few minutes. If a pulse returns, stop chest compressions and continue providing rescue breaths if needed (1 breath every 5 seconds).

KEEPING YOUR SKILLS SHARP: CPR PRACTICE

Review the steps and skills of one-rescuer CPR regularly (several times every year). If you learn CPR at work, try to practice it on a manikin with coworkers. If you learn CPR for a loved one at home, review practice videos and CPR prompt devices that use recorded instructions. Renew your CPR skills with an instructor at least every 2 years by taking an AHA refresher course.

The Heartsaver FACTS Course teaches you the skills of adult CPR. Other AHA courses add instruction on CPR, treatment of choking in infants and children, and other skills.

Never rehearse or practice CPR skills on another person! Chest compressions can be dangerous to a conscious, healthy person but lifesaving for the cardiac arrest victim.

FIGURE 8
Rescue breathing and compressions.

---

* Thanks to Allan Braslow, PhD, for coining the term *pump and blow* to describe chest compressions and rescue breathing.

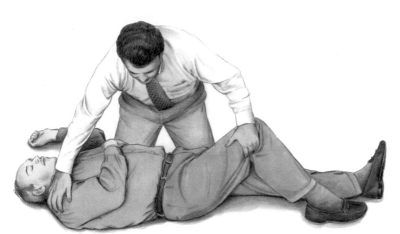

FIGURE 9A

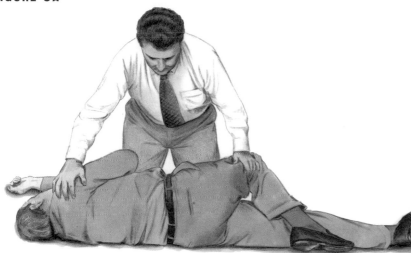

FIGURE 9B

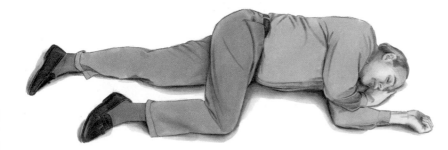

FIGURE 9C
The recovery position.

CRITICAL CONCEPTS: THE RECOVERY POSITION

HOW TO PLACE A PERSON IN THE RECOVERY POSITION IF UNCONSCIOUS BUT BREATHING

If there is no evidence of trauma, place the victim on his or her side in the *recovery position* (FIGURE 9C). The recovery position keeps the airway open. The following steps are recommended:

1. Kneel beside the victim and straighten the victim's legs.

2. Place the victim's arm that is nearest you in a "waving good-bye" position, that is, at right angles to the victim's body, elbow bent, palm up.

3. Place the victim's other arm across his or her chest, as pictured above, left. If the victim is small, bring this arm further across so that the back of the hand can be held against the victim's nearest cheek.

4. Grasp the victim's far-side thigh above the knee; pull the thigh up toward the victim's body (FIGURE 9A).

5. Place your other hand on the victim's far-side shoulder, and roll the victim toward you onto his or her side (FIGURE 9B). Begin moving the victim's uppermost hand toward the victim's nearest cheek (the hand must not get trapped under the body).

6. Adjust the upper leg of the knee you are holding until both the hip and knee are bent at right angles.

7. Tilt the victim's head back to keep the airway open. Bring the back of the uppermost hand under the victim's cheek. Use this hand to maintain head tilt. Use chin lift if necessary (FIGURE 9C).

Continue to check the victim:

8. Check breathing regularly ("look, listen, and feel").

9. If the victim stops breathing, turn the victim onto his or her back, be sure that 911 has been called and the AED is near, and begin the ABCs of CPR.

10. *Memory aid: Victim is waving good-bye while taking a nap.*

BARRIER DEVICES AND MASKS

When you perform CPR, you have almost no chance of becoming infected with viral diseases such as AIDS or hepatitis. To date no human has ever "caught" AIDS or hepatitis by mouth-to-mouth contact during CPR.

Many rescuers, however, prefer to avoid direct mouth-to-mouth contact with another person, especially a stranger. The AHA recommends that you learn to use a barrier device to avoid direct mouth-to-mouth contact with a victim. But a barrier device is *not* required to provide CPR. **Do not withhold rescue breathing from a cardiac arrest victim just because you have no barrier device.**

There are 2 types of barrier devices: face shields and face masks.

Face Shields

Face shields are clear plastic or silicon sheets placed over the victim's face to keep the rescuer's mouth from directly touching the victim. All face shields have an opening or tube in the center of the plastic sheet. This allows your rescue breaths to enter the victim's mouth. Face shields are small, flexible, and portable. A shield will fit easily on a key ring. If you keep it on your key ring, it is much more likely to be available when you need it.

Face Masks

Face masks (**FIGURE 10A**) are firmer, more rigid devices that fit over both the mouth and nose. Masks are much more effective than face shields, but they are bulkier, they cost more, and they're less likely to be available. Face masks and disposable gloves should be packed in every AED carrying case.

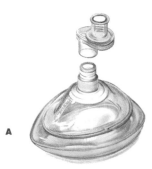
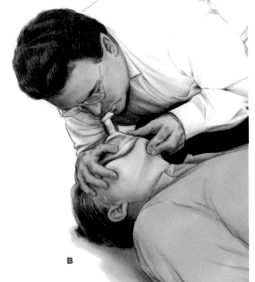

A

B

FIGURE 10
Face mask.

In the Heartsaver FACTS Course you will learn about the specific face mask you will use during rescue breathing and CPR. Correct use requires practice. Practice on a manikin several times. The most critical step in using a face mask is achieving a good seal around the mouth and nose because this prevents air leakage during rescue breaths (**FIGURE 10B**).

CHOKING: AIRWAY OBSTRUCTION BY A FOREIGN BODY

Choking is an alarming and dramatic emergency. The desperate efforts of the choking person to clear his or her airway heighten the emotional drama and increase the pressure on the rescuer to take the correct action.

FOUNDATION FACTS: CHOOSING A FACE MASK

Face masks should
- **Be easy to apply to the face**
- **Provide a good seal between mask and face**
- **Have a one-way valve with a bacterial barrier to keep the victim's exhaled air and body fluids away from the rescuer's mouth**
- **Be transparent so that the rescuer can see vomit or foreign material in the victim's airway**

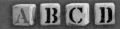

FOUNDATION FACTS: CAUSES OF AIRWAY OBSTRUCTION

There are 3 common ways an adult's airway may become obstructed. Each is treated differently.

1. Foreign body: **A foreign body (for example, food) may become lodged in the air passage and block the airway. If the victim is an adult, give abdominal thrusts (Heimlich maneuver) or chest thrusts and finger sweeps (discussed below).**

2. Relaxed tongue: **In an unconscious victim (for example, after a stroke or head trauma or in cardiac arrest), the tongue may fall back against the throat, blocking the airway. Use either the head tilt–chin lift maneuver or the jaw-thrust maneuver to lift the tongue away from the back of the throat. (SEE FIGURES 3 AND 6.)**

3. Swollen air passages: **This condition is a medical problem rather than a mechanical problem. Swelling and blockage of the airway are caused by conditions such as asthma, infection, or allergy. Positioning of the head or neck and using the Heimlich maneuver will not eliminate this form of airway obstruction. If the victim stops breathing, give rescue breaths. Critical narrowing of the airway is a life-threatening condition. This condition cannot be resolved without using medications, such as epinephrine, or surgery.**

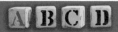

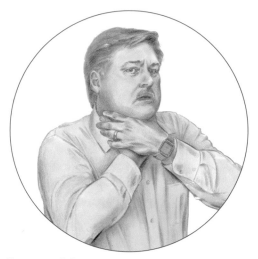

FIGURE 11
Universal sign of choking distress.

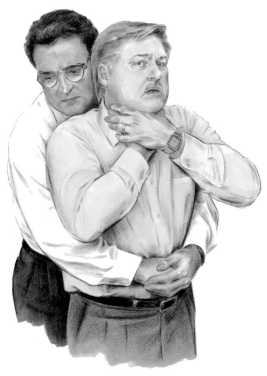

FIGURE 12
Conscious-choking maneuver.

How to Recognize Severe Airway Obstruction by a Foreign Body in a Conscious Victim

Foreign bodies may *partially* block the airway but still allow good air movement. These choking victims remain conscious, can cough forcefully, and usually can speak. Breath sounds may be noisy. These victims require no immediate action from you, but prepare to act if the airway obstruction worsens.

Victims with *severe* airway obstruction will remain conscious at first but will not be able to move enough air to cough forcefully. You must be prepared to help relieve the obstruction with abdominal thrusts.

To determine if a conscious victim has an obstructed airway, ask, "Are you choking?" In a conscious, choking person the following are *red flags* or major warning signs of severe airway obstruction that require you to act:

- *"Universal distress signal"* of choking: the victim clutches his or her neck with the thumb and index finger (**FIGURE 11**)
- Inability to speak (ask, "Are you choking?")
- Poor, ineffective coughs
- High-pitched sounds while inhaling
- Increased difficulty breathing
- Bluish skin color (cyanosis)
- Loss of consciousness if not treated immediately

NOTE ABOUT THE UNIVERSAL DISTRESS SIGNAL: You do not need to act if the victim can cough forcefully and speak. **Do not interfere** at this point because a strong cough is the most effective way to remove a foreign body. Stay with the victim and monitor his or her condition. If the partial obstruction persists, activate the EMS system.

First Aid for Airway Obstruction by a Foreign Body

Use the Heimlich maneuver (abdominal thrusts) to relieve severe airway obstruction caused by a foreign body. The Heimlich maneuver quickly forces air from the victim's lungs. This expels the blocking object like a cork from a bottle. Two approaches are used:

1. Use the **Heimlich maneuver** if the victim is *conscious* (but not speaking) and *standing* (**FIGURE 12**).

2. Use CPR skills **A (open the airway)** and **B (give rescue breaths)** plus **abdominal or chest thrusts (straddle the victim) and finger sweeps** if the victim is *unconscious* (**FIGURE 13**).

If the choking victim is *conscious* and *standing*: perform the Heimlich maneuver:

1. Make a fist with one hand.

2. Place the thumb side of the fist on the victim's abdomen, slightly above the navel and well below the breastbone.

3. Grasp the fist with the other hand and provide quick upward thrusts into the victim's abdomen.

4. Repeat the thrusts and continue until the object is expelled or the victim becomes unconscious.

If the foreign-body airway obstruction is not relieved, the victim will stop breathing. Then the brain and heart will lack oxygen-rich blood. The victim will lose consciousness and become unresponsive. When the victim loses consciousness, **activate the EMS system by calling 911 and get the AED.** Then perform the *unconscious-choking maneuver* described below.

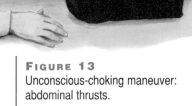

FIGURE 13
Unconscious-choking maneuver: abdominal thrusts.

If the choking victim becomes *unconscious*: perform finger sweep, straddle the victim, use the Heimlich maneuver:

1. Place the victim on his or her back.

2. Grasp the tongue and jaw with one hand. Perform a finger sweep with the index finger of the other hand (**FIGURE 14**).

3. Attempt rescue breathing.

4. If the chest does not rise, reposition the victim's head and try blowing again.

5. If the victim's chest still does not rise with your breaths, perform the Heimlich maneuver for an unconscious victim:

    *   Straddle the victim.

    *   Place the heel of one hand on the abdomen just above the navel and well below the breastbone.

    *   Place the heel of the other hand on top of the first.

    *   Give up to 5 quick abdominal thrusts.

6. Repeat finger sweeps, rescue breaths, and abdominal thrusts until the obstruction is cleared.

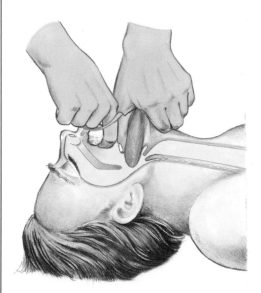

FIGURE 14
Unconscious-choking maneuver: finger sweep.

First Aid for Choking in Pregnant and Obese Victims: Conscious and Unconscious

When choking victims are in the later stages of pregnancy or are very obese, you must position your hands on the chest rather than on the abdomen to deliver thrusts.

Obese or Pregnant Choking Victim — Conscious:

1. Stand behind the victim and put your arms around the victim's chest.
2. Place your fist on the middle of the victim's breastbone between the nipples (take care to avoid the lower tip of the breastbone).
3. Grab your fist with your other hand and perform firm backward thrusts.
4. Repeat thrusts until the object is removed or the victim becomes unconscious.

Obese or Pregnant Choking Victim — Unconscious:

1. Place the victim on his or her back.
2. Grasp the victim's tongue and jaw with one hand. Perform a finger sweep with the index finger of the other hand (FIGURE 14).
3. Try to give rescue breaths.
4. If the victim's chest does not rise: reposition the victim's head and try again.
5. If the victim's chest still does not rise with your breaths, perform chest thrusts:
   - *Do not* straddle the victim. Work from the side.
   - Place the heel of one hand on top of the other. Then place the heel of the lower hand on the center of the breastbone at the nipple line (similar to chest compressions of CPR).
   - Position your body directly over your hands (similar to chest compressions of CPR).
   - Give up to 5 firm chest thrusts.
6. Repeat finger sweeps, breathing attempts, and chest thrusts until the obstruction is cleared.

SUMMARY

The ABCs of CPR are an important first aid skill that everyone should know. In your lifetime you will probably encounter at least one emergency in which your ability to perform the ABCs will help save someone's life or prevent an urgent problem from becoming a life-threatening emergency.

Problems with **A**irway are common. Everyone should know the steps to take for

- Opening the airway of an unconscious victim
- Rescuing a choking victim who is distressed but still conscious
- Rescuing a choking victim who becomes unconscious
- First aid for choking in pregnant or obese victims, both conscious and unconscious

Problems with **B**reathing occur in these emergencies:

- Respiratory and cardiac arrest
- Stroke and seizure victims
- Victims of head trauma
- Drowning and near-drowning victims
- Victims of medication overdoses and drug intoxication

To manage **B**reathing problems, you need to know how to open the airway and give rescue breaths.

Finally, *chest compressions* (for **C**irculation) are needed in emergencies in which the victim also has no pulse. The most common cause of loss of a pulse is sudden cardiac arrest due to VF. The actions of pumping are simple and easy to learn.

The next chapter covers the use of AEDs, a seemingly technical skill that is easier to learn, as a matter of fact, than the skills of CPR.

REVIEW QUESTIONS

1. You are helping someone who is unresponsive. Which of the following groups of actions includes major steps of CPR in the correct order?

   a. call 911, check for a pulse, open the airway, give 2 breaths if needed

   b. open the airway, give 2 breaths if needed, check for a pulse, call 911 if no pulse

   c. call 911, open the airway, give 2 breaths if needed, and check for a pulse

   d. give 2 breaths, check for a pulse, call 911, begin chest compressions

2. You hear a colleague cry out in the next room. You enter the room and find a man collapsed on the floor. Your first step in assessing the situation is to

   a. check for breathing

   b. check the pulse

   c. check for responsiveness

   d. open the airway

3. If the victim is unresponsive, you perform a head tilt–chin lift and look, listen, and feel for breathing. If the victim is not breathing, what should you do next?

   a. give 2 rapid breaths

   b. give 2 slow breaths

   c. give 1 slow breath

   d. give 1 rapid breath

   e. begin chest compressions

4. For step **C** of the **ABCs**, where should you feel for the pulse of an unconscious adult victim?

   a. the wrist

   b. the neck

   c. the thigh

   d. the upper arm

5. What is the correct ratio of compressions (pumping) to ventilations (blowing) when performing one-rescuer CPR on an adult victim?

   a. 15 compressions to 2 ventilations

   b. 10 compressions to 2 ventilations

   c. 5 compressions to 2 ventilations

   d. 5 compressions to 1 ventilation

6. Which of the following is the most critical step when using a mouth-to-mask device?

   a. achieving a good seal around the mouth and nose

   b. using a two-way valve

   c. using a nontransparent mask

   d. blowing rapidly with each breath

7. What is the best way to ensure a proper rescue breath?

   a. see a change in the victim's color

   b. check the victim's pulse regularly

   c. see the victim's chest rise during rescue breathing

   d. check the airway frequently

8. You try to give a rescue breath to a victim and find that you cannot blow in easily and the victim's chest docs not rise. What should you do immediately?

   a. use the Heimlich maneuver

   b. do a finger swccp

   c. reposition the head and try a rescue breath again

   d. give a more forceful breath

9. A conscious adult victim is clutching his throat and cannot speak, breathe, or cough. What should you do immediately?

   a. give abdominal thrusts

   b. give several back blows

   c. call 911

   d. check the airway

How did you do?

1. c; **2.** c; **3.** b; **4.** b; **5.** a; **6.** a; **7.** c; **8.** c; **9.** a

INTRODUCTION TO AUTOMATED EXTERNAL DEFIBRILLATORS

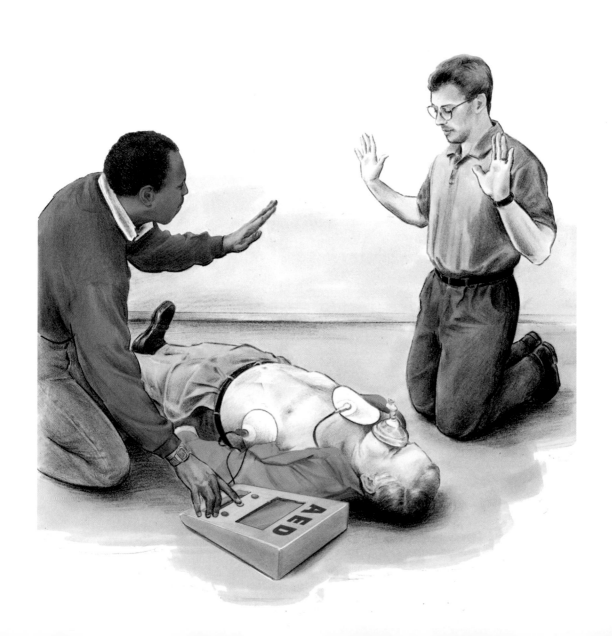

CONTENTS

3

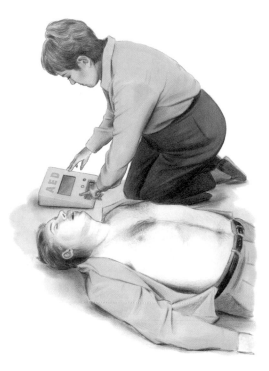

FIGURE 1
An automated external defibrillator.

LEARNING OBJECTIVES

After reading this chapter, you should be able to

1. Describe the purpose of an AED

2. List the 4 universal steps required to operate all AEDs

3. Describe the details of the 4 universal steps

4. Describe the proper procedure for attaching the AED electrode pads in the correct positions on the victim's chest

5. Explain why no one should touch the victim while the AED is analyzing, charging, or shocking the victim

6. List at least 3 special conditions that might change your actions when using an AED

7. Describe the proper actions to take when the AED indicates *"no shock indicated"* (or *"no shock advised"*)

8. Discuss how to maintain an AED

WHAT IS AN AUTOMATED EXTERNAL DEFIBRILLATOR?

An *automated external defibrillator* (AED) is a computerized defibrillator (**FIGURE 1**). An AED can

- Analyze the heart rhythm of a person in cardiac arrest

- Recognize a shockable rhythm

- Advise the operator (through voice prompts and lighted indicators) whether the rhythm should be shocked

If a shock is indicated, the AED charges to a preset energy level. When the operator presses a SHOCK button, the AED delivers a shock to the cardiac arrest victim.

AEDs are relatively inexpensive and need little maintenance. They can be operated easily with very little training. Because of their effectiveness and ease of use and care, they are now being placed on airplanes and in public buildings, homes, and worksites. With more rescuers and more AEDs available, defibrillation can occur within minutes of a cardiac arrest.

How an AED Analyzes the Heart Rhythm

AEDs contain computer chips that analyze the rate, size, and wave shape of the human cardiac rhythm. AEDs have been tested and are very accurate for use with adults.

AED electrode pads have 2 functions:

- To sense the cardiac electric signal and send it to the computer
- To deliver a shock through the electrodes if a shock is indicated

AEDs look at the victim's heart to see if it has a rhythm that can be shocked. If it does, the AED will tell you that a shock is advised. All AEDs must charge before they can deliver a shock. Some AEDs charge automatically. With some AEDs you have to press a CHARGE button before they will charge. You can then push another button to deliver the shock.

Overview: The 4 Universal Steps for Operating an AED

Like automobiles, AEDs are available in different models. There are small differences from model to model, but (like cars) all AEDs operate basically the same way. Do not be distracted by minor differences. Focus instead on the 4 universal steps you must perform with all AEDs. They are listed in the Critical Concepts box.

Special Conditions That May Require Additional Actions

When you arrive with an AED at the scene of a possible cardiac arrest, or if you are doing CPR and someone else arrives with an AED, quickly look for "special conditions" that may change how you use the AED. These are listed in the Critical Concepts box on the next page.

Place the AED Next to the Victim's Left Ear

Make sure you have enough room to perform CPR and to operate the AED. Do not attempt CPR in a bed, for example, or with the victim slumped over in a car or a chair. Place the victim on a firm surface, such as the floor. If possible, place the AED next to the victim's left ear. This allows you to easily reach the AED controls, place the adhesive electrode pads in the proper location, and direct CPR. However, this may not always be possible because of the circumstances and location of the collapse.

CRITICAL CONCEPTS:
4 UNIVERSAL STEPS
OF AED OPERATION

1. **POWER ON the AED first!**
2. **ATTACH the AED to the victim's chest with electrode pads.**
3. **ANALYZE the rhythm.**
4. **SHOCK (if a shock is indicated).**

CRITICAL CONCEPTS: SPECIAL SITUATIONS IN AED USE

1. Water: *Is the victim lying in water (for example, the wet surfaces around a swimming pool)?* Shocking on a wet surface may cause burns or shocks to the victim or rescuers.
   Actions:
   • Remove the victim from contact with water.
   • Drag the victim gently by the arms or legs, or use a blanket drag.
   • Dry the victim's chest quickly before attaching the AED.

2. Metal surface: *Is the victim lying on a metal surface?* Avoid shocking a victim who is lying on a metal surface. Because all metal conducts electric current, there is a small but unlikely risk of the electric charge shocking a rescuer or bystander near the victim.
   Action:
   • Remove the victim from contact with a metal surface.

3. Children: *Is the victim a child younger than 8 years?* AEDs have been tested and approved by the FDA only for children 8 years old (or older). In addition, the electric energy settings of AEDs are often too high for children under 8 years old.
   Action:
   • If the victim is younger than 8 years, do not use the AED.

4. Transdermal medications: *Do patch medications interfere with placement of electrode pads on the victim's chest?* Placing an AED electrode pad on top of a medication patch may block delivery of shocks or cause small burns to the skin.
   Action:
   • Remove the patch and wipe the area clean before attaching the AED.

5. Implanted pacemakers or defibrillators: *Does the victim have a pacemaker or implanted cardioverter-defibrillator?* These devices create a hard lump beneath the skin of the upper chest or abdomen (usually on the victim's left side). The lump is about half the size of a deck of cards and usually has a small overlying scar. Placing an AED electrode pad directly over an implanted medical device may reduce the effectiveness of defibrillation.
   Actions:
   • Do not place an AED electrode pad directly over an implanted device.
   • Place an AED electrode pad at least 1″ to the side of any implanted device.

FOLLOWING THE UNIVERSAL STEPS OF AED OPERATION

In Chapter 4 we will "put it all together" and blend your CPR skills with AED operation. This section covers specific details you should know about using an AED in a real situation. These details are summarized in the Critical Concepts box on the right. Remember, these steps start only *after* you have verified that the victim is unresponsive, is not breathing, and has no pulse and you have placed the AED near the victim's left ear. You will practice and rehearse real-life situations during the Heartsaver FACTS practice scenario sessions.

Step 1. POWER ON the AED first! (FIGURE 2)

a. **Open the AED.** This automatically turns the *power on* in some devices.

b. **Press the POWER ON button first.**
This is critical because sound alerts, lights, and voice prompts will tell you that the power is ON and will direct you through the steps of using the AED. Always turn the AED ON as the first step. Do *not* wait until you have opened the package of adhesive electrode pads or attached the electrode pads to the victim's chest.

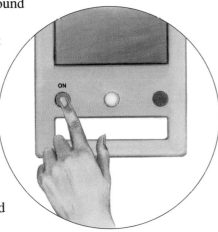

FIGURE 2
Operate AED; POWER ON first.

CRITICAL CONCEPTS: THE UNIVERSAL STEPS FOR AED OPERATION

1. **POWER ON the AED first (use prompts for guidance).**
   - **Open the carrying case or top of the AED.**
   - **Turn the power on (some devices will power up automatically when you open the lid or case).**

2. **ATTACH electrode pads to the victim's chest. (Stop CPR chest compressions just before attaching the pads.)**
   - **Attach AED connecting cables to the "box." (Some AED cables are already connected.)**
   - **Attach AED connecting cables to the chest electrode pads. (Some AED electrode pads are already connected.)**
   - **Peel the backing away from the electrode pads. Stop CPR.**
   - **Attach the adhesive electrode pads to the victim's bare chest.**

3. **ANALYZE the rhythm.**
   - **Press the ANALYZE button to start rhythm analysis (some AEDs do not require this step).**
   - **Always "clear" the victim during analysis. Be sure that no one is touching the victim, not even the person in charge of rescue breathing.**

4. **Press the SHOCK button if shock is indicated.**
   - **Clear the victim before delivering the shock: be sure no one is touching the victim.**
   - **Press the SHOCK button to deliver the shock when — and only when — the AED signals a shock is indicated.**

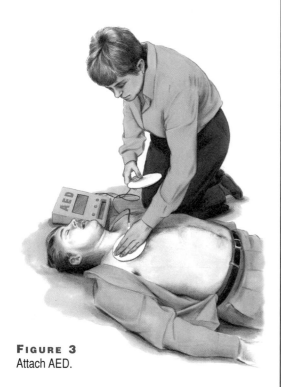

FIGURE 3
Attach AED.

Step 2. ATTACH adhesive electrode pads to the victim's chest (stop CPR chest compressions) (FIGURE 3).

a. ***Remove clothing from the victim's chest.*** Place 2 adhesive electrode pads directly on the skin of the victim's chest. The chest should be bare to the skin. Remove clothing and undergarments as needed, even for women. Do not hesitate — remember that you are trying to save the victim's life. Bandage scissors can be stored in the AED carrying case to cut clothing that is hard to remove.

b. ***Dry the victim's chest if necessary.*** *Be sure* the victim's chest is bare and wiped dry. This will help the AED electrode pads stick firmly so that they will not shift or fall off during defibrillation. Keep a cloth or gauze in the AED carrying case for drying.

c. ***Open the package of adhesive electrode pads in the AED carrying case.*** Some defibrillation electrode pads are preconnected to the cables. For others, join one end of the cable to the AED. Then attach the other end of the cable to the electrode pads.

d. ***Join ("snap") the connecting cables to the electrode pads (in some AEDs the cables are preconnected to the electrode pads).*** First put the electrode pads on the floor or the ground. Then snap the cables down on the pad connecting posts *before* you place the pads on the victim's chest.

e. ***Attach the adhesive electrode pads to the victim's chest (stop CPR chest compressions during this step to ensure proper pad placement).*** Peel away the protective plastic backing from the electrode pads to expose the adhesive surface. Attach the AED electrode pads, adhesive side down, directly to the skin of the victim's chest. Follow the example pictured on the pad packaging. It is not necessary to match position and cable alignment exactly, but try to place the pads like those in the example.

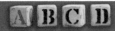

FIGURE 4
Chest-to-AED circuit.

f. **Proper pad locations.** The *first pad* goes on the *upper right side* of the victim's chest, to the right of the breastbone, between the nipple and collarbone. The second pad goes to the outside of the left nipple, with the top margin of the pad several inches below the left armpit. Follow the example on the package. The AED will operate even if pad placement is not exactly as pictured.

Step 3. ANALYZE the victim's rhythm (FIGURES 4, 5, 6).

a. **Stop CPR. Do not touch the victim.** When you are ready to analyze the victim's rhythm, stop CPR completely. *Do not touch the victim or have any physical contact with the victim* (FIGURE 5) (because it could interfere with AED analysis). Some AEDs start to analyze the rhythm as soon as the electrode pads are attached. Others require you to push an ANALYZE button to start rhythm analysis. From this point forward — whenever the machine is analyzing, preparing to shock, or actually delivering the shock to the victim — it is critical that you, your team members, and all bystanders avoid *all* contact with the victim.

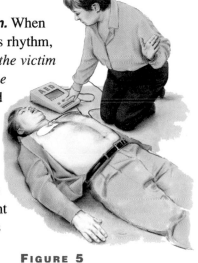

FIGURE 5
"Clear" during analysis.

b. **Announce, "Stand clear of the victim!"** The rescuer operating the AED should state clearly, *"Stand clear of the victim! Analyzing rhythm! Stand clear!"* You do not need to use these exact words, but make sure the message gets across. *No one should touch the victim during analysis or shock.* If anyone is touching the victim, refuse to push the ANALYZE or SHOCK buttons until contact with the victim stops.

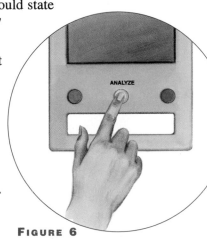

FIGURE 6
Clear/analyze.

FOUNDATION FACTS: MAKING THE CONNECTIONS

AEDs require that 4 objects be connected in a line: from the AED, to the connecting cable, to the AED electrode pads, to the victim's chest. Remember

1. The AED is joined to the
2. Connecting cables, which are joined to the
3. AED electrode pads, which are attached to
4. The victim's chest

AED manufacturers have not yet standardized these connections. Learn these details of your particular AED during the course. In newer AED models the electrode pads are preattached to the connecting cables, and the connecting cables are preattached to the AED. All the operator has to do is open the electrode pad package and attach the pads to the patient's chest.

Learn exactly how much of the AED "circuit" you must put together for your AED *before* you need it in an emergency. Remember that you can figure out the connections by recalling the 4 elements that must be joined: AED, cables, electrode pads, victim (FIGURE 4).

A B C D

FOUNDATION FACTS: THE HAIRY CHEST PROBLEM

If the victim has a hairy chest, the adhesive electrode pads may stick to the hair of the chest so that contact is not made with the skin on the chest. This will lead to a "check electrodes" or "check electrode pads" message on the AED. Try the following:

- Press down firmly on each pad. That may solve the problem.

- Quickly pull off the electrode pads. This will remove much of the chest hair. Dry the chest and apply a second set of electrode pads. See if the AED will now analyze.

- If you still cannot get a good connection, pull off the second set of electrode pads. Then shave the area for pad placement with a few strokes of the prep razor in the AED carrying case. Then open and apply a new (third) set of electrode pads.

Professional responders are given plastic disposable razors to quickly shave a suitable area of chest hair so that the electrode pads stick directly to the skin. Consider whether you are comfortable with the idea of shaving someone's chest after practicing the Heartsaver FACTS scenarios. Two of these razors should be packed in the AED storage case with 2 extra sets of electrode pads.

A B C D

Step 4. Charge the AED and deliver the SHOCK (if indicated) (FIGURE 7).

a. ***Stay clear while charging.*** When the AED recognizes a shockable rhythm, voice messages will prompt you to "stay clear." Most AED models begin charging automatically. You must make sure that no one is touching the victim. To prepare for shock delivery, announce and verify (with a visual check), *"I'm clear, you're clear, we're all clear."*

b. ***Push to shock.*** When charging is complete, the machine will advise you to *"push to shock."* Just before you press the SHOCK button, *make one last check to be sure that no one is touching the victim.* Then press the SHOCK button to deliver the shock to the victim.

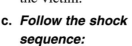

c. ***Follow the shock sequence:***
- *Analyze, shock*
- *Analyze, shock*
- *Analyze, shock*

FIGURE 7
Shock.

The number of shocks an AED delivers and the energy level for each shock are preset by the manufacturer. Let the AED follow the shock sequence it has been programmed to deliver. Follow the AED voice and visual prompts. Continue to follow the sequence of actions outlined in Chapter 4 until EMS personnel arrive. Transfer the care of the victim to EMS personnel after the AED has completed the shock cycles.

If "no shock indicated," check pulse. Then begin sequence of CPR.

a. ***Leave AED electrode pads attached. Check ABCs.*** If the victim's heart is no longer in VF, the AED will signal *"no shock indicated"* (or *"no shock advised"*) or *"check breathing and pulse."* Leave the AED electrodes attached to the victim's chest. Check for a pulse. Then follow the ABCs of CPR.

b. **If the victim is breathing** *adequately* **and has a pulse,** place the victim in the **recovery position** and monitor breathing until EMS personnel arrive.

c. **If the victim is not breathing but has a pulse,** give rescue breaths (1 breath every 5 seconds). Check the pulse frequently (**FIGURE 8**).

d. **If the victim is not breathing and has no pulse,** resume CPR.

e. **Care after shock.** Leave the AED electrode pads in place and the AED turned ON.

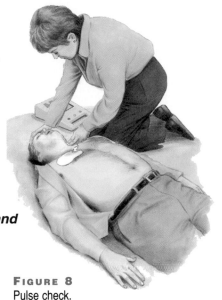

FIGURE 8
Pulse check.

CRITICAL CONCEPTS: AED MAINTENANCE

• **Become familiar with your AED and how it operates.**

• **Check the AED for any visible problems, such as open case or sign of damage.**

• **Check the "ready-for-use" indicator on your AED (if so equipped) daily.**

• **Perform any other user-based maintenance according to the manufacturer's recommendation.**

• **Check to see that the AED carrying case contains the following minimum accessories:**

  — **2 sets of *spare* defibrillator electrode pads (3 total)**

  — **2 pocket face masks**

  — **1 extra battery (if appropriate for your AED; some AEDs have batteries that last for years)**

  — **2 prep razors (supplied by manufacturers)**

  — **5 to 10 alcohol wipes**

  — **5 sterile gauze pads (4 x 4 inches), individually wrapped**

  — **1 absorbent cloth towel**

  Remember: **AED malfunctions are extremely rare. Most reported problems have been caused by failure to perform user-based maintenance of the AED.**

CRITICAL CONCEPTS: PAD PLACEMENT

Practice opening the electrode pad package and attaching the cables while your partner performs CPR, including rescue breathing and chest compressions. When you are ready to apply the electrode pads, remove the adhesive backing of the first pad. Then stop CPR chest compressions. Quickly apply the pads and allow the AED to analyze the rhythm. With some AEDs you may have to press the ANALYZE button. Other AEDs will automatically analyze as soon as the electrode pads are properly attached.

You may receive a voice prompt or alarm if the electrode pads are not securely attached to the chest or if the cables are not fastened properly. The voice warning will state "check pads" or "check electrodes," or words to that effect. Troubleshoot by checking the following:

1. If the victim has a hairy chest, try removing and reapplying the pads or shaving the chest (see "The Hairy Chest Problem" box).

2. Are the electrode pads stuck firmly and evenly to the skin of the chest?

3. Are the cables correctly connected to the adhesive electrode pads?

4. Are the cables correctly connected to the AED?

When you correct the problem, most AEDs will automatically go into the analyze mode.

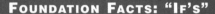

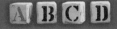

*Do **NOT** remove the electrode pads or turn the AED off until instructed to do so by EMS personnel.* The victim may "rearrest" and lose spontaneous respirations and pulse. If the AED is always ready for use, you and others on your rescue team can resume the AED action sequence as soon as it is needed.

AED MAINTENANCE AND TROUBLESHOOTING

Newer models of AEDs require almost no maintenance. They can check themselves to see if they are working and ready for use. But you and your coworkers who are trained to use an AED must still make sure your AED is ready for use at a moment's notice.

AED manufacturers provide specific recommendations about checking maintenance and readiness. See the handout *Manufacturer's Instructions and Guide to Maintenance* that your instructor will have. Your instructor will give you information about the type of maintenance your AED needs or refer you to a source of more information.

SUMMARY

Do not become confused by the details presented in this chapter. AEDs are simple, easy to use, and user friendly. Many people who take a Heartsaver FACTS course need only a few minutes to get the "big picture" of operating an AED and then spend time practicing:

- POWER ON the AED first. Listen to the voice and visual prompts.
- ATTACH the electrode pads (paying attention to the figures on pad location and stopping chest compressions).
- ANALYZE the rhythm (this may occur automatically).
- Press the SHOCK button if shock is indicated (clear the victim first).

These are the only defibrillation steps most lay rescuers using an AED will ever need to know. Performing these same steps during an actual VF arrest will get the job done.

Other lay responders, however, will appreciate the details about defibrillation presented in this chapter. If you are curious about the rich variety of "what if?" situations that can arise during defibrillation, this chapter will help answer your questions. It will also enrich your understanding of defibrillation.

REVIEW QUESTIONS

1. What is an AED?

   a. a heart monitor that tells you when to start CPR

   b. a device used to treat victims of cardiac arrest who fail to respond to 15 minutes of CPR

   c. a device to analyze the adult heart for a shockable rhythm and to deliver defibrillation shocks

   d. a device that electrically "paces" the heart at 60 to 80 beats per minute

2. In correct order, what are the 4 universal steps required to operate an AED?

   a. POWER ON, ATTACH the electrode pads to the victim's chest and to the AED, ANALYZE the victim's rhythm, and deliver a SHOCK if needed

   b. call 911, begin CPR, use the AED, and provide advanced life support

   c. move the victim to a safe place, attach the electrode pads to the victim's chest, attach the cables to the electrode pads, and attach the cables to the AED

   d. check for a pulse, POWER ON, deliver a shock, and then analyze the victim's rhythm

HOW DID YOU DO?

1. c; 2. a

ABCD: PUTTING CPR AND DEFIBRILLATION TOGETHER

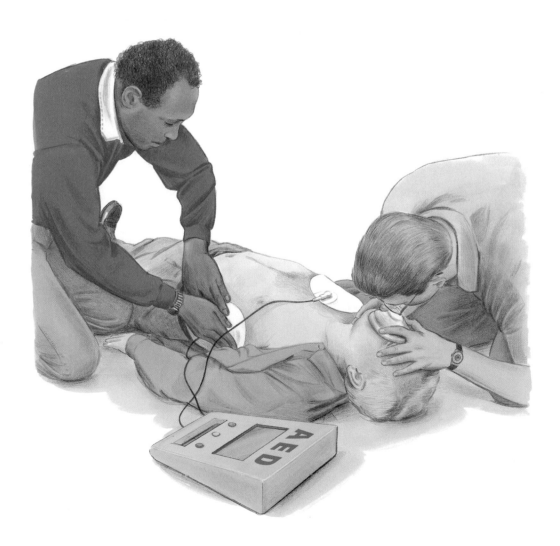

4

CONTENTS

Defibrillation

sounds

complicated,

but it is

actually

easier

than CPR.

LEARNING OBJECTIVES

After reading this chapter, you should be able to

1. List the criteria for when to start CPR and use the AED
2. Describe the 3 assessment steps for a collapsed person
3. Describe the roles for lay rescuers with an AED
4. Demonstrate how to manage the following collapsed victims with an AED when you are given a scenario:
   - No shock advised, no pulse
   - Shock advised, single shock, return of pulse and breathing
   - Shock advised, 3 shocks in a row, CPR for 1 minute, return of pulse after the fourth shock
5. Describe how you can help a victim of cardiac arrest even if no AED is available

INTRODUCTION

In this chapter you will learn to combine the skills of CPR (Chapter 2) with your knowledge of using an AED (Chapter 3). You will learn a simple algorithm (a set of steps) for most rescue situations you will encounter. The Heartsaver AED algorithm guides you whether you respond to a cardiac arrest as a single rescuer alone or with others who can help. The AEDs you will use will provide audio and visual prompts at every step, including CPR and defibrillation. You have only a few steps to memorize and a few decisions to make along the way. Your major learning task is to become familiar with the steps you will perform during the "pump and blow" of CPR and how to open, attach, and use the AED. The chapter ends with several practice scenarios to review what you have learned and to cover several possible outcomes of your rescue efforts.

MAINTAINING THE CHAIN OF SURVIVAL

Whether you respond to a cardiovascular emergency at home, at the worksite, or in the community, you can be the start of a strong Chain of Survival. The links in the Chain of Survival are early activation of the EMS system, early CPR, early defibrillation, and early advanced care. The call to 911 activates the EMS system and brings a professional emergency care team to the scene. The CPR you provide maintains the heart in a condition that favors successful defibrillation. When advanced EMS personnel arrive at the scene, they will help stabilize the victim and give additional treatments that increase the chance of successful resuscitation. This is especially true for victims who are not in ventricular fibrillation.

WHEN TO START CPR?
WHEN TO USE THE AED?

Here are 3 major cues for starting CPR and using the AED. You need to remember them. All 3 conditions must be present to start CPR and use the AED.

- *Unresponsiveness:* This prompts you to take 2 actions: call 911 and get the AED.

- *Not breathing:* This prompts you to give rescue breathing.

- *No pulse:* This prompts you to take 2 actions: use the AED and start chest compressions.

At this point you really don't have to make decisions. Just recognize the 3 conditions: ***unresponsive, not breathing, no pulse.*** Know the action you must take in response.

When the AED is turned on, attached to the victim, and placed in analyze mode, it will identify one of two conditions: *shockable rhythm present* or *shockable rhythm absent.* You respond to the AED prompts by "clearing" the victim, pressing the ANALYZE button (this is done automatically in some models), and pressing the SHOCK button when indicated. That's all there is to the use of the AED. Once you complete the use of the AED, you return to supporting the victim with CPR, rescue breathing, or the recovery position. EMS responders should arrive within a few short minutes.

ACTION SEQUENCE:
THE HEARTSAVER AED PROTOCOL

Combining CPR With Using an AED:
The Heartsaver AED Protocol

When you see a person who may be in cardiac arrest, act quickly but calmly. Follow the same sequences you learned for CPR (Chapter 2) and AED operation (Chapter 3). The Heartsaver FACTS Course teaches CPR and AED in 3 learning steps:

- *The steps of CPR*

- *The steps of AED operation*

- *The full action sequence of the Heartsaver AED protocol*

The Heartsaver AED Protocol

SUMMARY: THE HEARTSAVER AED PROTOCOL

A-B-C: The 4 Steps of CPR

1. Unresponsive?
   Call 911 — get the AED.

2. Airway: Perform head tilt – chin lift.

3. Breathing: *Look, listen, and feel.* Give 2 breaths if needed.

4. Circulation: Check pulse; start chest compressions if needed. (Stop during pad placement.)

D: The 4 Universal Steps of AED Operation

1. POWER ON the AED first!

2. ATTACH the AED to the victim's bare chest (AED, cables, pads).

3. ANALYZE rhythm.

4. SHOCK (if shock indicated).

UNRESPONSIVE? 911 — AED

Check unresponsiveness: Shout, *"Are you OK?"*
If unresponsive:
Call 911! Point to another witness: *"You! Go call 911!"*
(Start CPR while witness goes for the AED. If alone, you must go yourself.)
AED: Get the AED located next to the telephone:
". . . And get the AED next to the phone!"
(If alone, you must get the AED yourself.)

(Return to the side of the victim.)

START THE ABCDs:

A: **A**irway open: head tilt–chin lift; jaw thrust.

B: **B**reathing check *(look, listen, and feel):*

if no breathing, give **2 slow breaths.**

C: **C**irculation check — **no pulse** is the signal to

- **Start chest compressions/begin**

  rescue breathing

  plus

D: **D**efibrillation: **attach** and **operate** the AED

(To continue, see next section,
"The 5-Step AED Treatment Protocol.")

THE 5-STEP AED TREATMENT PROTOCOL

Attach and operate the AED:

1. **POWER ON the AED first:**

   - Open carrying case or top of AED; turn AED **ON**.

     — *POWER ON allows voice and visual prompts from the AED to guide the operator.*

     — *POWER ON may occur automatically in some AEDs by opening the lid.*

2. **ATTACH the AED to the victim:**

   - **Attach** AED connecting **cables** to the **AED**.

     — *May be preconnected in some AEDs.*

   - **Attach** AED connecting **cables** to the adhesive chest electrode **pads**.

     — *May be preconnected.*

   - **Attach** adhesive **pads** to victim's bare **chest** after peeling off backing.

     — *Stop chest compressions while placing AED electrode pads.*

3. **ANALYZE the rhythm:**

   - **Clear** the victim before and during analysis; check that no one is touching the victim, including the person doing rescue breathing.

   - **Press** the **ANALYZE** button to start rhythm analysis *(some brands of AEDs do not require this step).*

4. **"Shock" Sequence (if indicated):**

   - **"Clear."** Clear victim once more before pushing the SHOCK button.

   - **"SHOCK."** Press the SHOCK button to deliver the shock *(victim may display muscle contractions).*

   - **"Clear."** *Clear the victim again before each analysis and shock.*

   - **"ANALYZE."**

   - **"Clear."** *Clear the victim again before each analysis and shock.*

   - **"SHOCK."** Press the SHOCK button up to 2 more times if AED signals *"shock indicated."*

5. **"No Shock Indicated" Sequence:**

   Check **pulse:**

   - If **pulse:** check **breathing.**

     — If *inadequate* **breathing:** assist with rescue breathing (1 breath every 5 seconds).

     — If *adequate* **breathing:** place the victim in the recovery position.

   - If **no pulse:** resume CPR for 1 minute; then **recheck** pulse.

   - If **no pulse** after 1 minute, reanalyze rhythm: AED will indicate either *"shock indicated"* (go to step 4) or *"no shock indicated"* (repeat step 5).

Memorize the 2

action sequences:

"shock indicated"

and

"no shock indicated."

Memorize the "shock indicated" and "no shock indicated" sequences

We highly recommend that you memorize 2 simple action sequences: *"shock indicated"* and *"no shock indicated."* The sequence you follow is based on the AED's rhythm analysis and the clinical responses of the victim. The AED will lead you through the 2 sequences. We will refer to these sequences throughout the Heartsaver FACTS handbook and course.

As long as the "shock indicated" message occurs, follow this sequence:

- Clear
- **SHOCK**
- Clear
- **ANALYZE**
- Repeat up to 3 shocks if needed; then resume CPR.

Whenever the "no shock indicated" message occurs, follow this sequence:

- Check **pulse.**
- If **pulse,** check breathing. Inadequate: assist breathing. *Adequate:* place the victim in the recovery position.
- If **no pulse,** resume CPR for 1 minute; then recheck pulse.
- If **no pulse,** analyze rhythm; then repeat the sequences: *"shock indicated"* or *"no shock indicated."*

Remember the 3 Conditions That Must Be Present to Start CPR or Use the AED

Recognize the 3 conditions and know the action you must take in response.

To start CPR or use the AED, victim must be

1. Unresponsive — call 911 and get the AED
2. Not breathing — give rescue breaths
3. Pulseless — use the AED and start compressions

Applying the Two-Rescuer Heartsaver AED Action Sequence

Witnessed Arrest With Two People Responding

Chapters 2 and 3 show the one-rescuer scenario: a single person witnesses a collapse and must perform the entire Heartsaver AED action sequence. Another common scenario is the two-rescuer scenario: a witnessed arrest, such as at a worksite or a public place, with several bystanders. **Figures 1 through 14** demonstrate use of the Heartsaver AED action sequence for this scenario.

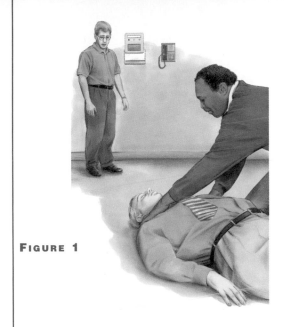

Figure 1

Two-Rescuer Heartsaver AED Action Sequence

- **Check unresponsiveness:** Shout, "Are you OK?" **(Figure 1)** If unresponsive:
- **Call 911!** Point to another witness: "You! Go call 911!"
- **AED:** Get the AED located next to the telephone: ". . . And get the AED next to the phone!" **(Figure 2)**

- The person who calls 911 gets the AED.
- The person who will use the AED stays with the victim.

  (These roles may be reversed in many circumstances.)

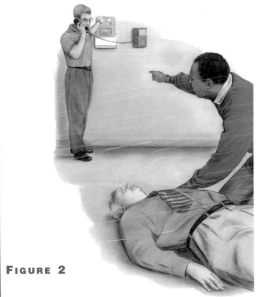

Figure 2

- The Heartsaver AED rescuer starts CPR during the call to 911.
- **A** — **Airway** open: head tilt–chin lift; jaw thrust **(Figure 3)**.
  - If trauma is suspected, use the jaw-thrust maneuver to open the airway.
  - Face mask is available in AED carrying case.
  - Face shield is more likely to be available to first rescuer.
- **B** — **Breathing** check *(look, listen, and feel)* **(Figure 3)**.

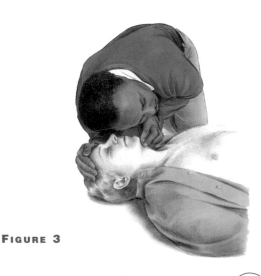

Figure 3

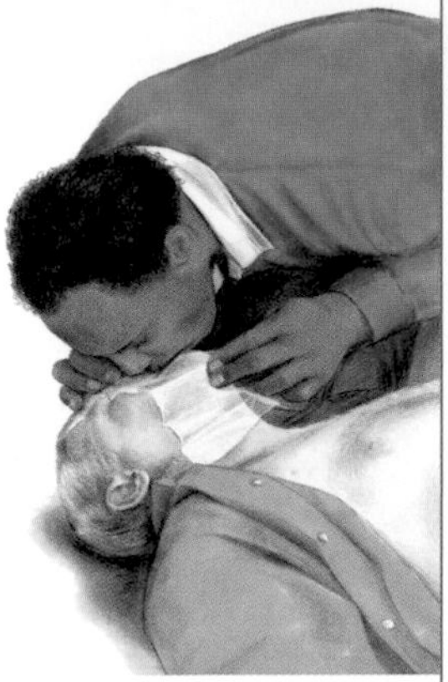

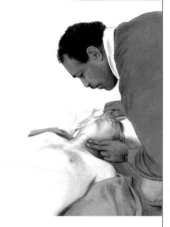

FIGURE 4

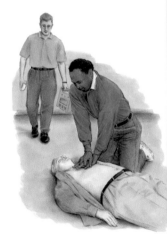

FIGURE 5

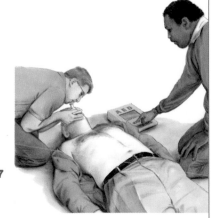

FIGURE 6

- If no breathing, give 2 slow breaths **(FIGURE 4)**.
  - Key: Rescuer must see chest rise with each breath.
  - Face masks are the preferred barrier device, but face shields are acceptable.
  - Face masks should have a one-way valve.

- **C — Circulation:** check for a pulse **(FIGURE 5)**. Finding no pulse is the signal to
- Start chest compressions, begin rescue breathing, attach the AED.
  - Pulse checks are notoriously inaccurate; if there is any doubt, do chest compressions and use the AED.

- Remove clothing covering the chest. The victim's chest should be bare for chest compressions and using the AED.
- Use the landmark "center of chest, right between the nipples" to locate hand compression point **(FIGURE 6)**.

- The 911 caller delivers the AED to the person doing CPR.
- The 911 caller begins doing CPR **(FIGURE 7)**. (It is acceptable to reverse these roles.)
- The preferred AED placement is next to the victim's left ear, but this may not be possible in all cases.

FIGURE 7

- Open the carrying case or top of the AED.
- **POWER ON** the AED first **(FIGURE 8)** (some devices will turn on automatically when the AED lid or carrying case is opened).

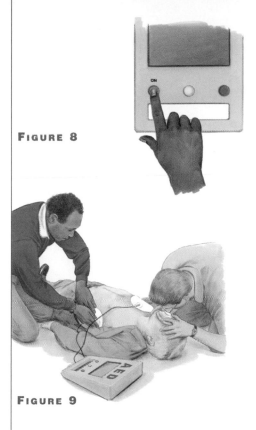

FIGURE 8

- **ATTACH** AED connecting *cables* to the *AED* (may be preconnected).
- **ATTACH** AED connecting *cables* to the adhesive *electrode pads* (may be preconnected).
- **ATTACH** adhesive *electrode pads* to the victim's bare *chest* **(FIGURE 9).**
  - If necessary, stop chest compressions while placing AED electrode pads.

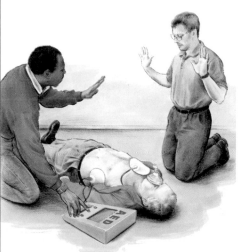

FIGURE 9

- **ANALYZE** the rhythm.
- Clear the victim before and during analysis **(FIGURE 10).**
- Check that no one is touching the victim, including the person doing rescue breathing.
- Press the **ANALYZE** button to start rhythm analysis **(FIGURE 11)** (some brands of AEDs do not require this step).

FIGURE 10

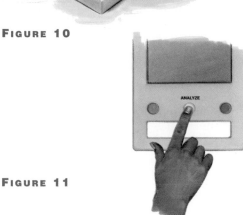

FIGURE 11

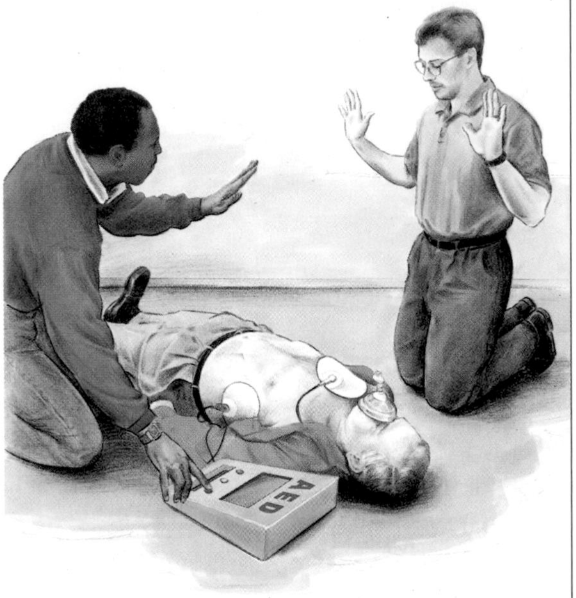

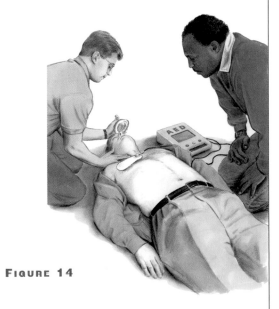

FIGURE 12

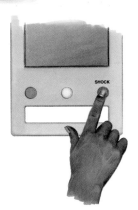

FIGURE 13

- *"Shock advised" :* Follow the *"shock indicated"* **sequence:**

  — Clear the victim once more before pushing the SHOCK button (**FIGURE 12**).

  — Press the SHOCK button to deliver shock if the AED signals *"shock advised"* (**FIGURE 13**) (victim may display muscle contractions; continue to clear).

  — Press the ANALYZE and SHOCK buttons up to 2 more times if AED signals *"shock advised"* or *"shock indicated."* (Clear the victim again before each analysis and shock.)

- Whenever the AED signals *"no shock indicated" :* Follow the *"no shock indicated"* **sequence:**

  — Check the pulse (**FIGURE 14**).

  — If pulse, check breathing. If breathing is inadequate, assist breathing. If breathing is adequate, place the victim in the recovery position.

  — If no pulse, resume CPR for 1 minute; then recheck pulse.

  — If no pulse, analyze rhythm.

  — Then follow *"shock indicated"* or *"no shock indicated"* steps above.

FIGURE 14

THE HEARTSAVER RESCUER WITH AN AED: THE RESCUE DIRECTOR

In this course you will be trained to be the *rescue director.* You have the skills both to do CPR and operate an AED. In many rescue situations you may be the only witness who has either of these abilities. Although your responsibility is great, the tasks are simple — tell other witnesses to *"call 911 — get the AED located by the telephone"* ; tell other rescuers to *"help with CPR."* You will ensure that actions are taken in the proper sequence as quickly as possible and that they are well coordinated.

The bottom line — you must make only **3 critical assessments:** *unresponsive? breathing? pulse?* You learned these assessments in basic CPR. After that you simply follow prompts from the AED.

The beauty of AED technology is its simple design. Almost anyone can operate an AED. As you will see in the training video and demonstrations by your instructor, AEDs give you a lot of guidance: voice prompts, tone and light signals, and visual icons and figures on the device and defibrillator pads. Defibrillation sounds complicated, but you will see during practice sessions that operating an AED is easy. It is actually easier than learning and performing CPR.

As you mentally rehearse during this class and future practice sessions, think of yourself as the rescue director. When you think through several sample scenarios, you will realize that **You Can Do It!** Other witnesses will appreciate your knowledge, skills, and confidence. They will be happy to follow your directions and help where they can.

You must make only 3 critical assessments: Unresponsive? Breathing? Pulse?

The Heartsaver AED Rescuer With Two or More People to Help

What happens when a cardiac arrest is witnessed by several people? They all want to help but may be unsure of what to do. In some worksites all employees will be trained as Heartsaver AED rescuers. Almost everyone will be knowledgeable and have a sense of what to do. The answer — *you direct them.* Unless you are alone, as a Heartsaver AED rescuer you should not leave the victim's side. If other witnesses are present, particularly other Heartsaver AED rescuers, *use them.* Direct them to perform one of these tasks:

- *Call 911.*

- *Get the AED.*

- *Do CPR: Do rescue breathing. Do chest compressions.*

You will practice these scenarios during the Heartsaver FACTS Course. The rescue tasks of calling 911, getting the AED, starting CPR, and operating the AED will be practiced in the 8 core scenarios, where the tasks will be divided several ways. In each scenario *the Heartsaver AED rescuer is the rescue director.* The Heartsaver AED rescuer will perform both the initial assessment and CPR and will operate the AED when it arrives.

Instructors may teach these roles another way: *whoever calls 911 and gets the AED will operate the AED.* This means that the second rescuer must be able to perform the initial ABCs and CPR. Either approach is acceptable. The preferred approach is for the AED rescuer always to remain with the victim.

THE HEARTSAVER AED RESCUER AND PROMPTS FROM THE AED

The AED is a remarkable electronic device. One of its most useful features is the audio voice prompts that provide feedback to the Heartsaver AED rescuer. During the Heartsaver FACTS Course you will have many opportunities to practice and learn the audio and visual prompts of the specific AED you will use. All AED models provide at least 4 types of voice messages:

- *Analysis indicator:* when the AED is analyzing the rhythm (*"analyzing; do not touch the victim"*).

- *Shockable rhythm indicator:* whether or not the AED identifies a shockable rhythm during analysis (*"shock indicated"* or *"no shock indicated"*).

- *Loose electrode indicator:* *"check electrodes"* sounds when there is any break in the connections between the victim's skin and the AED. Most often this break occurs where the electrode pad contacts the skin, but the break can also occur at the cable-to-pad connections or at the cable-to-AED connections.

- *Sequencing information:* AEDs provide sequencing steps (*"connect electrodes"* or *"check airway, check breathing, check pulse"* or *"perform CPR if no pulse"*).

SUMMARY

This is the "putting-it-all-together" chapter. A trained Heartsaver AED rescuer must know how to give CPR, how to use an AED, and how to use the two together. Although most lay rescuers will respond with others to a witnessed cardiac arrest, many arrests occur in the home with only a distraught loved one to provide the first minutes of care. This chapter demonstrates how easy it is to integrate the two skills — CPR and AED — for use by a single, well-trained provider — the Heartsaver AED rescuer.

The cases that follow were carefully selected and developed to provide an overview of the major types of emergencies you are likely to encounter. Review the cases and try to answer the questions. This "thinking" exercise will strongly reinforce the ideas and skills you learn in the Heartsaver FACTS Course. In the course you will actually rehearse similar scenarios multiple times.

....

A Heartsaver AED rescuer must know how to

- *Give CPR*

- *Use an AED*

- *Put CPR and AED together.*

You Can Do It!

....

STUDY CASES

The following **study cases** let you review different situations that you may face as a Heartsaver AED rescuer. Do the following:

- Carefully review each case.
- Consider the single **best** answer to the case question.
- Write your answer in the space provided.
- In the answer section, review the correct answer and why it is the best answer.
- If the answer and discussion are unclear, review the related section in this book.
- If you have further questions, ask your Heartsaver AED Course instructor.

CASE 1: RETURN OF PULSE, NOT BREATHING

Your 50-year-old spouse clutches his or her chest while eating dinner and collapses on the floor. You verify unresponsiveness, call 911, and get the AED from near the telephone. You then assess the ABCs and find that your spouse is pulseless and not breathing. You attach the AED. You clear for analysis; the AED advises a shock. You deliver a shock, and the machine displays a no-shock message. You reassess the ABCs. You can now feel your spouse's pulse, but your spouse is not breathing. What should you do next? Continue shocking? Start chest compressions? Start rescue breathing? Place victim in the recovery position?

What is your answer? _____

_____

Why? _____

Case 1 — Answer

The best answer is to support the breathing with rescue breathing (1 breath every 5 seconds; 12 breaths per minute). You do not need to do chest compressions because the pulse has returned. You should not place a victim in the recovery position unless he or she has both a pulse and adequate breathing. Continue rescue breathing until your spouse breathes adequately on his or her own or EMS personnel arrive. You should also check your spouse's pulse periodically to confirm that cardiac arrest did not recur.

Case 2: Cardiac Arrest at a Swimming Pool

A 52-year-old woman with a history of heart disease has been doing water aerobics in the community pool. Suddenly the class instructor sees her clutch her chest and gasp for air before she sinks beneath the water. Several people reach for the woman and drag her, wet and dripping, from the pool. The victim is not breathing and does not have a pulse. Another lifeguard runs to get the AED from the main lifeguard station. Should they shock her right away?

What is your answer? _____

_____

Why? _____

Case 2 — Answer

The best answer is *do not shock a victim who is lying in water, even as little as a wet surface*. Try to quickly move the woman to a dry surface, and dry her chest off with a towel. Shocking a victim while he or she is lying in water may cause some arcing of electric current between the electrodes or to the AED operator. This scenario is risky because rescuers are barefoot.

Case 3: Man With a Medication Patch on the Chest

An 82-year-old man has collapsed in his kitchen while getting a glass of water. His wife has called 911, and now you arrive on the scene. The man has no pulse and is not breathing. After removing the man's shirt, you discover that he is wearing a nitroglycerin patch on the left side of his chest. What should you do about this patch?

What is your answer? _____

_____

Why? _____

Case 3 — Answer

Do not place AED electrode pads over the nitroglycerin transdermal patch. If a victim has a medication patch on his or her chest, remove it and wipe the area clean before attaching the AED. Failure to do so may result in small burns to the victim's skin.

CASE 4: ELECTROCUTION OF A CHILD

You are a Heartsaver AED rescuer who arrives on the scene and finds a 6-year-old boy in cardiac arrest in the basement of a house under repair. Next to his hand is a live electric wire, which he pulled out of the wall. After assessing the boy and finding that he has no pulse, your partner begins to open the AED and turn the power on. You stop him. Why?

What is your answer? _____

_____

Why? _____

Case 4 — Answer

The best answer is that AEDs *are not authorized for use on children younger than 8 years of age.* The computer algorithms in the AED have been tested only with adult cardiac rhythms. Children less than 8 years old often are too small to tolerate the electric current delivered by an AED for adults. Defibrillation could damage the heart muscle. A VF rhythm could be shocked into asystole, which is even worse than VF. Future AEDs may have a pediatric shock setting. Unless specifically directed otherwise by a medical authority, rescuers should verify unresponsiveness, call 911, and apply the ABCs, including CPR.

CASE 5: VICTIM LYING ON A METAL SURFACE

A 51-year-old woman collapses on a freight elevator with a metal floor. Your partner, another police officer, has noted that the victim has no pulse and is not breathing. You get the AED from the trunk of the police cruiser, open the carrying case, and start to attach the AED pads to the woman's chest. Your partner stops you. Why?

What is your answer? —————————————————

—————————————————————————————

Why? —————————————————————

Case 5 — Answer

The best answer is that *you should avoid shocking a victim who is lying on a metal surface*. You should move the victim out of the elevator to a nonmetal surface. Because all metal conducts electric current, there is a small risk of the electric charge shocking a rescuer or bystander near the victim. If you're wearing rubber-soled shoes, the risk is virtually zero. If moving the victim is difficult or time-consuming, proceed with CPR and AED use.

CASE 6: MAN WITH RETURN OF PULSE AND BREATHING AFTER 2 SHOCKS

A 68-year-old executive collapses in his office. You and two coworkers are the company's emergency responders with the AED. You follow these steps:

- You confirm unresponsiveness.
- You send one coworker to call 911 and get the AED.
- You assess the ABCs; the patient is not breathing and has no pulse.
- You tell the other coworker to start CPR.
- You operate the AED (power-attach-analyze-shock) with loud statements to "clear."

After 2 shocks the AED screen displays "*no shock indicated,*" and the voice prompt states "check pulse." When you check the patient, you feel a strong pulse and see the victim breathe. What should you do next? (Choose one.)

A. Congratulate your coworker and remove the AED.

B. Remove the AED and place the victim in the recovery position.

C. Leave the AED attached and carefully observe the adequacy of the breathing and strength of the pulse.

D. Turn the AED off and resume CPR until the victim regains consciousness.

What is your answer? _____

_____

Why? _____

Case 6 — Answer

The correct answer is C.

You should always leave the AED power ON and the electrode pads attached to the victim's chest. Wait until EMS personnel arrive and give you further instructions. In this case the victim looks as if he has been successfully converted to a regular cardiac rhythm. Leave the AED attached. Closely observe how well the victim is breathing and whether his pulse continues to be strong.

This victim may have a second cardiac arrest ("refibrillation"). With close monitoring you will be able to detect a second arrest in seconds, and with the AED electrode pads still attached you'll be prepared to immediately analyze and shock. Monitor the victim until EMS personnel arrive. You may need to place the victim in the recovery position if he continues to breathe and has a pulse but remains unconscious.

Two important things to remember from this case: once you turn on the power and attach the pads to the victim's chest, (1) *leave the AED ON* and (2) *leave the electrode pads attached* until EMS personnel or other medical authorities tell you to turn the AED off.

REVIEW QUESTIONS

1. A victim's pulse is weak but present; however, her face has turned blue and she isn't breathing. You should attach the AED pads and start the shock cycle immediately.

   true   false

2. A victim has no pulse but has weak, sporadic, gasping breaths. He or she meets the criteria for use of an AED.

   true   false

3. The criteria for initiating CPR and using an AED are (choose one)
   a. unresponsive, weak pulse, no breathing
   b. unresponsive, no pulse, weak breathing
   c. unresponsive, weak pulse, weak breathing
   d. unresponsive, no pulse, no breathing

4. The correct sequence of actions to treat a person who suddenly collapses is (choose one)
   a. call 911, verify unresponsiveness, ABCD
   b. call 911, ABCD, verify unresponsiveness
   c. verify unresponsiveness, call 911, ABCD
   d. verify unresponsiveness, ABCD, call 911

5. You and two other rescuers respond to a 50-year-old man who is unresponsive, pulseless, and not breathing. What tasks do you assign the other rescuers while you set up the AED?
   a. one calls 911 and the other does CPR
   b. both help with setting up the AED and doing CPR
   c. both do CPR
   d. both leave to get additional first responders to help

6. After 3 shocks the victim is still pulseless. What should you do next?
   a. continue shocking immediately
   b. do not shock again until EMS arrives
   c. perform CPR for 1 minute and reanalyze
   d. remove the AED and transport the victim to the emergency department

7. You attach an AED to the chest of a 43-year-old victim who is unresponsive, not breathing, and pulseless. The AED advises "no shock." What would you do?
   a. shock anyway
   b. perform CPR for 1 minute and reanalyze
   c. perform CPR until EMS arrives
   d. remove the AED

HOW DID YOU DO?

1. false; **2.** true; **3.** d; **4.** c; **5.** a; **6.** c; **7.** b

CHAPTER 5

CPR AND DEFIBRILLATION: THE HUMAN DIMENSION

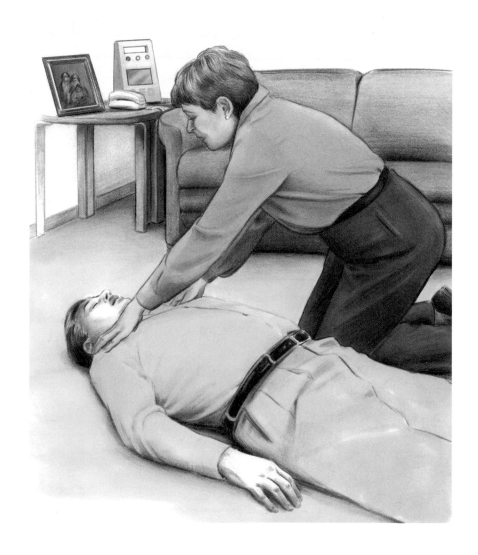

5

CONTENTS

Take pride

in your skills

as a Heartsaver

AED rescuer.

LEARNING OBJECTIVES

After reading this chapter, you should be able to

1. Explain how often CPR and defibrillation restore normal heartbeat and breathing in the out-of-hospital setting

2. Give 2 different definitions for "success" in lay rescuer resuscitation

3. State the importance of debriefing after a resuscitation attempt

4. Explain the role of the debriefing facilitator

5. Note the information your instructor gave you about whom to contact after you have attempted a resuscitation or used the AED in your location

THE HUMAN DIMENSION OF CPR: HOW OFTEN WILL CPR AND LAY RESCUER DEFIBRILLATION SUCCEED?

Since 1973 more than 40 million people have learned CPR. Many public health experts consider CPR training to be the most successful public health initiative of modern times. Millions of people have been willing to prepare themselves to take action to save the life of a fellow human being. Despite your best efforts, however, we know that the majority of times your efforts will not succeed. CPR attempts at home or in public help restart the heart and restore breathing only about 50% of the time, even in the most "successful" communities. Research tells us that training rescuers how to use an AED in citizen CPR courses will dramatically increase the number of survivors of cardiac arrest. Still, the exact degree of success is not known. The American Heart Association supports efforts to have nontraditional rescuers use AEDs through the public access defibrillation program.

Tragically even when their hearts restart, only about half of VF cardiac arrest victims admitted to the emergency department and the hospital survive and go home. This means that 3 of 4 times your CPR attempts will be unsuccessful. We think it is important to briefly discuss the range of possible emotional reactions from rescuers and witnesses to any resuscitation attempts, especially when your efforts appear to have made no difference.

TAKE PRIDE IN YOUR SKILLS AS A HEARTSAVER AED RESCUER

You should be proud of the fact that you are learning CPR and defibrillation skills. We hope you never have to use these skills. But emergencies happen. Now you can be confident that you will be better prepared to do the right thing for your family and loved ones, your coworkers, and your neighbors. Of course these emergencies can have negative outcomes. You, the equipment, and the emergency personnel who arrive to take over care may not succeed in restoring life. Some people have a cardiac arrest simply because they have reached the end of a well-lived life. Your success will not be measured by whether a cardiac arrest victim lives or dies. Your success will be measured by the fact that you tried. Simply by taking action, making an effort, and just trying to help you will be judged a success.

STRESS REACTIONS OF RESCUERS AND WITNESSES AFTER RESUSCITATION ATTEMPTS

A cardiac arrest is a dramatic and emotional event, especially if the victim is a friend or loved one. The emergency may involve disagreeable physical details, such as bleeding, vomiting, or poor hygiene. Any emergency can be an emotional burden, especially if the rescuer is closely involved with the victim. The emergency can produce strong emotional reactions in bystanders, lay rescuers, and EMS professionals. Failed attempts at resuscitation can impose even more stress on rescuers. This stress can result in a variety of emotional reactions and physical symptoms that may last long after the original emergency. These reactions are frequent and quite normal. There is nothing wrong with the rescuer or other witnesses.

It is **common** for a person to experience emotional aftershocks when he or she has passed through an unpleasant event. Usually such stress reactions occur immediately or within the first few hours after the event. Sometimes the emotional response may occur later.

Psychologists working with professional emergency personnel have learned that rescuers may experience grief, anxiety, anger, and sometimes guilt. Typical physical reactions include difficulty sleeping, fatigue, irritability, changes in eating habits, and confusion. Many people say that they are unable to stop thinking about the event.

Remember that these reactions are **common** and **normal.** They do not mean that you are "disturbed" or "weak." Strong

Your success will be measured by the fact that you tried.

Review and practice sessions will strengthen your skills, build your confidence, and increase the chance of an effective resuscitation effort.

reactions simply indicate that this particular event had a powerful impact on you. With understanding and the support of loved ones the stress reactions usually pass quickly.

TECHNIQUES TO PREVENT AND REDUCE STRESS IN RESCUERS, FAMILIES, AND WITNESSES

Psychologists have learned that the most successful way to reduce stress after rescue efforts is very simple: **Talk about it.** Sit down with other people who witnessed the event and talk it over. EMS personnel responding to public access defibrillation sites are encouraged to offer emotional support to lay rescuers and bystanders. More formal discussions should include not only the lay rescuers but also the professional responders.

In these discussions you will be encouraged to describe what happened. Do not be frightened about "reliving" the event. It is natural and healthful to do this. Describe what went through your mind during the rescue effort. Describe how it made you feel at the time. Describe how you feel now. Be patient with yourself. Understand that most reactions will diminish within a few days. Sharing your thoughts and feelings with your companions at work, fellow rescuers, EMS personnel, friends, or clergy will either prevent stress reactions or help with your recovery.

In some locations (for example, the homes of high-risk patients or at worksites) leaders of public access defibrillation programs may establish plans for more formal discussions or debriefings after resuscitations. Such sessions have been called **"critical incident stress debriefings,"** or CISDs.

Teams of specially trained persons are available to organize and conduct these debriefings. Such persons are usually associated with EMS services, employee assistance programs, community mental health centers, or public school systems. Other sources of psychological and emotional support can be local clergy, police chaplains, fire service chaplains, or hospital and emergency department social workers. Your course instructor will tell you what is planned for critical event debriefings in your program.

Critical event debriefings are a confidential group process. The facilitator leads and encourages persons involved in a stressful situation to express their thoughts and feelings about the event. You do not have to talk during the briefing, but if you do, what you say may help and reassure others. Rescuers and witnesses to an event can express and discuss shared feelings they experienced during and after a resuscitation attempt. These may be feelings of guilt, anxiety, or failure, especially if the resuscitation attempt had a negative outcome. Ideally the rescuers who were most involved in the resuscitation should be present for the debriefing. In some public access defibrillation programs, EMS personnel visit the lay rescuers who were involved in the resuscitation effort.

In some CPR courses instructors neglect this human dimension of CPR. Frequently this is because of time limitations and a full teaching agenda. The AHA encourages medical directors and Heartsaver FACTS Course instructors to discuss the emotional impact and stress that may follow resuscitation attempts.

PSYCHOLOGICAL BARRIERS TO ACTION

This course is preparing you to respond appropriately to a future emergency. Although you are preparing yourself by taking this course, chances are that you will never have to use your skills. Most laypeople have never been close to a victim of cardiac arrest and have seen CPR performed only on television or in the movies. Reality is quite different. During your Heartsaver FACTS Course and while reading this handbook, you may have had some troubling thoughts.

Here are some of the common concerns lay rescuers express about responding to sudden cardiac emergencies. *Will you really have what it takes to respond to a true emergency?* Any emergency involving a friend, family member, or loved one will produce severe emotional reactions. Parents, for example, have felt themselves paralyzed in the first few moments of an emergency in which their child is a victim. Will you be able to take action? Will you remember the steps of CPR and defibrillation?

What about the unpleasant and disagreeable aspects of doing CPR? There was a dramatic scene in the Michael Douglas movie *The Game* where an overweight, intoxicated man collapsed in front of a main character. When the young woman rushed forward to start CPR and mouth-to-mouth breathing, the unattractive stranger vomited into her face. Would you really be able to do mouth-to-mouth rescue breathing on a stranger? What if the victim is bleeding from facial injuries that occurred when he or she collapsed? Would this not pose a risk of disease for a rescuer without a CPR barrier device?

Both CPR and defibrillation require the rescuer to remove clothing from the victim's chest. Defibrillation electrodes cannot be attached unless the pads are placed directly on the skin of the chest. The rescuer must open the shirt or blouse of the cardiac arrest victim and remove the person's undergarments. Yet common courtesy and modesty inhibit many people from removing the clothing of strangers, especially in front of many other people in a public location.

Be proud of your new skills as a layperson who can perform CPR and operate an AED to save a life.

Feel free to

express your

concerns openly

after a stressful

resuscitation

attempt.

Television and the cinema have made many viewers familiar with defibrillation shocks. They know to expect the "jump" and muscle contractions whenever a character yells "clear." These shocks appear painful. Can you overcome your natural tendencies to not hurt others, even in an emergency when your actions could be lifesaving?

Often friends and relatives will be at the scene of an emergency. If you respond and take action, these people will look to you to perform precisely and confidently. Yet confidence will be hard to come by at such a rare and challenging event.

It is well known that these psychological barriers hinder a quick emergency response, especially by ordinary citizens who seldom face such an event. There are no easy solutions to help overcome these psychological barriers. Your instructor will encourage you to anticipate many of the scenes described above. Practice scenarios will include role playing and rehearsals. Think through how you would respond when confronted with such a circumstance. Mental practice, even without hands-on practice, is a good technique for improving future performance.

The Heartsaver FACTS Course presents a package already full of information. There is little time for an in-depth discussion of psychological barriers to action. The AHA Emergency Cardiovascular Care Committee encourages you to attend routine skills review and practice sessions at least every 6 months. The required renewal interval is **every 2 years.** These sessions will strengthen your skills, build your confidence, and increase the probability of a smooth and effective resuscitation effort. Most Heartsaver AED programs will establish review sessions to help you remain focused on the task at hand — the return of spontaneous circulation and the survival of your neighbor.

SUMMARY

Rapid changes in technology have given us AEDs that are simple to operate, safe to use, and effective. AEDs and innovative emergency medical leaders have opened the door for lay rescuers to perform not only CPR but also early defibrillation. Be proud of your initiative to take a CPR-AED course. Be proud of your new skills as a layperson who can operate a sophisticated medical device to save a life.

Despite all the excitement about AEDs and public access defibrillation, there are limitations to what you can do. Your efforts will not always succeed. What is important is taking action and trying to help another human being. Some people must overcome barriers to action if asked to respond to a dramatic emergency such as cardiac arrest. Many of these barriers will be reduced during the Heartsaver FACTS Course. Feel free to express your concerns openly during the course and in the small-group sessions.

All public access defibrillation programs that follow the AHA guidelines are encouraged to be aware of the mental and emotional challenge of rescue efforts. You will have support if you ever participate in a resuscitation attempt. You may not know for several days whether the victim lives or dies. If the person you tried to resuscitate does not live, take comfort from knowing that in taking action, you did your best.

The most successful way to reduce stress after rescue efforts is very simple:

Talk about it.

Your efforts will not always succeed. What is important is taking action and trying to help another human being.

REVIEW QUESTIONS

1. Fatigue, irritability, difficulty sleeping, guilt, loss of appetite, breathlessness, muscle weakness, anxiety, and depression are all signs of
   a. heart attack
   b. impending cardiac arrest
   c. stress response
   d. heart failure

2. The process of expressing one's feelings in a group meeting after a stressful situation such as a failed cardiac arrest is commonly called
   a. critical incident stress debriefing
   b. analysis
   c. biofeedback
   d. psychological ventilation

3. What role can the emergency professionals play after a stressful event?
   a. facilitators of a debriefing process
   b. observers of debriefing process
   c. passive participants
   d. no particular role

HOW DID YOU DO?
1. c; 2. a; 3. a

LEGAL AND ETHICAL ISSUES

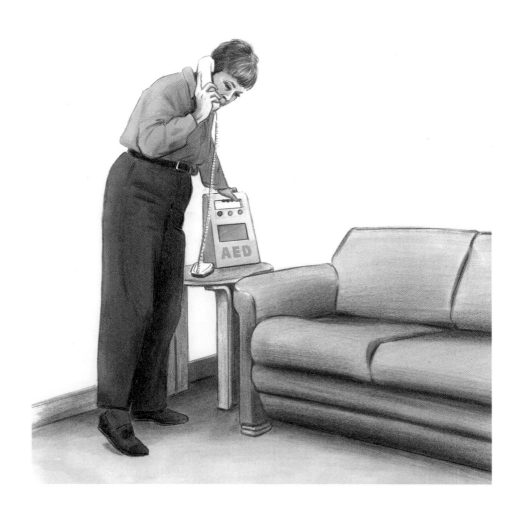

CONTENTS

6

Your participation

in the Heartsaver

FACTS Course

marks you as a

concerned citizen,

someone willing

to make the extra

effort to be

prepared.

LEARNING OBJECTIVES

After reading this chapter, you should be able to

1. Discuss the possibility of lawsuits and legal actions in relation to the performance of CPR
2. Explain the purpose of Good Samaritan laws
3. List conditions in which CPR can be stopped
4. Explain the purpose of advance directives
5. Discuss local and state laws related to AED use

OVERVIEW

This chapter reviews several ethical and legal topics about CPR and the use of AEDs by citizens in your community. Your participation in the new Heartsaver FACTS Course marks you as a concerned citizen, someone willing to make the extra effort to be better prepared.

LEGAL ASPECTS OF CARDIOPULMONARY RESUSCITATION

The American Heart Association has supported community CPR training for more than 3 decades. Citizen CPR responders have helped save thousands of lives. The AHA believes that the addition of training in the use of AEDs will dramatically increase the number of survivors of cardiac arrest.

Citizens can perform emergency CPR without fear of legal action. Chest compressions and rescue breathing require direct physical contact between rescuer and victim. Often these two people are strangers. Too often the arrest victim dies. In the United States people may take legal action when they perceive damage or think that one person has harmed another, even unintentionally. Despite this legal environment, CPR remains widely used and remarkably free of legal issues and lawsuits. Although attorneys have included rescuers who performed CPR in lawsuits, no **"Good Samaritan"** has ever been found guilty of doing harm while performing CPR.

All 50 states have Good Samaritan laws that grant immunity to anyone who attempts CPR in an honest, "good faith" effort to save a life. A person is considered a Good Samaritan if

- The person is genuinely trying to help
- The help is reasonable (you cannot engage in gross misconduct, for example, doing chest compressions on someone's neck)

- The rescue effort is voluntary and not part of the person's job requirements

Under most Good Samaritan laws, laypeople are protected if they perform CPR even if they have had no formal training.

Unless you are employed in a profession that expects you to perform CPR as part of your job responsibilities, you are under no **legal** obligation to attempt CPR on a victim of cardiac arrest. Failure to attempt CPR when there is no danger to the rescuer and the rescuer has the ability is considered an **ethical** violation by some commentators.

When to Stop CPR

Many citizens are troubled by the thought of attempting CPR on someone who never responds. How long do you keep doing CPR in such a situation? Stories are told, for example, about passengers in an overseas commercial aircraft having a cardiac arrest when the nearest airport is hours away. How long should you perform CPR for such an unfortunate person? The AHA recommends using common sense in such unusual circumstances. The general guidelines for stopping CPR are

- The victim responds and regains an adequate pulse and useful breathing.

- A trained professional responder takes over and assumes responsibility.

- You are too exhausted to continue, or continued CPR poses a danger to the rescuer. For example, during an in-flight cardiac arrest, do not continue CPR during landings. Stop CPR, return to your seat, and fasten your seatbelt. Resume CPR as soon as possible after touching the ground.

- A medical professional tells you to stop.

- Obvious signs of death become apparent.

What About "Do Not Start" CPR?

It is possible that you will encounter a victim of cardiac arrest who previously has expressed his or her wish to forego resuscitation attempts if cardiac arrest occurs. Friends or relatives of the victim may supply this information. Medic Alert® bracelets or wallet cards are often used as a way of communicating the victim's prearrest wishes. Many states have **"Do Not Attempt Resuscitation"** (DNAR) programs. Clear expressions of the victim's wishes should always be respected. This is discussed further in a later section.

Citizen CPR

responders have

helped save

thousands

of lives.

LIVING WILLS AND ADVANCE DIRECTIVES

The Patient Self-Determination Act of 1991 supports the right of a patient to make decisions about his or her medical care, including care at the end of life. An individual may express such preferences by preparing a **"living will."** The living will documents the person's wishes, providing instructions for family members, physicians, and other healthcare providers. Everyone, particularly persons entering their senior years, should prepare a living will.

Advance directives differ from living wills. Advance directives are prepared by the attending physician or other care provider rather than by the individual. Ideally the physician writes the advance directive using the patient's living will as a guide. However, advance directives are often written for patients after they are hospitalized with a terminal condition. Frequently patients are too ill to participate in the decision making. Physicians and families should talk with patients about their preferences regarding CPR in various clinical settings. For more information, contact your physician or hospital.

EMS NO-CPR PROGRAMS

A number of states have adopted **"EMS No-CPR"** programs. These programs allow patients to call 911 for emergency care and support at an end-of-life event, for example, shortness of breath, bleeding, or uncontrolled pain. At the same time patients are able to avoid unwanted resuscitation efforts. In a no-CPR program the patient, who usually has a terminal illness, signs a document requesting "no heroics" if there is a loss of pulse or if breathing stops. In some states this document allows the patient to wear a no-CPR identification bracelet. In an emergency the bracelet or other documentation signals rescuers that CPR efforts, including use of an AED, are prohibited.

If you find a person in apparent cardiac arrest (unresponsive, no pulse, not breathing) and see that he or she is wearing a no-CPR bracelet (or has some other indication of no-CPR status), respect the person's wishes. Call 911 and report the problem as a "collapsed, unresponsive person who is wearing a no-CPR bracelet." Say that you do not think CPR is indicated and that you will await the arrival of emergency personnel.

LEGAL ASPECTS OF AED USE

Defibrillators, including AEDs, are restricted medical devices. Most states have health practice acts that require a physician to authorize the use of any restricted medical device. Public access defibrillation programs that make AEDs available to lay rescuers are required to have a *medical authority.* In one sense the **medical authority** *prescribes* the AED for use by the lay responder and therefore makes the use of the AED **legal.**

In the United States fear of malpractice accusations and product liability lawsuits grows larger every year. Innovative programs to bring early CPR and early defibrillation into every community have fallen under the shadow of this fear. Physicians, trainers, program directors, corporation heads, and legal counsel for many groups have often refused to support early defibrillation programs for fear of being involved in a lawsuit. Without medical authority, lay rescuers cannot use an AED. Yet physicians are extremely reluctant to support programs that place defibrillators in homes, worksites, and public places if it exposes them to legal risk. Likewise, lay rescuers, even with physician authorization, fear being sued if they try to help someone by using an AED and "something goes wrong."

To solve this problem, many states are changing existing laws and regulations. Many legislators are amending Good Samaritan laws to include the use of AEDs by lay rescuers. This means that lay rescuers will be considered Good Samaritans when they attempt CPR and defibrillation on someone in cardiac arrest. As a Good Samaritan you cannot be sued for any harm or damage that occurs during the rescue effort (except in cases of gross negligence).

In most public access defibrillation legislation, immunity from lawsuits is granted only when specific recommendations are fulfilled. These recommendations state that the rescuer must

- Have formal training in CPR and use of an AED (AHA Heartsaver FACTS Course or equivalent)

- Use treatment protocols such as the CPR-AED algorithm that are approved by a medical authority

- Perform routine checks and maintenance on the AED

- Notify local EMS authorities of the placement of the AED so that EMS personnel, particularly the EMS dispatch system, are aware that you are in a setting in which an AED is available

- Report actual use of the AED to EMS authorities (usually by calling 911)

Citizens can perform CPR without fear of legal action. No "Good Samaritan" has ever been found guilty of doing harm while performing CPR.

The patient's

wishes about

CPR should

always

be respected.

During the course your instructor will briefly discuss the method of legal immunity used in your state and what you should do to report any clinical event you might be involved in. You also will need to know who the medical authority is (often the medical director of your EMS system or the medical advisor to your worksite).

SUMMARY

There has never been a lawsuit in which a lay rescuer was found **guilty** of doing harm in attempting CPR on a victim of cardiac arrest. There has never been a lawsuit in which a professional responder was found **guilty** of doing harm in using an AED on a cardiac arrest victim. Good Samaritan laws exist in every state to give immunity to lay rescuers who try to help a person experiencing a medical emergency. The lay rescuer only has to act voluntarily in a **good faith** effort to help another person. (**Good faith** means the rescuer does not have a professional duty to respond.) The rescuer's efforts must make common sense and must be reasonable. For example, a lay rescuer cannot attempt to help in a manner that exceeds his or her skills or violates training.

The right of patients to self-determination of health care means that a patient can choose not to receive CPR or resuscitation efforts. This right should be respected. To ensure this right, some people use a living will to document their wish to forego resuscitation attempts in a cardiac arrest. A number of states have established "Do Not Attempt Resuscitation," or DNAR, programs. Patients may use Medic Alert®–type bracelets or wallet cards as a means of communicating their wishes before a cardiac arrest.

Because AEDs are restricted medical devices, a licensed physician must authorize the use of AEDs. A number of states have added AED use to their Good Samaritan laws so that a lay rescuer will be immune from legal action. Such legal action is highly unlikely. So far no lawsuit related to public-responder defibrillation is known to have been filed.

The American Heart Association recommends that course instructors provide a handout that summarizes your state's laws or regulations related to layperson use of AEDs.

REVIEW QUESTIONS

1. Heartsaver certification is required before a rescuer can perform CPR.
    true   false

2. CPR can be stopped in all of the following circumstances **except**

    a. the victim recovers (regains pulse and breathing)

    b. another trained person takes over

    c. you have called 911 and the EMS professionals have been dispatched

    d. you are too exhausted to continue

3. AED use is often defined by

    a. state laws or regulations

    b. the Constitution

    c. individuals

    d. contracts

HOW DID YOU DO?

1. false; **2.** c; **3.** a

HEARTSAVER AED LEARNING RESOURCES

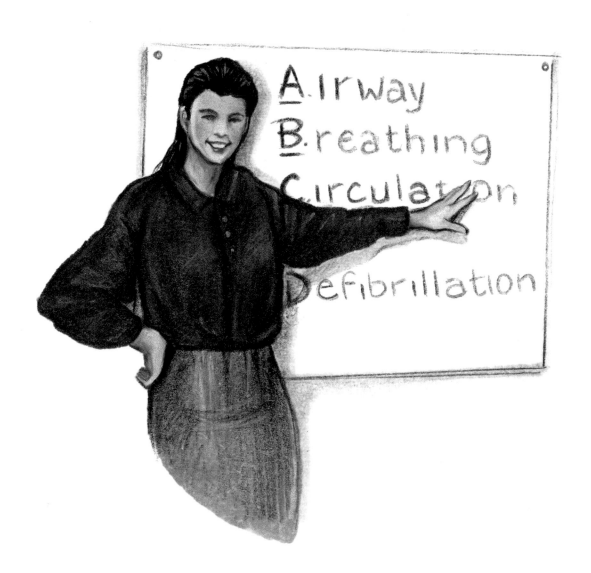

CONTENTS

7

HEARTSAVER AED SAMPLE COURSE AGENDA
(Slightly modified agendas may be used at specific courses.)

Introduction (instructor lecture with slides plus video)	**30 minutes**

- Welcome and introduction — 5 minutes
- Overview video: *EZ AED* — 10 minutes
- Overview of the Chain of Survival and automated external defibrillation — 15 minutes
  — Sudden cardiac death
  — Chain of Survival
  — Importance of early defibrillation
  — What is an AED?
  — How does an AED work?

Instruction in CPR and Relief of FBAO **(videos plus instructors: "watch-then-practice")**	**1 hour 15 minutes**

- Watch-then-practice: mouth-to-mouth breathing — 15 minutes
- Watch-then-practice: mouth-to-mask breathing — 15 minutes
- Watch-then-practice: chest compressions — 15 minutes
- Watch-then-practice: CPR (mouth-to-mask plus chest compressions) — 15 minutes
- Watch-then-practice: relief of FBAO (clearing the obstructed airway in the conscious and unconscious victim) — 15 minutes

Break — **15 minutes**

AED Instruction (instructor demonstrates — then practice)	**30 minutes**

- Instructor demonstrates operation and maintenance of AED — 15 minutes
  — Turning device on
  — Skin preparation
  — Location of pads
  — Pad placement
  — Analyze mode
  — Delivery of shock
  — No shock indicated
- Instructor demonstrates one-rescuer AED scenario: 1 shock; pulse and breathing return
- Participants practice Heartsaver AED algorithm (single-shock scenario) — 15 minutes

Scenario-based Practice (instructor-led hands-on)	**35-45 minutes**

- Practice and review: 8 critical scenarios (groups of 4; 8 rotations) — 45 minutes

Practical Evaluation **(individual demonstration of practical skills; written examination)**	**25-40 minutes**

- Practical evaluation — 20 minutes
- Written evaluation — 20 minutes

Total time: — **3½ to 4 hours**

HEARTSAVER AED RESCUER TREATMENT ALGORITHM
EMERGENCY CARDIAC CARE PENDING ARRIVAL OF EMERGENCY MEDICAL PERSONNEL
INCLUDING GUIDELINES 2000 CHANGES

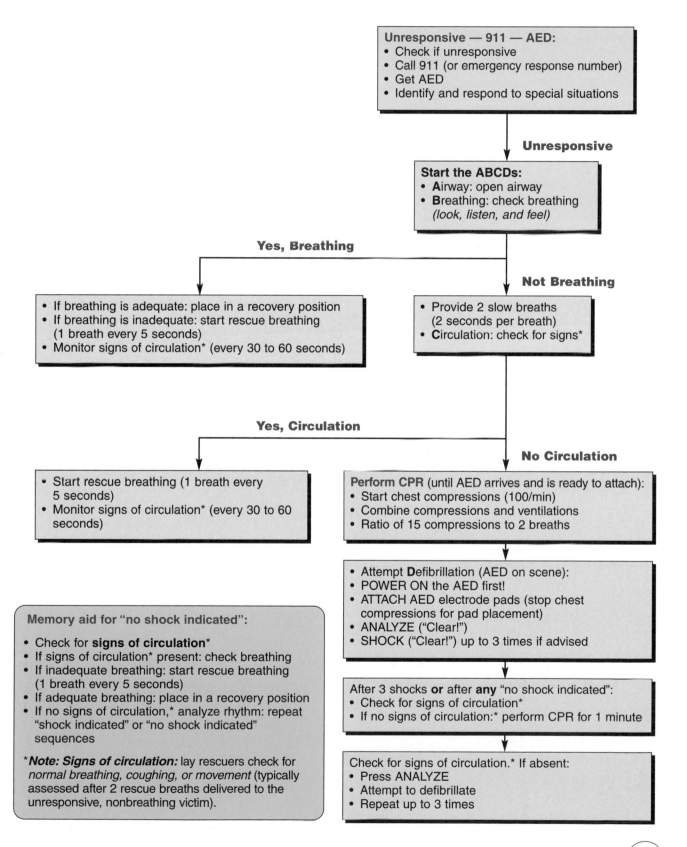

Unresponsive — 911 — AED:
- Check if unresponsive
- Call 911 (or emergency response number)
- Get AED
- Identify and respond to special situations

Unresponsive

Start the ABCDs:
- **A**irway: open airway
- **B**reathing: check breathing *(look, listen, and feel)*

Yes, Breathing

Not Breathing

- If breathing is adequate: place in a recovery position
- If breathing is inadequate: start rescue breathing (1 breath every 5 seconds)
- Monitor signs of circulation* (every 30 to 60 seconds)

- Provide 2 slow breaths (2 seconds per breath)
- **C**irculation: check for signs*

Yes, Circulation

No Circulation

- Start rescue breathing (1 breath every 5 seconds)
- Monitor signs of circulation* (every 30 to 60 seconds)

Perform CPR (until AED arrives and is ready to attach):
- Start chest compressions (100/min)
- Combine compressions and ventilations
- Ratio of 15 compressions to 2 breaths

Memory aid for "no shock indicated":

- Check for **signs of circulation***
- If signs of circulation* present: check breathing
- If inadequate breathing: start rescue breathing (1 breath every 5 seconds)
- If adequate breathing: place in a recovery position
- If no signs of circulation,* analyze rhythm: repeat "shock indicated" or "no shock indicated" sequences

***Note: Signs of circulation:** lay rescuers check for *normal breathing, coughing, or movement* (typically assessed after 2 rescue breaths delivered to the unresponsive, nonbreathing victim).

- Attempt **D**efibrillation (AED on scene):
- POWER ON the AED first!
- ATTACH AED electrode pads (stop chest compressions for pad placement)
- ANALYZE ("Clear!")
- SHOCK ("Clear!") up to 3 times if advised

After 3 shocks **or** after **any** "no shock indicated":
- Check for signs of circulation*
- If no signs of circulation:* perform CPR for 1 minute

Check for signs of circulation.* If absent:
- Press ANALYZE
- Attempt to defibrillate
- Repeat up to 3 times

Heatsaver AED Course
Adult 1-Rescuer CPR
Performance Criteria Reflecting
Guidelines 2000 Changes

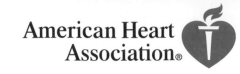

American Heart Association®

Fighting Heart Disease and Stroke

Participant Name _____ Date _____

Performance Guidelines	Performed
1. Establish that the victim is unresponsive. Phone 911 (or other emergency response number).	
2. Open the airway (head tilt–chin lift or, if trauma is suspected, jaw thrust). Check for normal breathing (look, listen, and feel).*	
3. If normal breathing is absent, give 2 slow breaths (2 seconds per breath), ensure adequate chest rise, and allow for exhalation between breaths.	
4. Check for signs of circulation (normal breathing, coughing, or movement in response to the 2 rescue breaths). If signs of circulation are present but there is no normal breathing, provide rescue breathing (1 breath every 5 seconds, about 10 to 12 breaths per minute).	
5. If no signs of circulation are present, begin cycles of 15 chest compressions (about 100 compressions per minute) followed by 2 slow breaths.*	
6. After 4 cycles of compressions and breaths (15:2, about 1 minute), recheck for signs of circulation.* If no signs of circulation are present, continue 15:2 cycles, beginning with chest compressions. If signs of circulation return but breathing does not, continue rescue breathing (1 breath every 5 seconds, or about 10 to 12 breaths per minute).	

*If the victim is breathing or resumes normal breathing and no trauma is suspected, place in the recovery position.

Comments _____

_____

_____

_____

_____

Instructor _____

Circle one: Complete   Needs more practice

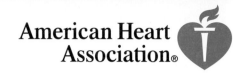

Heartsaver AED Course
Adult 2-Rescuer CPR
Performance Criteria Reflecting
Guidelines 2000 Changes

Fighting Heart Disease and Stroke

Participant Name _____ Date _____

Performance Guidelines	Performed
1. Establish that victim is unresponsive. One rescuer should first phone 911 (or other emergency response number).	

Rescuer 1	
2. Open the airway (head tilt–chin lift or, if trauma is suspected, jaw thrust). Check for normal breathing (look, listen, and feel).*	
3. If normal breathing is absent, give 2 slow breaths (2 seconds per breath), ensure adequate chest rise, and allow for exhalation between breaths.	
4. Check for signs of circulation (normal breathing, coughing, or movement in response to the 2 rescue breaths). If signs of circulation are present but there is no normal breathing, provide rescue breathing (1 breath every 5 seconds, about 10 to 12 breaths per minute).	

Rescuer 2	
5. If no signs of circulation are present, begin cycles of 15 chest compressions (rate of about 100 compressions per minute) followed by 2 slow breaths by rescuer 1.*	
6. After 4 cycles of compressions and breaths (15:2, about 1 minute), rescuer 1 provides 2 breaths and rechecks for signs of circulation.* If no signs of circulation are present, continue 15:2 cycles of compressions and ventilations, beginning with chest compressions, until more skilled rescuers (with an AED) arrive.	

*If the victim is breathing or resumes normal breathing and no trauma is suspected, place in the recovery position.

Comments _____

_____

_____

Instructor _____

Circle one: Complete   Needs more practice

Heartsaver AED Course
Adult FBAO in Responsive Victim
(and Responsive Victim Who Becomes Unresponsive)
Performance Criteria Reflecting
Guidelines 2000 Changes

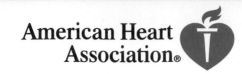

American Heart Association®

Fighting Heart Disease and Stroke

Participant Name _____ Date _____

Performance Guidelines	Performed
1. Ask "Are you choking?" If yes, ask "Can you speak?" If no, tell the victim you are going to help.	
2. Give abdominal thrusts (chest thrusts for victim who is pregnant or obese). Avoid pressing on the bottom of the breastbone (xiphoid).	
3. Repeat thrusts until foreign body is expelled (obstruction relieved) or victim becomes unresponsive.	

Adult Foreign-Body Airway Obstruction —
Victim Becomes Unresponsive
The following is for clarification only.

4. Phone 911 or other emergency response number (or send someone to do it). Return to the victim.	
5. Attempt CPR (each time you open the airway, look for a foreign object in the mouth; if you see it, remove it).	

Comments _____

_____

_____

Instructor _____

Circle one: Complete   Needs more practice

Heartsaver AED Course
Provider CPR and AED
Performance Criteria Reflecting
Guidelines 2000 Changes

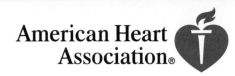

American Heart
Association®

Fighting Heart Disease and Stroke

Participant Name _____ Date _____

Performance Guidlines	Performance	
CPR Skills	**Satisfactory**	**Remediate**
1. Establish unresponsiveness — direct coworker to call 911 and get the AED.		
2. Open airway (head tilt–chin lift or jaw thrust) — check breathing (look, listen, and feel).		
3. If no breathing, give 2 slow breaths (**2** seconds per breath) that cause the chest to rise.		
4. Check **signs of circulation (no signs of circulation).** Start chest compressions (ratio of 15 to 2 breaths at **100** compressions per minute).		
AED Skills (AED arrives after 2 cycles of CPR)	**Satisfactory**	**Remediate**
5. Place the AED next to the victim's left ear; start time-to–first shock clock. POWER ON the AED.		
6. ATTACH pads in proper positions (as pictured on each of the AED electrodes, sternum, and apex).		
7. Clear victim and press ANALYZE (if present). (AED advises shock and charges.)		
8. Clear victim and press SHOCK button. End time-to–first shock clock. (May repeat 1 to 2 more analyze-shock cycles. End when AED gives *"no shock indicated"* message.)		
9. Check **signs of circulation (signs of circulation present).**		
10. Continue to check breathing and **signs of circulation** until EMS arrives. (Use of recovery position acceptable. Leave AED attached.)		
Critical Actions	**Satisfactory**	**Remediate**
• Assess responsiveness.		
• Call 911; get the AED.		
• Open the airway.		
• Provide 2 breaths (must cause the chest to rise).		
• Check **signs of circulation.**		
• Begin chest compressions (must have proper hand placement).		
• POWER ON the AED.		
• ATTACH pads to patient's bare chest in proper location.		
• Clear victim before ANALYZE and SHOCK (avoid contact with victim).		
• Check breathing and **signs of circulation** after *"no shock indicated"* message.		
• Time from start to first shock is less than 90 seconds.		

FREQUENTLY ASKED QUESTIONS ABOUT CPR

1. Can rescuers catch AIDS or hepatitis or other diseases during CPR?

It is extremely unlikely that a rescuer will become infected with either the AIDS or hepatitis virus as a result of doing mouth-to-mouth breathing or touching the victim. After more than 35 years of performing mouth-to-mouth breathing, there has never been a documented case of AIDS or hepatitis transmitted to a rescuer. You can use a face mask or a face shield as a barrier device. These devices are placed over the victim's mouth and nose to help block viruses and bacteria.

More important, about 70% to 80% of respiratory and cardiac arrests occur in the home, where the rescuer usually knows the victim and knows about the victim's health. A primary reason to learn CPR is for the benefit of your family and friends.

2. What are some possible hazards of CPR?

Poorly performed CPR can cause injuries. Follow performance guidelines at all times. Frequent manikin practice helps improve future performance. Some possible problems in performing CPR:

- Incorrect hand position for chest compression may lead to rib fractures, fractures of the end of the breastbone (xiphoid), and bruising or bleeding of the liver, lung, or spleen.
- Bouncing chest compressions may cause the rescuer's hands to move off the center of the sternum (breastbone).
- Compressing the chest too deeply may cause internal injury.
- Not compressing the sternum deeply enough may cause poor blood flow to the brain and other vital organs.
- Using breath volumes that are too great, breathing too rapidly, or not having the airway opened completely — any of these may cause you to blow large amounts of air into the stomach and cause stomach stretching (gastric distention).
- Gastric distention increases the chances the victim will vomit and may decrease the effectiveness of ventilation.

3. **How do I open the airway of a victim who may have a neck injury, such as the victim of an automobile accident?**

   Jaw thrust *without* head tilt is the first step in opening the airway in a victim with suspected neck injury.

4. **What should I do if the victim vomits?**

   You should turn the victim's head and body to the side so that the victim will not choke on the vomited material. Then clear the airway by sweeping the mouth. A cloth (corner of clothing, handkerchief, etc) over your fingers can be used to sweep out the mouth. Then reposition the victim and continue CPR.

5. **How will I know if CPR is effective?**

   A second rescuer can monitor the carotid pulse (in the neck) while you do chest compressions. A good, strong carotid or brachial pulse (in the upper arm) should be present with each compression. Rescue breathing can be checked by looking for chest rise with each lung inflation. Remember, too much volume will cause stomach distention.

6. **How will I know if pulse and breathing return?**

   The return of a pulse, with or without breathing, may be dramatic or subtle. The victim may take a big gasp of air, begin moving, or even start to regain consciousness. If breathing is present, keep the airway open and regularly check pulse and breathing. Place the victim in the recovery position to maintain an open airway. If breathing is absent, perform rescue breathing 10 to 12 times per minute (once every 5 seconds) for the adult.

7. **What should I do about a "neck breather" in need of CPR?**

   Neck breathers are persons who have had their voice box (larynx) removed by surgery and have a permanent opening (stoma) that connects the airway or windpipe (trachea) directly to the skin. The opening is at the base of the front of the neck.

   To tell whether the victim's breathing has returned, place your ear over the opening in the neck. If rescue breathing is required, do direct mouth-to-stoma rescue breathing. For more information, contact the International Association of Laryngectomees, c/o the American Cancer Society, 1599 Clifton Rd. NE, Atlanta, GA 30329.

8. **If a victim is found on a bed, should I move him or her to the floor so that I have a hard surface under the victim's spine?**

Victims receiving CPR should be moved to a firm surface. Make sure that the head and neck are supported and not left to dangle. If you are alone and cannot move the victim, leave the victim on the bed and find something flat and firm to slide under the back to provide a hard surface.

9. **What do I do for an adult who I think may be having a heart attack?**

First have the victim rest quietly and calmly. Both angina (severe pain around the heart) and heart attack are caused by too little oxygen-rich blood to the heart muscle. So keep activity to a minimum. If chest discomfort lasts more than a few minutes, the most important thing to do is activate the EMS system. (Phone First!)

10. **If I find a victim and I am alone, should I telephone for help first or should I immediately begin CPR?**

For the adult victim, phone first and then begin CPR. If you have access to an AED through a public access defibrillation program, first call 911, get the AED, and return to the victim. Provide CPR and use the AED as you learned in Heartsaver FACTS training. Continue until EMS professionals arrive. The sooner EMS arrives, the better the chance for survival of the adult because of the special skills of EMS personnel and devices carried by EMS units. (Phone First!) Children have respiratory arrests more often than cardiac arrests. So for a child, begin CPR first. If after about 1 minute the child has not regained spontaneous pulse and breathing, take the least time possible and phone for help. (Phone Fast!)

11. **What should I do if the victim is wearing dentures?**

Leave the dentures in place if possible. This will help you make an airtight seal around the victim's mouth. Remove the dentures only if they are so loose or ill-fitting that they get in your way or obstruct the victim's airway.

12. **What should I do to prevent stomach swelling (gastric distention)?**

Distention of the stomach (air getting into the stomach) is most likely to occur if you blow too hard with rescue breathing or if the airway is partially obstructed. So control the force and speed of rescue breaths. Breathe slowly into the victim for 1½ to 2 seconds each time, and check that you do not continue to blow in after the chest rises.

13. What if the victim of complete airway obstruction is pregnant or very obese?

Treat the pregnant or obese victim of choking the same way as any other victim — unless it is impossible to perform safe or effective abdominal thrusts because the pregnancy is advanced or the obesity is extreme. In these cases, perform chest thrusts instead of abdominal thrusts. But perform these chest thrusts from the side of the unconscious victim.

14. How will I know when to start the obstructed airway sequence in a conscious choking victim?

With good air exchange the victim can cough forcefully, although frequently the victim wheezes between coughs. As long as good air exchange continues, encourage the victim to keep coughing and breathing. At this point do not interfere with the victim's attempts to expel the foreign body. With complete airway obstruction, the victim is unable to speak, breathe, or cough. The victim also may clutch his or her neck (universal distress signal). If the victim cannot speak, begin the obstructed airway sequence.

15. Should I handle a drowning victim differently from any other victim?

Handle drowning victims exactly as you would any other victim. If rescue breaths do not inflate the chest, begin the obstructed airway sequence.

- Reposition the head and attempt rescue breathing.
- If still unable to give rescue breaths, straddle the thighs of the unconscious victim and give 5 abdominal thrusts (the Heimlich maneuver).
- Use tongue-jaw lift and sweep the mouth with your finger.
- Try again to give rescue breaths.

16. How long can I stop CPR to move the victim?

Do not interrupt CPR for more than a few seconds except for special situations, such as transporting the victim. If you have to move a victim up or down a stairway, perform CPR at the head or foot of the stairs. Then interrupt CPR, move quickly to the next flat area, and resume CPR.

17. How often should I review or refresh my skills in CPR?

The national ECC Committee recommends retraining at least every 2 years to refresh CPR skills. Your local AHA may recommend more frequent renewal of skills. If you are also trained in AED use through the Heartsaver FACTS or Heartsaver AED Courses, review at least every 2 years or refresh your skills according to local protocols.

FREQUENTLY ASKED QUESTIONS ABOUT AEDs

1. Why does a person having a heart attack need an AED?

When a heart attack becomes a full cardiac arrest, the heart most often goes into uncoordinated electric activity called *fibrillation*. The heart twitches ineffectively and cannot pump blood. The AED delivers electric current to the heart muscle, momentarily *stunning* the heart, stopping all activity. This gives the heart an opportunity to resume beating effectively.

2. What does AED stand for?

AED stands for *automated external defibrillator*.

3. How does an AED work?

A microprocessor inside the defibrillator interprets (analyzes) the victim's heart rhythm through adhesive electrodes (some models of AEDs require you to press an ANALYZE button). The computer analyzes the heart rhythm and advises the operator whether a shock is needed. AEDs advise a shock to only ventricular fibrillation and fast ventricular tachycardia. The electric current is delivered through the victim's chest wall through adhesive electrode pads.

4. Why is it important to call 911 first when a person collapses?

While early defibrillation is the single most important treatment for VF cardiac arrest, other treatments are also needed. Even if there is an AED available on the scene, a victim of cardiac arrest needs effective CPR with oxygen, intravenous (IV) medicines, often endotracheal intubation, and rapid transport to an emergency department. These other links in the Chain of Survival optimize a victim's chances of survival and recovery. In addition, not every cardiac emergency is due to VF. Victims of non-VF emergencies need other skills and treatments from the EMS professionals.

5. Will an AED always resuscitate someone in cardiac arrest?

The AED treats only a heart that is fibrillating. In non-VF cardiac arrests the heart does not respond to electric current but needs medications and breathing support instead. Also, AEDs are less successful when the victim has been in cardiac arrest for longer than a few minutes, especially if no CPR was provided.

6. What does CPR do if what the victim really needs is defibrillation?

CPR provides some circulation of oxygen-rich blood to the victim's heart and brain. This circulation delays both brain death and the death of heart muscle. CPR buys time until the AED can arrive and makes VF more likely to respond to defibrillation shocks.

7. Is an AED safe to use?

An AED is safe to use by anyone who has been trained to operate it. The AHA recommends that anyone who lives or works where an AED is available for use by lay rescuers participate in a Heartsaver AED or Heartsaver FACTS Course. AEDs, in fact, are so user-friendly that untrained rescuers can generally succeed in attaching the pads, pressing ANALYZE (if required), and delivering shocks. Untrained rescuers, however, may not know when to use an AED, and they may not use an AED safely, posing some danger of electric shock to themselves and others. Also, untrained rescuers would not know how to respond to the victim when the AED prompts *"no shock indicated."* An operator needs only to follow the illustrations on the electrode pads and the control panel, and listen and follow the voice prompts (for example, "Do not touch the victim"). An AED will deliver a shock only when a shock is advised and the operator pushes the SHOCK button. This prevents a shock from being delivered accidentally.

8. Will I get zapped if I shock a victim in the rain or near water?

It is remotely possible to get shocked or to shock bystanders if there is standing water around and under the victim. Try to move the victim to a dry area and cut off wet clothing. Also be sure that the skin has been toweled off so that the electrode pads will stick to the skin. At the moment of pressing the SHOCK button you must make sure that no one, including the AED operator, touches any part of the victim.

9. Can an AED make mistakes?

An AED will almost never decide to shock an adult victim when the rhythm is non-VF. AEDs "miss" fine VF about 5% of the time. The internal computer uses complex analysis algorithms to determine whether to shock. If the operator has attached the AED to an adult victim who is *not breathing and pulseless* (in cardiac arrest), the AED will make the correct "shock" decision more than 95 times out of 100 and a correct *"no shock indicated"* decision more than 98 times out of 100. This level of accuracy is greater than the accuracy of emergency professionals.

10. **Why do you stop CPR as the electrode pads are placed and analysis occurs?**

    For the AED to analyze accurately, the victim must be motionless. Sometimes there will be an agonal respiration (a gasping breath that can occur when the heart is stopped) that causes some movement. AEDs can recognize this extra *motion* and indicate *"motion detected"* to the operator. This warns the operator to assess carefully for extra movements from the victim or from the other people at the scene.

11. **Why should a lay rescuer continue CPR after the arrival of EMS professionals?**

    It is helpful to EMS professionals to be able to set up their equipment, including the defibrillator, while lay rescuers continue CPR. The EMTs will take over CPR and reconfirm that the victim is in cardiac arrest.

12. **Why does it seem that the victim goes without CPR for so long during defibrillation, and why does the AED shock so many times?**

    After prescribed periods of CPR, the machine analyzes the victim's rhythm. The machine requires the victim to be motionless while it decides to shock and delivers the shock. Sometimes the victim does not change from VF to non-VF at once. These victims require multiple shocks. If repeated shocks are needed, the shocks are "stacked" in sets of 3 to increase their effectiveness.

13. **In addition to using the AED, how else might a layperson help at the scene of a sudden cardiac arrest?**

    Lay rescuers are most often going to be asked to *call 911 and get the AED*. The lay rescuer could assemble the pocket face mask and begin providing mouth-to-mask ventilations. Responders might provide CPR or continue defibrillation if a workplace defibrillator is being used. Support and direction to the bystanders, friends, and family are appropriate. When EMS personnel arrive, the lay rescuer can provide directions and help obtain information about the victim.

14. What actions should a CPR responder take after he or she has used an AED on a person in cardiac arrest?

There should be some type of debriefing for the employees or lay rescuers involved. Also, collect the *voice-rhythm-shock* record from the AED's event documentation system. The AHA recommends strongly that AEDs used in a public access or home responder setting have both rhythm and voice event documentation. AEDs can record and store (at a minimum) the following information:

- Victim rhythm throughout the resuscitation
- Response of the AED (*shock* versus *no shock; shockable* rhythm versus *nonshockable* rhythm)
- Event and interval timing
- Audio recording of the voices and actions recorded at the scene of a cardiac arrest

SELF-TEST QUESTIONS

Please take the following self-test. If you are unsure of the answer, take the time to review the material on the pages listed below the item.

1. **Before you try to resuscitate a victim by performing CPR, you should confirm**

    a. brain damage

    b. dilated pupils

    c. unresponsiveness and absence of breathing and pulse

    d. shallow breathing

    Answer, pp. 18-20, 47, 50

2. **The most common cause of airway obstruction in the unconscious victim is**

    a. food

    b. tongue

    c. mucus

    d. dentures

    Answer, p. 20

3. **The first thing that should be done for a collapsed victim of illness or accident is**

    a. examine the victim's mouth for foreign bodies

    b. determine unresponsiveness

    c. perform the Heimlich maneuver

    d. open the airway

    Answer, pp. 18, 48

4. **If the airway seems obstructed after the first attempt to give rescue breaths to an unconscious victim, you should**

    a. reposition the head and attempt rescue breaths again

    b. begin chest compressions

    c. go on to check the pulse

    d. check for foreign-body airway obstruction

    Answer, p. 27

CHAPTER 7

5. **The method used for opening the airway is**

   a. head tilt with chin lift

   b. turning the head to one side

   c. striking the victim on the back

   d. wiping out the mouth and throat

   Answer, pp. 19, 20

6. **You can tell if an unconscious victim is breathing by**

   a. checking if the pupils of the eyes are dilated

   b. checking if the skin is cool and clammy

   c. checking the pulse

   d. looking, listening, and feeling for air movement

   Answer, pp. 19, 21

7. **If breathing seems absent after opening the airway, you should**

   a. begin chest compressions

   b. determine pulselessness

   c. check pupils

   d. give 2 rescue breaths

   Answer, pp. 19, 47, 48, 52

8. **Gastric distention (swelling of the stomach) during CPR is caused by**

   a. rapid and forceful ventilation

   b. inadequate exhalation by the unconscious victim

   c. excessive fluids in the stomach

   d. too much chest compression force

   Answer, pp. 21, 94

9. **To perform chest compressions on an adult, you place one hand on top of the other with the heel of the lower hand pressing the breastbone at**

   a. the upper end

   b. the nipple line

   c. the clavicle

   d. the tip

   Answer, p. 22

10. **To determine if there is an obstructed airway in a conscious victim, you should**

    a. ask the victim, "Are you choking?"

    b. shake the victim

    c. reposition the victim

    d. perform abdominal thrusts

    Answer, p. 26

11. **To perform the Heimlich maneuver on an unconscious victim, you should**

    a. stand behind the victim with your hands grasping the waist

    b. kneel beside the victim's chest

    c. kneel beside the victim's feet

    d. straddle the victim at thigh level

    Answer, p. 27

12. **If a victim is coughing forcefully with a partial airway obstruction, you should**

    a. check the pulse

    b. give abdominal thrusts

    c. sweep out the mouth

    d. not interfere

    Answer, p. 26

13. **Foreign-body airway obstruction in the adult usually develops during**

    a. sleep

    b. eating

    c. a heart attack

    d. exercise

    Answer, pp. 13, 25

14. **When you arrive at the side of the victim, you should place the AED near**

    a. the right foot

    b. the left ear

    c. the left abdomen

    d. the right abdomen

    Answer, pp. 35, 37, 52

15. **One AED pad is placed on the right chest above the right nipple, below the right collarbone and to the right of the breastbone. Where is the other one placed?**

    a. over the left nipple

    b. below the left collarbone

    c. 1 inch to the left of the breastbone

    d. several inches below the left armpit

    Answer, pp. 38, 39

16. **Immediately after applying the AED pads you should**

    a. clear the bystanders and ANALYZE

    b. recheck the pulse

    c. recheck breathing

    d. push the SHOCK button

    Answer, pp. 39, 49

17. **If you use the AED to shock a victim and then receive a "no shock indicated" message, you should immediately**

    a. defibrillate

    b. check the pulse

    c. perform CPR

    d. press the ANALYZE button

    Answer, pp. 40, 49, 50

18. **You use the AED and deliver a shock. On the next analysis you see a "no shock indicated" message. You immediately check the carotid pulse (absent); open the airway; and look, listen, and feel for breathing (absent). Next you should**

    a. defibrillate immediately

    b. remove the AED and wait for EMS

    c. resume CPR

    d. press the ANALYZE button again

    Answer, p. 41

19. **You use the AED and deliver a shock. There is a "no shock indicated" message. There is a pulse and adequate breathing. You should**

    a. leave the AED attached and monitor pulse and breathing

    b. detach the AED and wait for EMS

    c. perform CPR for 1 minute and reanalyze

    d. press the ANALYZE button again

    Answer, p. 41

20. **You use the AED, shock the victim, and then receive a "no shock indicated" message. There is a pulse but no breathing. You should**

    a. provide rescue breathing

    b. detach the AED and wait for EMS

    c. perform CPR for 1 minute and reanalyze

    d. press the ANALYZE button again

    Answer, pp. 41, 49, 50

Part

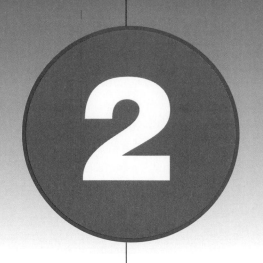

2

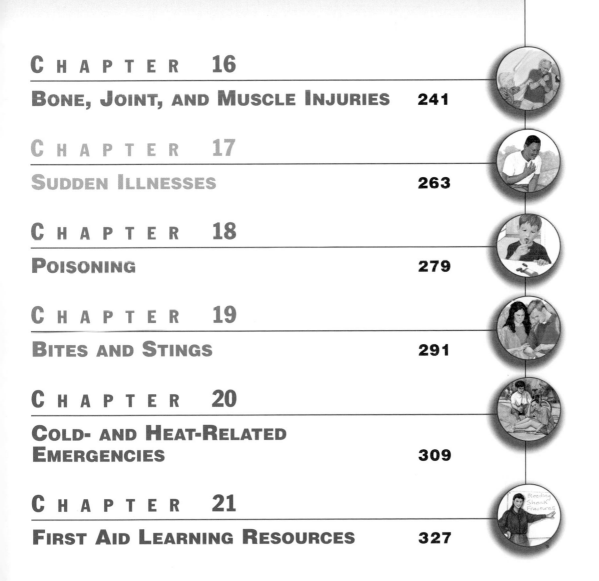

FIRST AID FUNDAMENTALS

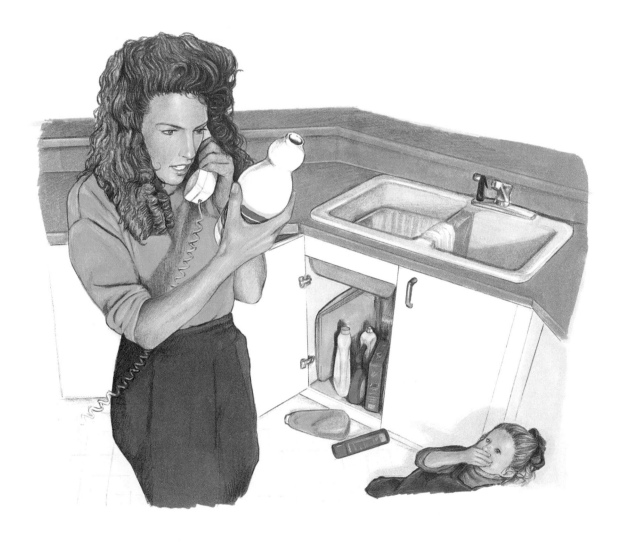

CONTENTS

8

LEARNING OBJECTIVES

After reading this chapter you should be able to

1. Identify the need for knowing how to perform first aid

2. Define first aid

3. Describe legal concerns of first aid

4. Identify the steps of bystander intervention

5. Identify the things to look for in a scene survey

6. List dispatcher's questions that the caller should be prepared to answer

7. Recommend precautions against bloodborne and airborne diseases

8. Describe how to rescue a victim in the following situations:
   - Water
   - Ice
   - Electrical emergency
   - Hazardous materials incident
   - Motor vehicle collision
   - Fires
   - Confined space

9. Describe how to provide care for multiple victims

10. Move victims in emergency and nonemergency situations using
    - One-person moves
    - Two/three-person moves

NEED FOR FIRST AID TRAINING

It's better to know first aid and not need it, than to need it and not know it. Everyone should be able to perform first aid, since most people will eventually find themselves in a situation requiring it, either for another person or for themselves.

What a bystander does can mean the difference between life and death. However, most injuries do not require lifesaving efforts. In their lifetimes, most people will see only one or two situations involving life-threatening conditions. While saving lives is important, knowing what to do for less severe injuries also demands attention and first aid training.

LEGAL CONSIDERATIONS

Giving first aid to others involves certain legal and ethical issues.

Consent

Before giving first aid, you must have the victim's consent. Touching another person without his or her permission or consent is unlawful (known as battery), and could be grounds for a lawsuit. Likewise, giving first aid without the victim's consent is unlawful.

Expressed Consent Consent must be obtained from every conscious, mentally competent (able to make a rational decision) adult of legal age. Tell the victim your name and that you have first aid training, and explain what you will be doing. Permission from the victim may be expressed either verbally or with a nod of the head.

Implied Consent Consent is implied with an unconscious victim in a life-threatening condition. It is assumed that an unresponsive victim would consent to lifesaving interventions. Consent also is implied when the first aider begins care and the victim does not resist.

With a child in a life-threatening situation, if the parent or legal guardian is not available for consent, there is implied consent. Do not withhold first aid from a minor just to obtain parental or guardian permission.

Abandonment

Abandonment means terminating the care of a victim without ensuring continued care at the same level or higher. Once you begin first aid in an emergency, you must not leave a victim who needs continuing first aid until another competent and trained person takes responsibility for the victim.

Negligence

Negligence means not following the accepted standards of care that results in further injury to the victim. Negligence involves

1. Having a duty to act
2. Breaching that duty (substandard care)
3. Inflicting injury and damage

Duty to Act No one is required to render first aid unless he or she has a legal duty. Duty to act may occur in the following situations:

CRITICAL CONCEPTS: WHAT IS FIRST AID?

First aid is the immediate care given to an injured or suddenly ill person. First aid does not take the place of proper medical treatment. It consists only of giving assistance until medical care, if needed, is obtained, or until it is clear the person will recover without medical care. Most injuries and illnesses do not require medical care.

First aid may mean the difference between life and death, between rapid recovery and long hospitalization, or between temporary disability and permanent injury. First aid is not just for other people—it can be for yourself as well.

Being able to recognize a serious medical emergency and knowing how to get help may mean the difference between life and death. Without first aid training, people may not recognize the signs of a serious problem such as a heart attack. First aid knowledge will also help you to avoid panic in an emergency.

- When employment requires it. If your employer designates you as responsible for rendering first aid to meet OSHA (Occupational Safety and Health Administration) requirements and you are called to an accident scene, you have a duty to act. Other examples of occupations involving the giving of first aid include law enforcement officers, park rangers, athletic trainers, lifeguards, and teachers, all of whose job descriptions designate them to give first aid.

- When a preexisting responsibility exists. You may have a preexisting relationship with other persons that demands you be responsible for them, which means you must give first aid should they need it. Examples include a parent for his or her child and a driver for a passenger.

Duty to act means following guidelines for standards of care. Standards of care ensure good-quality care and protection for injured or suddenly ill victims.

Breach of Duty Generally, a first aider breaches (breaks) his or her duty to a victim by failing to provide the type of care that would be provided by a person with the same or similar training. One's duty can be breached by acts of omission or acts of commission. An act of omission is the failure to do what a reasonably prudent person with the same or similar training would do in the same or similar circumstances. An act of commission is doing something that a reasonably prudent person would not do under the same or similar circumstances. Forgetting to put a dressing on a wound is an act of omission; cutting a snakebite site is an act of commission.

Injury and Damages Inflicted In addition to physical damage, injury and damage can include physical pain and suffering, mental anguish, medical expenses, and sometimes loss of earnings and earning capacity.

Good Samaritan Laws

Good Samaritan laws encourage people to assist others in distress by granting them immunity from lawsuits. Although the laws vary from state to state, Good Samaritan immunity generally applies when the rescuer is (1) acting during an emergency; (2) acting in good faith, which means that he or she has good intentions; (3) acting without compensation; and (4) not guilty of any malicious misconduct or gross negligence toward the victim (deviating from rational first aid guidelines).

Many legal experts believe that Good Samaritan laws have given first aiders a false sense of security when they erroneously believe that the law protects them from lawsuits regardless of their actions. Good Samaritan laws are not a substitute for competent first aid or for keeping within the scope of your training.

Good Samaritan laws exist in all 50 states. Many protect lay-persons providing first aid. You should be familiar with the Good Samaritan law in your state.

Fear of lawsuits has made some people wary of getting involved in emergency situations. However, first aiders are rarely sued, and courts usually rule in their favor.

ACTION AT AN EMERGENCY

Bystander Intervention

The bystander is a vital link between the emergency medical service (EMS) and the victim. Typically, it is a bystander who identifies a situation as an emergency and acts to help the victim. A bystander must perform the following actions quickly and reliably:

Recognize the Emergency To help in an emergency, the bystander first has to notice that something is wrong.

Decide to Help Everyone will at some time have to decide whether to help another person. Bystanders are unlikely to make a quick decision to get involved at the time of an emergency unless they have considered, in advance, the possibility of helping. The most important time to make the decision to help is before you ever encounter an emergency.

Deciding to help involves an attitude about people, about emergencies, and about one's ability to deal with emergencies. Some people need time to develop this attitude.

Contact EMS If Needed Laypeople often make inappropriate decisions concerning EMS. They may delay contacting EMS until they are absolutely sure that it is an emergency, or they may bypass EMS and transport the victim to medical care in a private vehicle. Such actions can have negative effects on the victim. It is important to know when the EMS should be called and to act promptly.

Assess the Victim The bystander must decide whether a life-threatening condition is present and what kind of help a victim needs immediately.

Provide First Aid Often the most critical life-support measures are effective only if they are started immediately by someone who is already present on the scene—usually a bystander.

The bystander is a vital link between the emergency medical service (EMS) and the victim.

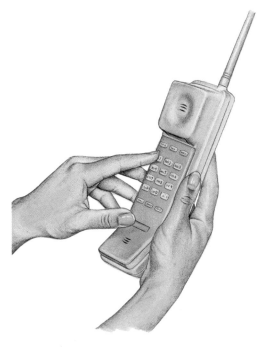

FIGURE 1
For help, phone 911 or the local emergency number.

Scene Survey

As you approach an emergency scene, scan the area for immediate dangers to yourself or to the victim. You cannot help another person if you also become a victim. Always ask yourself: Is the scene safe to enter?

Also in the first 10 seconds, try to determine the cause of the injury. Be sure to tell this to EMS personnel when you call for help, and when they arrive, so they can anticipate the extent of the injuries.

Determine how many people are injured. There may be more than one victim, so look around and ask about others who might be involved.

In a serious situation, **call EMS first.** Do not call your doctor, the hospital, a friend, relatives, or neighbors for help before you call the EMS. Calling anyone else first wastes valuable time.

If the situation is not an emergency, call your doctor. However, if you are in any doubt as to whether the situation is an emergency, call EMS.

How to Call EMS

In most communities, to receive emergency assistance of every kind, you simply phone 911 (**FIGURE 1**). You should know whether this is true in your community. Emergency telephone numbers are usually listed on the inside front cover of telephone directories. Keep these numbers near or on every telephone. Call "0" (the operator) if you do not know the emergency number.

When you call EMS, be ready to give the dispatcher the following information. Speak slowly and clearly:

1. The victim's location: Give the address, names of intersecting roads, and other landmarks, if possible. This information is the most important you can give. Also, tell the victim's specific location (eg, "in the basement").

2. Your phone number and name: This shows that yours is not a false call and allows a dispatch center that does not have an enhanced 911 system to call back for additional information if needed.

3. What happened: State the nature of the emergency (eg, "My husband fell off a ladder and is not moving").

4. The number of people who need help and any special conditions.

5. The victim's condition (eg, "My husband's head is bleeding") and any first aid that you have tried (such as pressing on the site of the bleeding).

Do not hang up the phone unless the dispatcher instructs you to do so. Enhanced 911 systems can track a call, but some communities lack this technology. The EMS dispatcher may tell you how best to care for the victim. If you send someone else to call, have the person report back to you so that you can be sure the call was made.

Disease Precautions

First aiders should understand the risk of infectious disease, which can range from mild to life threatening. First aiders should know how to reduce the risk of contamination to themselves and to others. Precautionary measures are important to help protect against infection from viruses and bacteria.

Bloodborne Disease

Some diseases are caused by microorganisms that are borne (carried) in a person's bloodstream. Contact with blood infected with such microorganisms may lead to infection. Of the many bloodborne pathogens, three pose significant health threats to first aiders: hepatitis B virus (HBV), hepatitis C virus, and human immunodeficiency virus (HIV).

Hepatitis B Hepatitis is a viral infection of the liver. Types A, B, and C are most common. Each is caused by a different virus.

Hepatitis B starts as an inflammation of the liver and usually lasts 1 to 2 months. In a few people the infection is very serious; in some, mild infection continues for life. The virus may stay in the liver and can lead to severe damage (cirrhosis) and liver cancer. Medical treatment that begins immediately after exposure may prevent infection from developing.

The vaccine for hepatitis B is recommended for all infants and for adults who may have contact with carriers of the disease or with blood. Medical and laboratory workers, police, intravenous drug users, people with multiple sexual partners, and those living with someone who has lifelong infection are at high risk of contracting hepatitis B (and hepatitis C as well). Vaccination is the best defense against HBV. There is no chance of developing hepatitis B from the vaccine. Federal laws require employers to offer a series of three vaccine injections free to all employees who may be at risk of exposure.

Without vaccination shots, exposure to hepatitis B may produce symptoms within 2 weeks to 6 months after exposure. People with hepatitis B infection may be symptom free, but that does not mean they are not contagious. These people may infect others through exposure to their blood. Symptoms of hepatitis B resemble those of the flu and include fatigue, nausea, loss of appetite, stomach pain, and sometimes a yellowing of the skin.

CRITICAL CONCEPTS: WHEN TO CALL EMS

In the following instances, calling EMS is definitely the right thing to do:

- Severe bleeding
- Drowning
- Electrocution
- Possible heart attack
- Breathing difficulty or no breathing
- Choking
- Altered mental status
- Poisoning
- Attempted suicide
- Some seizure cases (most do not require EMS assistance)
- Critical burns
- Paralysis
- Spinal injury
- Imminent childbirth

CRITICAL CONCEPTS: PROTECTION FROM BLOODBORNE DISEASE

In most cases, you can control the risk of exposure to bloodborne pathogens by wearing the proper personal protective equipment and by following some simple procedures.

PERSONAL PROTECTIVE EQUIPMENT

Personal protective equipment (PPE) blocks entry of an organism into the body. The most common type of protection is gloves. The Food and Drug Administration (FDA), the Centers for Disease Control and Prevention (CDC), and the Occupational Safety and Health Administration (OSHA) have stated that vinyl and latex gloves are equally protective. All first aid kits should have several pairs of gloves.

Protective eyewear and a standard surgical mask may be necessary in some emergencies, but first aiders ordinarily will not have or need such equipment.

Mouth-to-barrier devices are recommended for use during rescue breathing. No case of bloodborne disease transmission to a rescuer as a result of performing unprotected CPR on an infected victim has been documented. Nevertheless, a mouth-to-barrier device should be used whenever possible (FIGURE 2).

UNIVERSAL PRECAUTIONS OR BODY SUBSTANCE ISOLATION?

Individuals who are infected with HBV or HIV might not show symptoms and might not even know that they are infectious. For that reason, all human blood and body fluids should be considered infectious, and precautions should be taken to avoid contact. The body substance isolation (BSI) technique assumes that all body fluids pose a possible risk. EMS personnel routinely follow BSI procedures, even if blood or body fluids are not visible.

OSHA requires any company with employees who are expected to give first aid in an emergency to follow universal precautions, which assume that all blood and certain body fluids pose a risk for transmission of HBV and HIV. OSHA considers an employee who assists another with a nosebleed or a cut to fall under the definition of "Good Samaritan." However, such acts are not considered occupational exposure unless the employee who provides the assistance is a member of a first aid team or is designated or expected to render first aid as part of his or her job. In essence, OSHA's requirement excludes unassigned employees who perform unanticipated first aid.

Whenever there is a chance that you could be exposed to bloodborne pathogens, your employer must provide appropriate PPE, which might include eye protection, gloves, gowns, and masks. The PPE must be accessible, and your employer must provide training to help you choose the right PPE for your work.

While EMS personnel follow BSI procedures and OSHA requires designated worksite first aiders to follow universal precautions, what should a typical first aider do? It makes sense for first aiders to follow BSI procedures and assume that all blood and body fluids are infectious and follow appropriate protective measures.

COPING WITH EMERGENCIES

When an injury occurs, first aiders can protect themselves and others against bloodborne pathogens by following these steps:

1. Wear appropriate PPE, such as gloves.
2. If you have been trained in the correct procedures, use absorbent barriers to soak up blood or other infectious materials.
3. Clean the spill area with an appropriate disinfecting solution, such as diluted bleach.
4. Discard contaminated materials in an appropriate waste disposal container.

Hepatitis C Hepatitis C is caused by a different virus from HBV, but these diseases have much in common. Like hepatitis B, hepatitis C affects the liver and can lead to long-term liver disease and liver cancer. Hepatitis C varies in severity and may even cause no symptoms at the time of infection. Currently, there is no vaccine or effective treatment for hepatitis C.

HIV Estimates are that over 1.5 million people in the United States are infected with HIV but have no symptoms. A person who is infected with HIV can infect others, and HIV-infected people almost always develop acquired immunodeficiency syndrome (AIDS), which interferes with the body's ability to fight off other diseases. No vaccine is available to prevent HIV infection, which eventually proves fatal. The best defense against AIDS is to avoid becoming infected.

Personal Protection Wearing PPE and handwashing provide optimal personal protection. If you have been exposed to blood or body fluids, follow these steps:

1. Remove your gloves and wash your hands and contaminated body area immediately with soap and water. Rub your hands together vigorously for at least 10 to 15 seconds (work up a lather), then rinse your hands and dry them with a paper towel.

2. Use a paper towel to turn off the faucet so that you do not recontaminate yourself or others.

3. If you cannot wash immediately with soap and water, use antiseptic towelettes and wash with soap and water as soon as possible.

4. Flush your eyes, nose, and other mucous membranes with water if they have been exposed.

5. If the exposure happens while you are at work, report the incident to your supervisor. Otherwise, contact your personal physician. Early action can prevent the development of hepatitis B and enable affected workers to track potential HIV infection.

Airborne Disease Infective organisms (eg, bacteria, viruses) that are introduced into the air by coughing or sneezing are said to be "airborne." Droplets of mucus that carry those bacteria or viruses can then be inhaled by other individuals. The rate of tuberculosis (TB) has increased recently and is receiving much attention. TB is caused by bacteria and sometimes settles in the lungs and can be fatal. In most cases a first aider cannot know whether a victim has TB. Assume that any person with a cough,

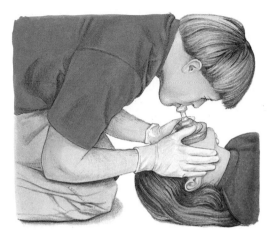

Figure 2
Pocket face mask with one-way valve.

FYI: Glove Removal

Proper glove removal is as important as wearing gloves to protect against infection. Follow this procedure:

1. Grip one glove near the cuff and peel it down until it comes off inside out. Cup it in the palm of your gloved hand.

2. Place two fingers of your bare hand inside the cuff of the remaining glove.

3. Peel that glove down so that it also comes off inside out and over the first glove.

4. Properly dispose of the gloves.

5. Wash your hands with soap and water.

especially one who is in a nursing home or a shelter, may have TB. Other symptoms include fatigue, weight loss, chest pain, and coughing up blood. If a surgical mask is available, wear it or wrap a handkerchief over your nose and mouth.

RESCUING AND MOVING VICTIMS

Victim Rescue

Water Rescue Reach-throw-row-go identifies the sequence for attempting a water rescue. The first and simplest rescue technique is to reach for the victim. Reaching requires a lightweight pole, ladder, long stick, or any object that can be extended to the victim. Secure your footing and have a bystander grab your belt or pants for stability. Secure yourself before reaching for the victim.

You can throw anything that floats, such as an empty picnic jug, empty fuel or paint can, life jacket, floating cushion, piece of wood, inflated spare wheel—whatever is available. If there is a rope handy, tie it to the object so that you can pull the victim back in or, if you miss, you can retrieve the object and throw it again. The average untrained rescuer has a throwing range of about 50 feet.

If the victim is out of throwing range and there is a rowboat, canoe, motorboat, or boogie board nearby, you can try to row to the victim. Maneuvering these craft requires skill learned through practice. Wear a personal flotation device (PFD) for your own safety. To avoid capsizing, never pull the victim in over the side of a boat; pull him or her over the stern (rear end).

If these three reach-throw-row techniques are impossible and you are a capable swimmer trained in water lifesaving procedures, you can go to the drowning victim by swimming. Note that entering even calm water to make a swimming rescue is difficult and hazardous. All too often, a would-be rescuer becomes a victim as well.

Ice Rescue If a person has fallen through the ice near the shore, extend a pole or throw a line with a floatable object attached to it. When the person has hold of the device, pull him or her toward the shore or the edge of the ice.

If the person has fallen through the ice away from the shore and you cannot reach him or her with a pole or a throwing line, lie flat and push a ladder, plank, or similar object ahead of you. You can also tie a rope to a spare tire and the other end to an anchor point, lie flat, and push the tire ahead of you. Pull the person ashore or to the edge of the ice.

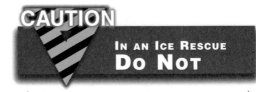

CAUTION

IN A WATER RESCUE
DO NOT

- swim to and grasp a drowning person unless you are trained in lifesaving.

CAUTION

IN AN ICE RESCUE
DO NOT

- go near broken ice without support.

Confined Spaces A confined space is any area not intended for human occupancy that may contain or accumulate a dangerous atmosphere. Examples of confined spaces are tanks, vessels, vats, bins, vaults, trenches, and pits.

An accident in a confined space demands immediate action. If an entrant into a confined space signals for help or becomes unconscious, follow these steps to help:

1. Call for immediate help

2. Do not rush in to help

3. If you are the attendant, do not enter the confined space unless you are relieved by another attendant and you are part of the rescue team

4. When help arrives, try to rescue the victim without entering the space

5. If rescue from the outside cannot be done, allow trained and properly equipped (respiratory protection plus safety harnesses or lifelines) rescuers to enter the space and remove the victim

6. Activate the local EMS

7. Give first aid, rescue breathing, or CPR if necessary and if you are trained

Electrical Emergency Rescue Electrical injuries can be devastating. Even just a mild shock can cause serious internal injuries. A current of 1,000 volts or more is considered high voltage, but even the 110 volts of household current can be deadly.

When a person gets an electric shock, electricity enters the body at the point of contact and travels along the path of least resistance (nerves and blood vessels). The current travels rapidly, generating heat and causing destruction.

Most indoor electrocutions are caused by faulty electrical equipment or careless use of electrical appliances. Before you touch the victim, turn off the electricity at the circuit breaker, fuse box, or outside switch box or unplug the appliance if the plug is undamaged.

If the electrocution involves high-voltage power lines, the power must be turned off before anyone approaches a victim. If you approach a victim and feel a tingling sensation in your legs and lower body, stop. You are on energized ground, and an electrical current is entering one foot, passing through your lower body, then leaving through the other foot. If that happens, raise

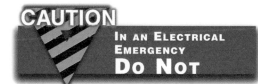

CAUTION

IN AN ELECTRICAL EMERGENCY

DO NOT

- touch an appliance or the victim until the current is off.
- try to move downed wires.
- use any object, even dry wood (eg, a broomstick, tools, chair, stool) to separate the victim from the electrical source.

one foot off the ground, turn around, and hop to a safe place. Wait for trained personnel with the proper equipment to cut the wires or disconnect them.

If a power line has fallen over a car, tell the driver and passengers to stay in the car. A victim should try to jump out of the car only if an explosion or fire threatens, and then without making contact with the car or the wire.

Hazardous Materials Incidents At almost any highway accident scene, there is the potential danger of hazardous chemicals. Clues that indicate the presence of hazardous materials include

- Signs on vehicles (eg, "explosive," "flammable," "corrosive")
- Spilled liquids or solids
- Strong, unusual odors
- Clouds of vapor

Stay well away and upwind from the area. Only people who are specially trained in handling hazardous materials and who have the proper equipment should be in the area.

Motor Vehicle Incidents

In most states, you are legally obligated to stop and give help when you are involved in a motor vehicle incident. If you come upon an incident shortly after it happens, the law does not require you to stop, although it might be argued that you have a moral responsibility to render any aid that you can.

1. Stop your vehicle in a safe place. If the police have taken charge, do not stop unless you are asked to do so.
2. Turn on your flashing hazard lights.
3. Direct bystanders to warn other drivers and to set up warning flares or reflectors.
4. Try to enter an involved vehicle through a door. If the doors are jammed, try to get someone inside the car to roll down a window. As a last resort, break a window to gain access. Once inside, place the vehicle in park, turn off the ignition, and set the parking brake.
5. For unresponsive victims and those who might have spine injuries, use your hands to immobilize their heads and necks.
6. Treat any life-threatening injuries.

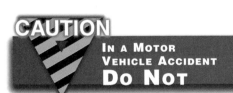

CAUTION

IN A MOTOR VEHICLE ACCIDENT DO NOT

- rush to get victims out of a car that has been in an accident. Most vehicle crashes do not involve fire, and most vehicles stay upright.

7. Whenever possible, wait for EMS personnel to extricate the victims, since they have training and the proper equipment. In most cases, keep the victims stabilized inside the vehicle.

Fires

Should you encounter a fire inside a structure, you should

1. Get all the people out fast

2. Call the local emergency telephone number (usually 911)
    Then—and only then—if the fire is small and if your own escape route is clear, should you fight the fire yourself with a fire extinguisher. You might be able to put out the fire or at least hold damage to a minimum.

    If clothing catches fire, tear it off away from the face. Keep the victim from running, since that fans the flames. Wrap a rug or a woolen blanket around the victim's neck to keep the fire from the face or throw a blanket on the victim. In some cases, you might be able to smother the flames by throwing the victim to the floor and rolling him or her in a rug.

    To use a fire extinguisher, aim directly at whatever is burning and sweep across it. Extinguishers expel their contents quickly, in 8 to 25 seconds for most home models containing dry chemicals.

Triage: What to Do with Multiple Victims

You might encounter emergency situations in which there are two or more victims. This is often the case in multiple-car collisions or disasters. After making a quick scene survey, decide who must be cared for and transported first. This process of prioritizing injured victims is called triage. The term "triage" comes from the French word trier, meaning "to sort." The goal is to do the greatest good for the greatest number of victims.

Triage: Finding Life-Threatened Victims

A variety of systems are used to identify care and transportation priorities. To find the people who need immediate care for life-threatening conditions, first tell all victims who can get up and walk to move to a specific area. Victims who can get up and walk rarely have life-threatening injuries. These victims (the "walking wounded") are classified as delayed priority (see below). Do not force a victim to move if he or she complains of pain.

Find the life-threatened victims by performing only the initial survey on all remaining victims. Go to motionless victims first.

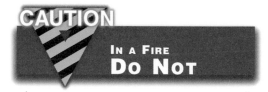

CAUTION

IN A FIRE
DO NOT

- let a victim run if clothing is on fire.
- get trapped while fighting a fire. Always keep a door behind you so that you can exit if the fire gets too big.

You must move rapidly (spend less than 60 seconds with each victim) from one victim to the next until all have been assessed. Classify victims according to the following care and transportation priorities:

1. *Immediate care.* Victims who have life-threatening injuries but can be saved:

    • Airway or breathing difficulties (not breathing or breathing at a rate slower than 8 per minute or faster than 24 per minute)

    • Weak or no pulse

    • Uncontrolled or severe bleeding

    • Unresponsive or unconscious

2. *Urgent care.* Victims who do not fit into the immediate or delayed categories. Care and transportation can be delayed up to 1 hour.

3. *Delayed care.* Victims with minor injuries. Care and transportation can be delayed up to 3 hours.

4. *Dead.* Victims who are obviously dead, mortally wounded, or unlikely to survive because of the extent of their injuries, age, or medical condition.

    Do not become involved in treating the victims at this point, but ask knowledgeable bystanders to care for immediate life-threatening problems (ie, rescue breathing, bleeding control).

    Reassess victims regularly for changes in their condition. Only after those with immediate life-threatening conditions receive care should those with less serious conditions be given care.

    You will usually be relieved from triage responsibility when more highly trained emergency personnel arrive on the scene. You may then be asked to provide first aid, to help move victims, or to help with ambulance or helicopter transportation.

Moving Victims

A victim should not be moved until he or she is ready for transportation to a hospital, if required. All necessary first aid should be provided first. A victim should be moved only if there is an immediate danger:

• There is a fire or danger of fire

• Explosives or other hazardous materials are involved

• It is impossible to protect the incident scene from hazards

• It is impossible to gain access to other victims in the situation (eg, a vehicle) who need lifesaving care

A cardiac arrest victim is usually moved unless he or she is already on the ground or floor, because CPR must be performed on a firm surface.

CAUTION

WHEN MOVING VICTIMS DO NOT

■ move a victim unless you absolutely have to. That might happen if the victim is in immediate danger or must be moved to shelter while waiting for EMS personnel to arrive.

■ make the injury worse by moving the victim.

■ move a victim who could have a spinal injury.

■ move a victim without immobilizing the injured part.

■ move a victim unless you know where you are going.

■ leave an unresponsive victim alone.

■ move a victim when someone could be sent for help. Wait with the victim and send someone else for help.

■ try to move a victim by yourself if other people are available to help.

Emergency Moves The major danger in moving a victim quickly is the possibility of aggravating a spinal injury. In an emergency, every effort should be made to pull the victim in the direction of the long axis of the body to provide as much protection to the spinal cord as possible. If victims are on the floor or ground, you can drag them away from the scene by one of various techniques.

Nonemergency Moves All injured parts should be stabilized before and during moving. If rapid transportation is not needed, it is helpful to practice first on another person who is about the same size as the injured victim.

ONE-PERSON MOVES

1. *Human crutch* (one person helps victim to walk). If one leg is injured, help the victim to walk on the good leg while you support the injured side (FIGURE 3A).

2. *Cradle carry.* Use for children and lightweight adults who cannot walk (FIGURE 3B).

3. *Fireman's carry.* If the victim's injuries permit, longer distances can be traveled if the victim is carried over your shoulder (FIGURE 3C).

4. *Pack-strap carry.* This method is also good for longer distances (FIGURE 3D).

5. *Piggyback carry.* Use this method when the victim cannot walk but can use the arms to hang onto the rescuer (FIGURE 3E).

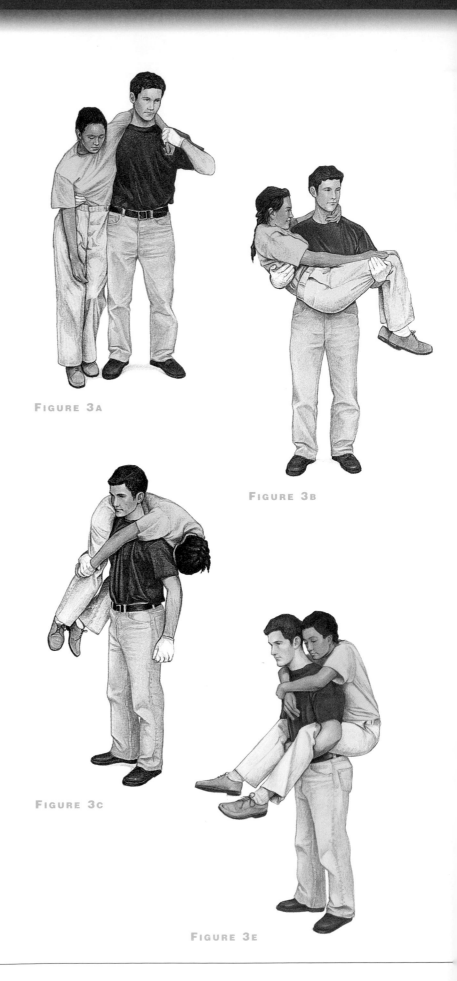

FIGURE 3A

FIGURE 3B

FIGURE 3C

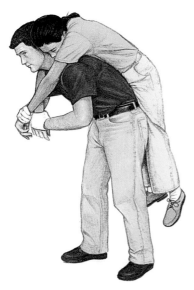

FIGURE 3D

FIGURE 3E

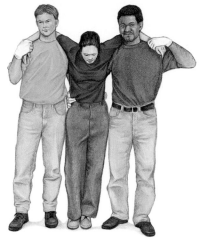

FIGURE 4A

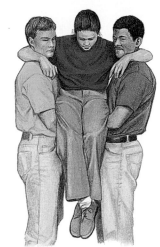

FIGURE 4B

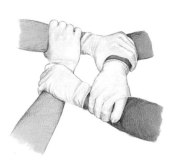

FIGURE 4C

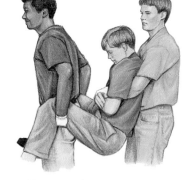

FIGURE 4D

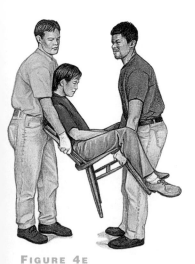

FIGURE 4E

FIGURE 4F

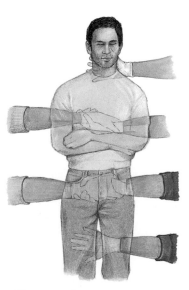

FIGURE 4G

SKILL SCAN

TWO/THREE-PERSON MOVES

1. *Two-person assist.* Similar to human crutch (FIGURE 4A).
2. *Two-handed seat carry* (FIGURE 4B).
3. *Four-handed seat carry.* The easiest two-person carry when no equipment is available and the victim cannot walk but can use his or her arms to hang onto the two rescuers (FIGURE 4C).
4. *Extremity carry* (FIGURE 4D).
5. *Chair carry.* Useful for a narrow passage or up or down stairs. Use a sturdy chair that can take the victim's weight (FIGURE 4E).
6. *Hammock carry.* Three to six people stand on alternate sides of the injured person and link hands beneath the victim (FIGURE 4F, FIGURE 4G).

First Aid Kits

Following are the recommended items that should be stocked inside a first aid kit in the workplace, at home, and for travel. First aid kits should be

- Impact-resistant and made of durable material to protect against moisture, dust, and contamination
- Portable and easily carried by a handle
- Of sufficient size to store the equipment listed
- Clearly marked as being a first aid kit by words and/or symbols
- Regularly inspected for completeness, content condition, and updating

Workplace First Aid Kit*	
Equipment	Minimum Quantity
1. Adhesive strip bandages (1" x 3")	20
2. Triangular bandages (muslin, 36" – 40" x 36" – 40" x 52" – 56")	4
3. Sterile eye pads (2 $\frac{1}{8}$" x 2 $\frac{5}{8}$")	2
4. Sterile gauze pads (4" x 4")	6
5. Sterile nonstick pads (3" x 4")	6
6. Sterile trauma pads (5" x 9")	2
7. Sterile trauma pads (8" x 10")	1
8. Sterile conforming roller gauze (2" width)	3 rolls
9. Sterile conforming roller gauze (4.5" width)	3 rolls
10. Waterproof tape (1" x 5 yards)	1 roll
11. Porous adhesive tape (2" x 5 yards)	1 roll
12. Elastic roller bandages (4" and 6")	1 each
13. Antiseptic skin wipes, individually wrapped	10
14. Medical-grade exam gloves (medium, large, extra large), conforming to FDA requirements	2 pairs per size
15. Mouth-to-barrier device, either a face mask with a one-way valve or a disposable face shield	1
16. Disposable instant activating cold packs	2
17. Resealable plastic bags (quart size)	2
18. Padded malleable splint (SAM splint, 4" x 36")	1
19. Emergency blanket, Mylar	1
20. Paramedic shears (with one serrated edge)	1
21. Splinter tweezers (about 3" long)	1
22. Biohazard waste bag (3.5 gallon capacity)	2
23. First aid and CPR manual and list of local emergency telephone numbers	1

* This list does not include over-the-counter ointments, topicals, or internal medicines; consult the workplace's medical director for these.

Home First Aid Kit**

1. Acetaminophen, ibuprofen, and aspirin tablets: for headaches, pain, fever, and simple sprains or strains of the body. (Aspirin should not be used for relief of flu symptoms or given to children.)
2. Ipecac syrup and activated charcoal: for treatment after ingestion of certain poisons. (Use only on the advice of a poison control center or the emergency department.)
3. Elastic wraps: for wrapping wrist, ankle, knee, and elbow injuries
4. Triangular bandage: for wrapping injuries and making an arm sling
5. Scissors with rounded tips
6. Adhesive tape and 2″ gauze: for dressing wounds
7. Disposable, instant activating ice bags: for icing injuries and treating high fevers
8. Bandages of assorted sizes: for covering minor cuts and scrapes
9. Antibiotic ointment: for burns, cuts, and scrapes
10. Gauze in rolls and in 2″ and 4″ pads: for dressing wounds
11. Bandage closures, 1/4″ and 1″: for taping cut edges together
12. Tweezers: to remove small splinters and ticks
13. Safety pins: to fasten splints and bandages
14. Rubber gloves: to protect your hands and reduce the risk of infection when treating open wounds
15. First aid manual
16. List of emergency phone numbers

Travel First Aid Kit**

1. Aspirin, acetaminophen, or ibuprofen: for headaches, pain, fever, and simple sprains or strains of the body. (Aspirin should not be used for relief of flu symptoms or given to children.)
2. Antihistamine/decongestant cough medicine
3. Anti-nausea/motion sickness medication
4. Bandages of assorted sizes, including adhesive bandages (eg, Band Aids™)
5. Adhesive tape and 2″ gauze: for dressing wounds
6. Elastic wraps: for wrapping wrist, ankle, knee, and elbow injuries
7. Triangular bandage: for wrapping injuries and making an arm sling
8. Scissors with rounded tips
9. Rubber gloves: to reduce the risk of infection
10. Disposable, instant activating ice bags: for icing injuries and treating high fevers
11. Antifungal cream (tolnaftate 1% or clotrimazole 1%): good for athlete's foot or ringworm
12. Antibacterial ointment
13. Antibiotic ointment: for burns, cuts, and scrapes
14. Thermometer with case
15. Sunscreen: SPF 15 or higher
16. Insect repellent: those that contain 35%-55% DEET with stabilizer
17. Antidiarrheal medications (eg, Pepto Bismol™, Imodium AD™) tablets or liquid; follow directions carefully.
18. Anti-malaria medications (if indicated)
19. Water-purifying pills or liquid (tincture of iodine or halazone tablets) or mechanical filtration devices, such as Katadyne™ water purifier
20. Steroidal cream, such as hydrocortisone cream: for insect bites
21. Tweezers: to remove small splinters and ticks
22. Safety pins: to fasten splints and bandages

**Recommended by the American College of Emergency Physicians.

······························

First aid is the

immediate care

that is given to an

injured or

suddenly ill

person until the

person receives

appropriate

medical treatment.

······························

SUMMARY

First aid is the immediate care that is given to an injured or suddenly ill person until the person receives appropriate medical treatment. Everyone should have first aid training, because most people will eventually find themselves in a situation requiring it. Being able to recognize a medical emergency and knowing how to get help and how to care for the victim until help arrives are critical.

For ethical and legal reasons, a first aider must have expressed or implied consent before caring for a victim. When giving first aid, one should follow accepted standards of care to avoid being negligent. Good Samaritan laws generally protect first aiders who act in good faith.

Intervening in an emergency involves recognizing it, deciding to help, calling EMS when needed, assessing the victim, and giving first aid. Survey the scene before calling EMS to check for dangers, and quickly check the nature of the injury or illness to report to EMS.

Because you might be in contact with a victim's blood or other body fluids when giving first aid, you must take precautions to protect yourself from the risk of infectious disease such as hepatitis or HIV. Use personal protective equipment such as gloves and face masks. Follow the Body Substance Isolation procedures and guidelines for handwashing and cleaning contaminated areas.

In some first aid situations it is necessary to rescue or move a victim before giving care. Rescuing a victim from the water, a fall through ice, an electrocution, a scene that is contaminated with hazardous materials, a motor vehicle collision, a fire, or a confined space poses risks. Know what to do and what not to attempt.

In situations in which there are multiple victims, follow a process of triage to classify victims and give care first to those with life-threatening injuries who can still be saved.

As a general rule, victims with significant injuries should not be moved before EMS personnel arrive—unless there is an immediate danger requiring moving them. Since movement may aggravate a spinal or other injury, use an accepted emergency move to minimize this risk.

REVIEW QUESTIONS

Background Information

Directions: Circle Yes if you agree with the statement, and circle No if you disagree.

Yes   No   1. In most locations, an ambulance can arrive within minutes. This quick response means that most people do not need to learn to perform first aid.

Yes   No   2. Correct first aid can mean the difference between life and death.

Yes   No   3. Most injuries do not require lifesaving first aid efforts.

Yes   No   4. Call for an ambulance and/or seek medical care for all injured victims.

Yes   No   5. In most situations, before you give first aid, the victim must give you consent (permission).

Yes   No   6. If you ask a victim whether you can help, and she or he says no, you can ignore the response and give first aid.

Yes   No   7. Employers can designate people as first aiders. This means that they must give first aid to injured employees while on the job.

Yes   No   8. First aiders who help injured victims are often sued.

Yes   No   9. Good Samaritan laws protect first aiders (nonmedical personnel) in all states.

Yes   No   10. Everyone will at some time have to decide whether to help another person.

Yes   No   11. Deciding whether to help others should be done before encountering an emergency.

Yes   No   12. A scene survey should be done before first aid is given to an injured victim.

Yes   No   13. For a severely injured victim, first call the victim's doctor before calling for an ambulance.

Yes   No   14. Most communities use the 911 telephone number for emergencies.

Yes   No   15. First aiders should assume that blood and all body fluids are infectious.

Yes   No   16. If you have been exposed to blood while on the job, report it to your supervisor; if off the job, report it to your personal physician.

Yes   No   17. First aid kits should contain disposable medical exam gloves.

Scenario 1. You are driving slowly, looking for a house number in an unfamiliar residential area. You are attempting to deliver an important package to a customer. You see an elderly woman lying at the bottom of porch stairs outside of a house. You see no one else in the neighborhood, and you are alone. You quickly but safely stop your vehicle in front of the victim's house. When you get nearer to the victim, you notice that her skin appears bluish and she is motionless.

Yes   No   18. Do you have to stop to help her?

19. If you stop and help, which type of consent would apply in this case?

a. expressed   b. implied

Yes   No   20. If she does not respond to your tapping on her shoulders and shouting "Are you okay?" can you leave her and assume that someone else who is more competent or is a family member will arrive shortly to help her?

Yes   No   21. Rather than check the victim's breathing and pulse, you proceed to care for the broken leg. By doing so, have you failed to provide appropriate first aid?

Yes   No   22. If the woman were your mother under your custodial care, would you be obligated to give first aid to her?

Scenario 2. You are rushing parts to one of your best customers to fix a broken machine. Since "time is money," the customer is losing a lot for each hour the machine is down. It's beginning to rain. Suddenly, you see a motorcyclist skidding off the country highway and ending up in a barbed wire fence alongside the highway. You see no other traffic. You have a cellular telephone in your car.

23. Name the five actions that a bystander can take at an emergency.

a. _____

b. _____

c. _____

d. _____

e. _____

24. A scene survey consists of looking for what three things?

a._____

b._____

c._____

25. When talking with an EMS dispatcher, what information should you expect to give?

a._____

b._____

c._____

d._____

26. How would you protect yourself against bloodborne pathogens?

a._____

b._____

c._____

How did you do?

1. No; 2. Yes; 3. Yes; 4. No; 5. Yes; 6. No; 7. Yes;
8. No; 9. No; 10. Yes; 11. Yes; 12. Yes; 13. No;
14. Yes; 15. Yes; 16. Yes; 17. Yes; 18. No; 19. b;
20. No; 21. Yes; 22. Yes

23. **a.** recognize the emergency
    b. decide to help
    c. contact the EMS if needed
    d. assess the victim
    e. provide first aid
24. **a.** hazards
    b. mechanism of injury
    c. number of victims
25. **a.** victim's location
    b. victim's condition
    c. your phone number and name
    d. what happened and the number of victims
26. **a.** wear personal protection
    b. afterward, wash with soap and water
    c. report to your supervisor if at work, or to a physician if otherwise

VICTIM ASSESSMENT

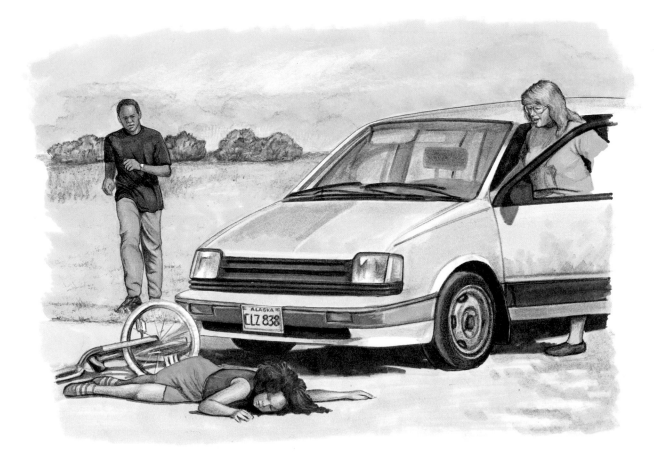

CONTENTS

Victim assessment

is an important

first aid skill.

After reading this chapter you should be able to

1. Identify and practice the steps of an initial assessment
2. Identify and practice the steps of a physical exam
3. Identify and practice the steps of obtaining a victim's history

VICTIM ASSESSMENT

Victim assessment is an important first aid skill. It requires an understanding of each assessment step and decision making.

Every time you encounter a victim, first check out the scene. If the scene is not surveyed, a potentially dangerous situation could result in further injury to the victim or to you and others. The scene survey is performed to determine the safety of the scene, the victim's cause of injury or nature of illness, and the number of victims.

The scene survey is followed by the initial victim assessment. During the initial victim assessment, the first aider identifies and corrects immediate life-threatening conditions involving problems with the victim's airway, breathing, and circulation. Victims with immediate life-threatening conditions can die within minutes without quick recognition and correction of their problems. Determining the type of injury or illness is also part of the initial assessment.

A physical examination and medical history follow the initial assessment. These assessments can reveal information that will help in identifying the injury or illness and its severity, as well as the appropriate first aid to give. Detailed information is gained about the victim's injury (eg, painful ankle, bleeding nose) or chief complaint (eg, chest pain, itchy skin).

If two or more people are injured, attend to the quiet one first. A quiet victim might not be breathing or have a heartbeat. A victim who is talking, crying, or alert, obviously is breathing.

INITIAL ASSESSMENT

The goal of the initial assessment is to determine whether there are life-threatening problems that require quick care. This assessment involves evaluating the victim's airway, breathing, and circulation. The following step-by-step process should not be changed. It takes less than a minute to complete, unless first aid is required at any point. At this stage, the victim's problem will most likely be identified as being an injury or an illness.

Begin the initial assessment with a check for responsiveness. If there is a possibility of a spinal cord injury, have another person hold the victim's head to minimize movement and avoid causing further damage (**FIGURE 1**).

Check for responsiveness by speaking to the victim. If the person can talk, breathing and heartbeat are present. If the victim does not respond, tap his or her shoulder and ask, "Are you okay?" If there is no response, consider the victim as being unresponsive.

The level of responsiveness is one of the most important indicators of the victim's overall condition. This can vary from alert to unresponsive. The AVPU scale is used to describe the level of responsiveness.

The AVPU Scale

A = Alert and aware
V = Responds to verbal stimulus
P = Responds to painful stimulus
U = Unresponsive

A: Alert. The victim's eyes are open, and he or she can answer questions clearly. A victim who knows the date (time), where he or she is (place), and his or her own name (person) is said to be alert.

V: Responsive to verbal stimulus. The victim might not be oriented to time, place, and person but does respond in some meaningful way when spoken to.

P: Responsive only to painful stimulus. The eyes do not open, and the victim does not respond to questions. The victim does respond to your pinching of the muscle between the neck and shoulder.

U: Unresponsive to any stimulus. The eyes do not open, and the victim does not respond to pinching of the muscle between the neck and shoulder.

RECOGNIZING THREATS TO LIFE

A: Airway

The airway must be open for breathing. If the victim is speaking or crying, the airway is open. If a responsive victim cannot talk, cry, or cough forcefully, then the airway is likely obstructed and must be checked and cleared. In this case, abdominal thrusts (Heimlich maneuver) can be given to clear an obstructed airway in a responsive adult victim. Obstructed airway problems have been discussed in earlier chapters.

In an unresponsive victim who is lying face up, the most common obstruction is the tongue. Snoring is evidence of this. If there is no suspected spinal cord injury, use the head tilt–chin lift method to open the airway. If a spinal cord injury is likely, use the jaw-thrust method to prevent further injury.

Once the victim's airway is clear of obstruction, the initial assessment can be continued.

B: Breathing

A breathing rate between 12 and 20 times per minute is normal for adults. Victims who are having difficulty moving air and who are breathing less than 8 times per minute or more than 24 times per minute need care. Note any breathing difficulties or unusual breathing sounds such as wheezing, crowing, gurgling, or snoring.

If the victim is unresponsive, after opening the airway, check for breathing. Do this by watching for the victim's chest to rise

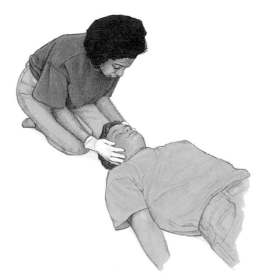

FIGURE 1
Immobilizing the head with the hands.

and fall while placing your ear next to the victim's mouth. "Look, listen, and feel" for about 5 seconds to check for breathing. If the victim is not breathing, keep the airway open and breathe two slow breaths into the victim. Whenever possible, use a mouth-to-barrier device (face mask or face shield).

C: Circulation

After checking for airway and breathing problems and correcting any problems, check the victim's circulation. "Circulation" refers to checking the victim's pulse and skin and searching for severe bleeding.

Pulse A normal adult pulse beats at a rate of 60 to 100 times per minute. If the victim is unresponsive, check the neck (carotid) artery **(FIGURE 2).** Check the pulse by locating the appropriate artery and feeling it for about 10 seconds. If the victim does not have a pulse, CPR must be started.

Severe Bleeding Check for severe bleeding by looking over the victim's entire body for blood (blood-soaked clothing or blood pooling on the floor or the ground). Bleeding requires the application of direct pressure or a pressure bandage. Avoid contact with the victim's blood, if possible, by using medical exam gloves or extra layers of dressings or cloth. Control any bleeding with pressure as described in Chapter 10.

Skin Condition A quick check of the victim's skin can also provide information about the circulatory status. Check skin temperature, color, and condition (eg, moist, dry). Skin color, especially in light-skinned people, reflects the circulation under the skin as well as oxygen status. In darkly pigmented people, changes might not be readily apparent but can be assessed by the appearance of the nail beds, the inside of the mouth, and the inner eyelids. When the skin's blood vessels constrict or the pulse slows, the skin becomes cool and pale or cyanotic (blue-gray color). When the skin's blood vessels dilate or blood flow increases, the skin becomes warm.

You can get a rough idea of temperature by putting the back of your hand or wrist on the victim's forehead. If the victim has a fever, you should be able to feel it. Abnormal skin temperature will feel hot, cool, cold, or clammy (cool and moist).

D: Disability

In Part One of this book, the letter "D" in the mnemonic "ABCD" represented "defibrillation" when assessing a cardiac arrest victim. When defibrillation is not needed, the "D" represents "disability," which refers to checking for a spinal cord injury.

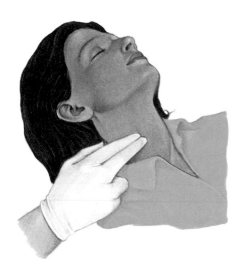

FIGURE 2
Palpating the carotid pulse.

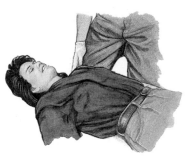

FIGURE 3A

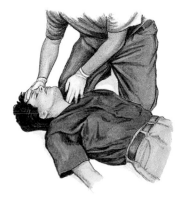

FIGURE 3B

INITIAL ASSESSMENT

1. **Responsive?** (FIGURE 3A)
2. **A = Airway open?** (FIGURE 3B)
3. **B = Breathing?** (FIGURE 3C)
4. **C = Circulation?**
   a. **Carotid pulse?** (FIGURE 3D)
   b. **Hemorrhage/severe bleeding?** (FIGURE 3E)
   c. **Condition of skin?** (not shown)
      color
      temperature
      moisture
5. **D = Disability?** (FIGURE 3F)
   spinal cord response

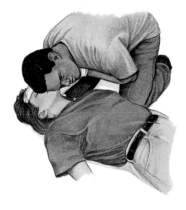

FIGURE 3C

FIGURE 3D

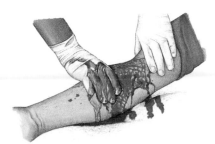

FIGURE 3E

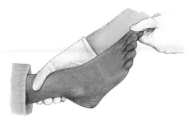

FIGURE 3F

Check for a spinal injury, especially if the victim has been injured in a fall, a motor vehicle crash, or other incident that could produce a spinal injury. Assume that a victim with a head injury has a spinal injury until proven otherwise. To assess a victim for a spinal injury

1. Check sensation by squeezing the victim's fingers and toes
2. Check movement by having the victim wiggle his or her fingers and toes
3. Have the victim perform a hand squeeze and a foot push

If you suspect a spinal injury, do not move the victim. See Chapter 14 for the best way to immobilize a suspected spinal injury.

E: Expose the Injury

Clothing can hide an injury. How much clothing you should remove varies, depending on the victim's condition and injuries. The general rule is to remove as much clothing as necessary to determine the presence or absence of a condition or an injury. Keep in mind that most injured victims are susceptible to hypothermia. If the removal of certain items of clothing might prove embarrassing to the victim or to bystanders, explain what you intend to do and why.

PHYSICAL EXAM AND SAMPLE HISTORY

The initial assessment is followed by a physical examination and the SAMPLE history. Up to this point, the initial assessment has been the same for ill and injured victims. Also, whether the victim has an injury or an illness, the steps in the physical exam and SAMPLE history are similar.

Injured Victim

The physical exam and SAMPLE history of the injured victim take place immediately after the initial assessment. They start with a reconsideration of the mechanism (cause) of injury (this was done previously, during the scene survey). This allows you to determine which procedures you are going to take in checking an injured victim.

Injured Victim With a Significant Mechanism of Injury For an injured victim with a significant mechanism of injury, do the following in this order: stabilize the head to keep it from moving, monitor the ABCs, perform a physical examination, and obtain a SAMPLE history.

In addition to the significant mechanisms of injury, assume that a victim with a head injury may have a spinal cord injury

---

FOUNDATION FACTS: Significant Mechanisms (Causes) of Injury

- Falls of more that 15 feet for adults, 10 feet for children, or 3 times the victim's height
- Vehicle collisions involving ejection, a rollover, high speeds, a pedestrian, a motorcycle, or a bicycle
- Unresponsive or altered mental status
- Penetrations of the head, chest, or abdomen (eg, stab and gunshot wounds)

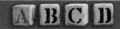

until proven otherwise. About 15% to 20% of head injury victims also have a spinal injury.

Assess a responsive victim for a spinal cord injury by asking

- Can you feel me squeezing your fingers and toes?
- Can you wiggle your fingers and toes?
- Can you squeeze my hand and push your foot against my hand?

For an unresponsive victim, test the spinal cord by stroking the bottom of the foot firmly toward the big toe with a key or similar sharp object. This is known as the Babinski reflex test. The normal response is an involuntary reflex that makes the big toe go down (except in infants). If the spinal cord or brain is injured, an adult's and child's toes will flex upward.

If you suspect a spinal cord injury, do not move the victim's head or neck. Stabilize the victim against any movement, and be sure to tell him or her not to move.

Physical Examination A good physical exam is very important for the injured victim who is unresponsive or has a significant mechanism of injury.

Check the victim's head, neck, chest, abdomen, pelvis, and extremities. To evaluate these areas, look and feel for the following signs of injury: deformities, open injuries, tenderness, and swelling. The mnemonic "DOTS" is helpful in remembering the signs of injury: **D**eformities occur when bones are broken, causing an abnormal shape. **O**pen wounds break the skin. **T**enderness is sensitivity to touch. **S**welling is a response of the body that makes the area look larger than usual.

Head Have someone stabilize the victim's head and neck to keep it from moving. Look and feel for DOTS over the entire head. Look for leakage of blood or fluid (cerebrospinal fluid) from the nose or ears.

Eyes Check the pupils of the eyes for equality and reactivity to light. (PEARL: **P**upils **E**qual **A**nd **R**eact to **L**ight.) The pupils are normally equal in size. To check for reactivity to light, use a flashlight or cover and then uncover the victim's eyes with your hand. (Pupils normally quickly constrict in response to light.) Unequal pupils occur normally in 2% to 4% of the population, but in others, the pupils should be of equal size when the brain is not injured.

Neck Look and feel for DOTS. (See page 142.)

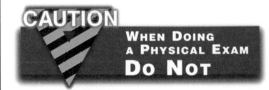

CAUTION

WHEN DOING A PHYSICAL EXAM DO NOT

- aggravate injuries or contaminate wounds.
- move a victim with a possible spinal injury.

The information

in a SAMPLE

history can

affect the first

aid you give.

Chest Look and feel the entire chest for DOTS. Squeeze or compress the sides together for rib pain.

Abdomen Look and feel for DOTS. Gently press all four abdominal quadrants for rigidity and tenderness, using the pads of your fingers. If the victim is complaining of pain in a particular area, ask the victim to point to it; press that area last.

Pelvis Look and feel for DOTS. Gently squeeze the hips inward together and gently press the hips downward.

Extremities Look and feel the entire length and girth of each extremity (arms and legs) for DOTS. Check the Circulation, Sensation, and Movement (use the mnemonic "CSM" as a way of remembering) of each extremity. Check for circulation in the arms by feeling for the pulse on the victim's thumb side of the wrist (radial) pulse and check the circulation of the legs by feeling for the pulse between the inside of the ankle bone and the Achilles tendon (posterior tibial pulse). To check for sensation, ask the victim whether he or she can feel you pinching his or her fingers and toes. To check for movement, ask the victim to wiggle his or her fingers and toes, to squeeze your hand with his or her hands, and to push his or her feet against your hand. Compare one extremity against the other for any differences.

SAMPLE History The information in a SAMPLE history can affect the first aid you give. It is called a SAMPLE history because the letters in the word "SAMPLE" stand for the elements of the history.

For an unresponsive victim, the SAMPLE history information may come from family, friends, or bystanders.

Injured Victim with No Significant Mechanism of Injury The victim without a significant mechanism of injury receives a physical examination based on areas that the victim complains about and areas that you think might be injured on the basis of the mechanism of injury. If the victim has no significant mechanism of injury and no immediately life-threatening injuries, the steps of physical exam and the SAMPLE history are simplified.

Determine the chief complaint—the problem as the victim describes it. For example, one victim might complain of a cut finger while another tells you about pain from twisting an ankle. Begin the physical examination at the site of the injury or the chief complaint, using the mnemonic "DOTS." Your assessment focuses on just the areas that the victim tells you are painful or that you suspect may be injured. After the physical exam, conduct a SAMPLE history.

Suddenly Ill Victim

With a responsive ill victim, obtaining the victim's SAMPLE history is followed by a physical examination focused on the victim's chief complaint (symptoms). With an unresponsive ill victim, a rapid physical examination is performed first, followed by gathering the victim's SAMPLE history.

Responsive Ill Victim A responsive ill victim's SAMPLE history is gathered first before the physical examination. The victim should be the main source of information; additional sources of information could include family, friends, and bystanders.

The main reason for talking to the victim is to find out his or her chief complaint—the one thing that seems most seriously wrong with him or her. After finding out what is wrong, get the rest of the SAMPLE history. This information can affect the first aid you give.

After obtaining the SAMPLE history, perform a physical examination. For a responsive ill victim, a physical examination is based on the victim's chief complaint. For example, if the victim's complaint is chest pain, the physical exam focuses on that area. After the physical examination, provide first aid based on what you found.

Unresponsive Ill Victim For an unresponsive ill victim, the sequence of assessment is different than that for a responsive ill victim. Since you cannot obtain a SAMPLE history from the victim, you begin with the physical exam. After this, gather as much of the SAMPLE history as you can from any family, friends, or bystanders.

Another difference between what you do for responsive and unresponsive ill victims is the type of physical exam that you perform. For a responsive victim, you can focus the physical exam on what the victim has complained about. Because an unresponsive ill victim can't tell you where the problem is, you will need to do a rapid physical examination of the entire body.

The physical exam of an unresponsive ill victim will be almost the same as the physical exam of an injured victim. You rapidly check the victim's head, neck, chest, abdomen, pelvis, and extremities. As you check each area, look for deformities, an open wound, tenderness, and swelling (DOTS). For the specific physical examination steps, see the earlier section "Injured Victim with a Significant Mechanism of Injury." Medic Alert® identification tags also provide important information **(FIGURE 4).**

Since an unresponsive ill victim cannot talk, interview bystanders as a possible source of SAMPLE history.

SAMPLE History

Description	Sample Questions
S = Symptoms	"What's wrong?" (known as the chief complaint)
A = Allergies	"Are you allergic to anything?"
M = Medications	"Are you taking any medications? What are they for?"
P = Past medical history	"Have you had this problem before? Do you have other medical problems?"
L = Last oral intake	"When did you last eat or drink anything? What was it?"
E = Events leading up to the illness or injury	Injury: "How did you get hurt?" Illness: "What led to this problem?"

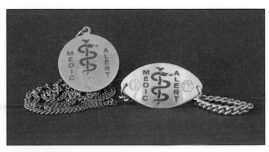

FIGURE 4
Medic Alert® identification tag.

D-O-T-S

Examine an area by looking and feeling for deformity, open wounds, tenderness, and swelling (DOTS).

D = **Deformity** (FIGURE 5A)

O = **Open wounds** (FIGURE 5B)

T = **Tenderness** (FIGURE 5C)

S = **Swelling** (FIGURE 5D)

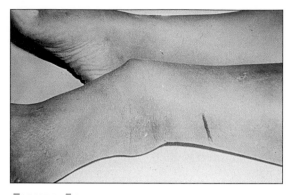

FIGURE 5A

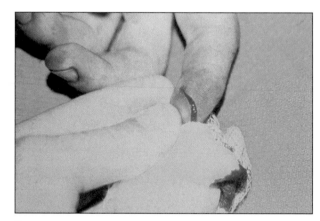

FIGURE 5B

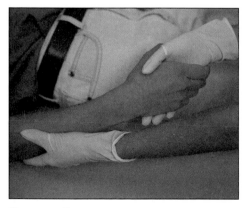

FIGURE 5C

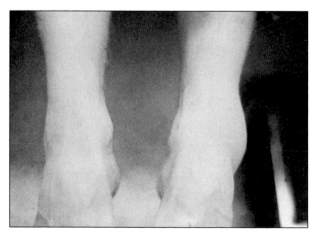

FIGURE 5D

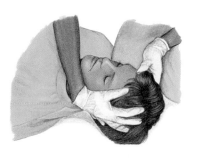

FIGURE 6A

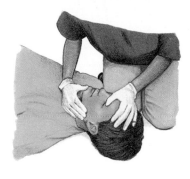

FIGURE 6B

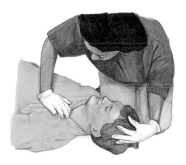

FIGURE 6C

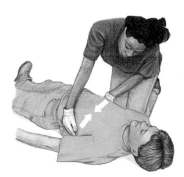

FIGURE 6D

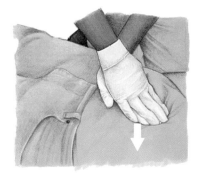

FIGURE 6E

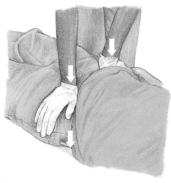

FIGURE 6F

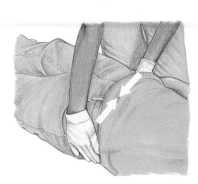

FIGURE 6G

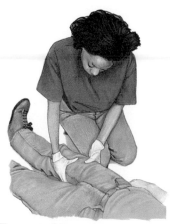

FIGURE 6H

PHYSICAL EXAM: INJURY

Briefly inspect by looking and feeling

1. **Head: DOTS, cerebrospinal fluid** (FIGURE 6A)
2. **Eyes: PEARL (Pupils are Equal And React to Light)** (FIGURE 6B)
3. **Neck: DOTS** (FIGURE 6C)
4. **Chest: DOTS, squeeze chest** (FIGURE 6D)
5. **Abdomen: DOTS, gently press abdomen** (FIGURE 6E)
6. **Pelvis:**

   a. Gently press downward (FIGURE 6F)

   b. Gently squeeze inward (FIGURE 6G)
7. **Extremities: DOTS arms and legs; check CSM (Circulation, Sensation, Movement)** (FIGURE 6H)

ONGOING ASSESSMENT

The initial assessment, physical examination, and SAMPLE history are done quickly so that injuries and illnesses can be identified and given first aid and, if necessary, transportation can be started. After the most serious problems have been cared for, an ongoing assessment is necessary.

Recheck the victim's responsiveness, airway, breathing, and circulation and the effectiveness of first aid. Do this at least every 15 minutes for an alert victim, who has no serious injury or illness, and at least every 5 minutes for a victim who is unresponsive; has difficulties with airway, breathing, or circulation, including major blood loss; or has a significant mechanism of injury. When in doubt, repeat the ongoing assessment every 5 minutes or as frequently as possible.

VICTIM ASSESSMENT

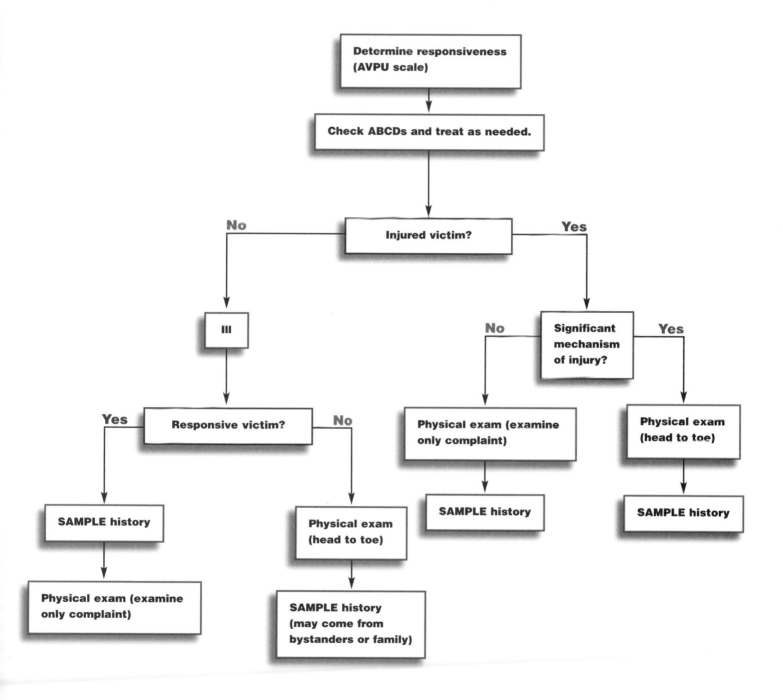

Determine responsiveness (AVPU scale)

↓

Check ABCDs and treat as needed.

↓

No ← Injured victim? → **Yes**

- No branch:

  III

  ↓

  Yes ← Responsive victim? → **No**

  - Yes: SAMPLE history → Physical exam (examine only complaint)
  - No: Physical exam (head to toe) → SAMPLE history (may come from bystanders or family)

- Yes branch:

  No ← Significant mechanism of injury? → **Yes**

  - No: Physical exam (examine only complaint) → SAMPLE history
  - Yes: Physical exam (head to toe) → SAMPLE history

SUMMARY

In all first aid situations, you need to assess the victim of injury or sudden illness after checking the scene. The initial assessment, in which you check for and give care for any life-threatening conditions, is followed by a physical examination and medical history. The overall assessment is important for how you proceed to provide care and contact EMS as needed.

The initial assessment begins with a check for responsiveness, using the AVPU scale. You then check the ABCs: airway, breathing, and circulation. The airway should be open, the victim should be breathing, and the victim should have a pulse and not be bleeding severely. Give care for any life-threatening problems that you find. Check the victim for D (disability) by checking for a spinal injury. Finally, to conclude the assessment, (E) expose the injured area by removing clothing that may obscure the injury.

Unless you are caring for a life-threatening condition, proceed to the physical examination and history. Your approach depends on the injury or illness. For any significant mechanism of injury, stabilize the victim's head first and monitor the ABCs while you perform a complete exam and obtain a history. If there is no significant mechanism of injury, perform the exam on the basis of the victim's complaint. With a responsive suddenly ill victim, obtain the history first. With an unresponsive ill victim, begin with the exam but try to obtain a history from other people who are present.

The physical exam includes a check of the head, neck, chest, abdomen, pelvis, and extremities. Use the DOTS approach to check for deformities, open injuries, tenderness, and swelling. For the extremities, check CSM: circulation, sensation, and movement.

Obtain the history using the mnemonic "SAMPLE," asking about signs and symptoms, allergies, medications used, past medical history, last oral intake, and events leading up to the illness or injury.

After you have cared for any serious problems that are found in the initial assessment or examination, continue with an ongoing assessment while waiting for EMS personnel or transporting the victim to medical care. Check the ABCs at least every 15 minutes for an alert victim without serious injury or illness and at least every 5 minutes for a victim who is unresponsive or has a major injury or problem with the airway, breathing, or circulation.

REVIEW QUESTIONS

Directions: Circle Yes if you agree with the statement, and circle No if you disagree.

Yes **No** 1. The purpose of an initial assessment is to find life-threatening conditions.

Yes **No** 2. Crying or screaming victims should be treated before quiet ones.

Yes **No** 3. Most injured victims require a complete victim assessment.

Yes **No** 4. In a physical exam, you usually begin at the head and work down the body.

Yes **No** 5. The mnemonic "AVPU" is useful for determining the victim's level of responsiveness.

Yes **No** 6. The mnemonic "DOTS" helps in remembering what to collect about the victim's history that may be useful.

Yes **No** 7. For all injured and suddenly ill victims, look for a Medic Alert® identification.

Yes **No** 8. The mnemonic "SAMPLE" can remind you how to examine an area for signs of an injury.

Scenario: During a midmorning break, a coworker screams that somebody has collapsed in the hallway. As a company-designated first aider, you push your way through a crowd of people gathered around the victim. You recognize one of the older employees, who is lying on the floor motionless. You notice that he wears a Medic Alert® identification bracelet.

9. After confirming that the scene is safe, you next check for

    a. breathing

    b. pulse

    c. broken bones

    d. responsiveness

10. If he is unresponsive, you

    a. open his airway and check for breathing

    b. feel for a neck pulse

    c. look and feel for broken bones

    d. look at his Medic Alert® ID tag

11. If he is unresponsive and breathing, what do you do next?

    a. perform a physical exam

    b. check for disability (spinal injury)

    c. obtain the victim's history

12. For injured victims, which usually comes first?

    a. physical exam

    b. victim's history

13. The physical exam on an adult should be started at the victim's

    a. head

    b. chest

    c. feet

14. Which of these would the Medic Alert® identification bracelet help to identify?

    a. allergies

    b. medications

    c. medical history

    d. all of these

15. When checking his eyes, you should look for

    a. color of the iris

    b. reaction of pupils to light

    c. equal or unequal size of the pupils

    d. both **b** and **c**

HOW DID YOU DO?

1. Yes; 2. No; 3. No; 4. Yes; 5. Yes; 6. No; 7. Yes;
8. No; 9. d; 10. a; 11. b; 12. a; 13. a; 14. d; 15. d

BLEEDING AND SHOCK

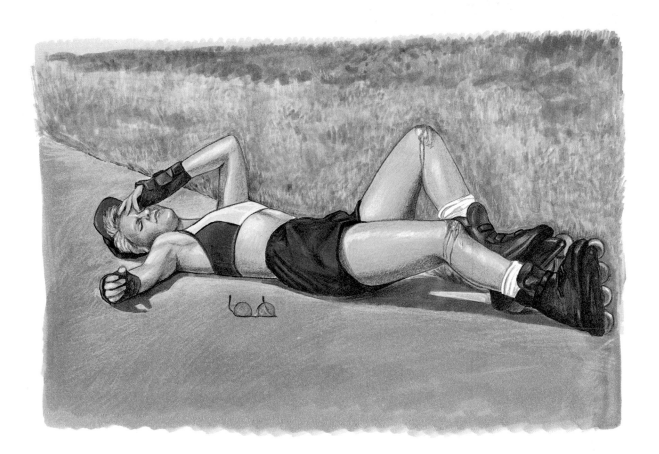

CONTENTS

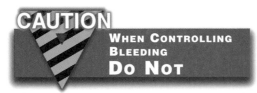

CAUTION

WHEN CONTROLLING BLEEDING

DO NOT

- touch a wound with your bare hands.

- use direct pressure on an eye injury, a wound with an embedded object, or a skull fracture.

- remove a blood-soaked dressing.

- remove an impaled object.

- apply a pressure bandage so tightly that it cuts off circulation.

- use a tourniquet. They are rarely needed and can damage nerves and blood vessels. Use of a tourniquet may cause the loss of an arm or leg.

LEARNING OBJECTIVES

After reading this chapter, you should be able to

1. Describe the types of external bleeding

2. Describe and practice how to control external bleeding

3. Recognize the signs and symptoms of internal bleeding

4. Describe how to care for internal bleeding

5. Describe the three types of shock

6. Describe how to care for shock

7. Describe anaphylaxis

8. Describe how to care for anaphylaxis

EXTERNAL BLEEDING

External bleeding occurs when blood comes out of an open wound. The term **hemorrhage** refers to a large amount of bleeding in a short time.

Types of External Bleeding

In **arterial bleeding,** blood spurts (up to several feet) from the wound. Arterial bleeding is the most serious type of bleeding because blood is lost at a fast rate and blood loss is usually great. Arterial bleeding also is less likely to clot because blood can clot only when it is flowing slowly or not at all. However, unless a very large artery has been cut, it is unlikely that a person will bleed to death before the flow can be controlled. Nevertheless, **arterial bleeding is dangerous and must be controlled.**

In **venous bleeding,** blood from a vein flows steadily or gushes. Venous bleeding is easier to control than arterial bleeding. Most veins collapse when cut. Bleeding from deep veins, however, can be as massive and as hard to control as arterial bleeding.

In **capillary bleeding,** blood oozes from capillaries. This is the most common type of bleeding. It usually is not serious and can be controlled easily. Quite often, this type of bleeding will clot and stop by itself.

Regardless of the type of bleeding or the type of wound, the first aid is the same. First, and most important, you must control the bleeding.

Controlling External Bleeding

1. Protect yourself against disease by wearing medical exam gloves. If medical exam gloves are not available, use several layers of gauze pads, plastic wrap, a plastic bag, or waterproof material. You can even have the victim apply

BLEEDING

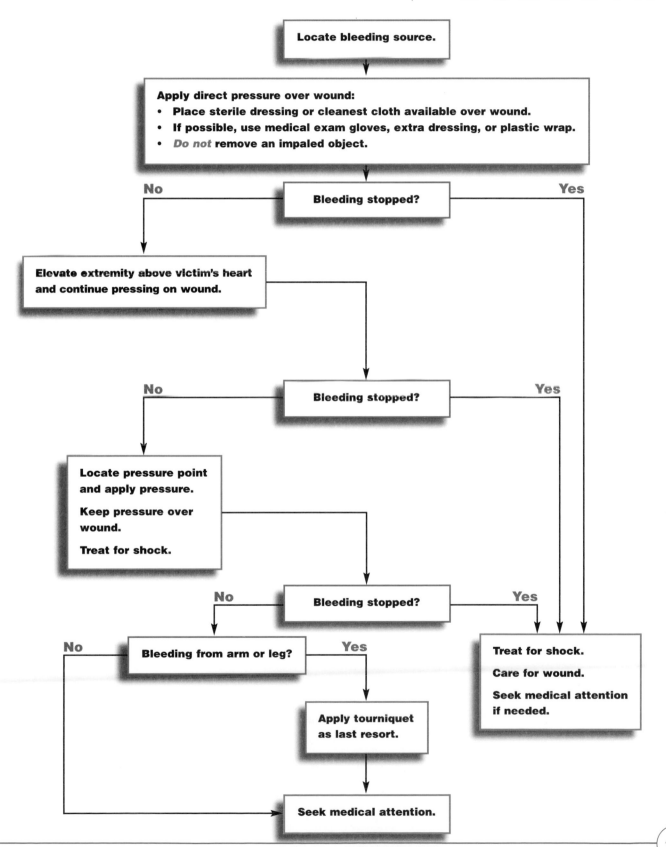

Locate bleeding source.

Apply direct pressure over wound:
- Place sterile dressing or cleanest cloth available over wound.
- If possible, use medical exam gloves, extra dressing, or plastic wrap.
- *Do not* remove an impaled object.

No | Bleeding stopped? | **Yes**

Elevate extremity above victim's heart and continue pressing on wound.

No | Bleeding stopped? | **Yes**

Locate pressure point and apply pressure.

Keep pressure over wound.

Treat for shock.

No | Bleeding stopped? | **Yes**

No | Bleeding from arm or leg? | **Yes**

Apply tourniquet as last resort.

Treat for shock.

Care for wound.

Seek medical attention if needed.

Seek medical attention.

Protect

yourself

against disease

by wearing

medical

exam gloves.

pressure on the wound with his or her own hand. If you must use your bare hands, do so only as a last resort. After the bleeding has stopped and the wound has been cared for, vigorously wash your hands with soap and water.

2. Expose the wound by removing or cutting the clothing to see where the blood is coming from.

3. Place a sterile gauze pad or a clean cloth (eg, a handkerchief, washcloth, or towel) over the entire wound and apply direct pressure with your fingers or the palm of your hand. The gauze or cloth allows you to apply even pressure. **Direct pressure stops most bleeding.** Be sure the pressure remains constant, is not too light, and is applied to the bleeding source. Do not remove blood-soaked dressings; simply add new dressings over the old ones.

4. **If bleeding does not stop in 10 minutes, the pressure may be too light or in the wrong location.** Press harder over a wider area for another 10 minutes. If the bleeding is from an arm or leg, elevate the injured area above heart level, while still applying pressure, to reduce blood flow. Elevation allows gravity to make it difficult for the body to pump blood to the affected extremity. However, elevation alone will not stop bleeding; it must be used in combination with direct pressure over the wound.

5. If the bleeding continues, apply pressure at a pressure point to slow the flow of blood, in combination with direct pressure over the wound. A pressure point is where an artery is near the skin's surface and where it passes close to a bone, against which it can be compressed. Two pressure points on both sides of the body are the most accessible: the brachial point in the upper inside arm and the femoral point in the groin. Using pressure points requires skill, and unless the exact location of the pulse point is used, the pressure-point technique is useless. Most bleeding, however, can be stopped by direct pressure over the wound.

6. After the bleeding stops, or to free you to attend to other injuries or victims, use a pressure bandage to hold the dressing on the wound. Wrap a roller gauze bandage tightly over the dressing and above and below the wound site.

7. When direct pressure cannot be applied (eg, in the case of a protruding bone, skull fracture, or embedded object), use a doughnut-shaped (ring) pad to control bleeding. To make a ring pad, wrap one end of a narrow bandage (roller or cravat

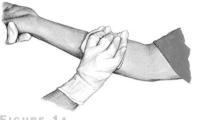

FIGURE 1A

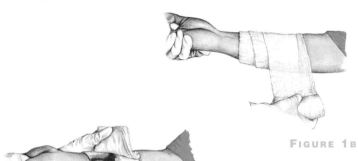

FIGURE 1B

FIGURE 1C

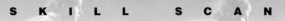

BLEEDING CONTROL

1. **Direct pressure stops most bleeding. Wearing medical exam gloves, place a sterile gauze pad or clean cloth over wound. If bleeding does not stop in 10 minutes, press harder over a wider area** (FIGURE 1A).

2. **A pressure bandage can free you to attend to other injuries or victims** (FIGURE 1B).

3. **Do not remove a blood-soaked dressing. Add more dressings on top** (FIGURE 1C).

4. **If medical exam gloves are not available, use another barrier or extra gauze pads or cloths** (FIGURE 1D).

5. **If bleeding persists, use elevation to help reduce blood flow. Combine with direct pressure over the wound** (FIGURE 1E).

6. **If bleeding still continues, apply pressure at a pressure point to slow blood flow. Locations are**
   - brachial (FIGURE 1F).
   - femoral (FIGURE 1G).
   Use with direct pressure over the wound.

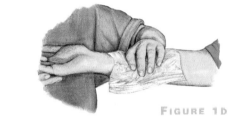

FIGURE 1D

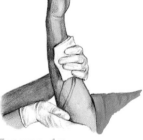

FIGURE 1E

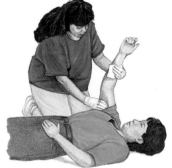

FIGURE 1F

FIGURE 1G

bandage) several times around the four fingers of one of your hands to form a loop. Pass the other end of the bandage through the loop and then wrap it around and around until the entire bandage is used and a ring has been made.

INTERNAL BLEEDING

Internal bleeding occurs when the skin is not broken and blood is not visible. **It can be difficult to detect but can be life threatening.** Internal bleeding comes from traumatic injuries or from nontraumatic disorders such as ulcers. The signs and symptoms of internal bleeding may occur soon after the injury or may take days to appear:

- Bruises or contusions of the skin
- Painful, tender, rigid, bruised abdomen
- Fractured ribs or bruises on the chest
- Vomiting or coughing up blood
- Stools that are black or contain bright red blood

Care for Internal Bleeding

For severe internal bleeding, follow these steps:

1. Monitor the ABCDs.
2. Expect vomiting. If vomiting occurs, keep the victim lying on the left side for drainage.
3. Treat for shock by raising the victim's legs 8″ to 12″ (except with victims with suspected head or spinal injuries, stroke, unconsciousness, or breathing difficulties) and cover the victim with a coat or blanket to keep warm.
4. Seek immediate medical attention.

Bruises are a form of internal bleeding but are not life threatening. To treat bruises, see Chapter 9.

SHOCK

Shock refers to circulatory system failure, which happens when oxygenated blood is not provided in sufficient amounts for every body part. Because every injury affects the circulatory system to some degree, first aiders should automatically treat injured victims for shock. To understand shock, think of the circulatory system as having three components: a working pump (the heart), a network of pipes (the blood vessels), and an adequate amount of fluid (the blood) pumped through the pipes. Damage to any of those components can deprive tissues of blood and produce the condition known as shock.

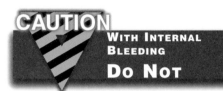

CAUTION

WITH INTERNAL BLEEDING

DO NOT

- give a victim anything to eat or drink. It could cause nausea and vomiting, which could result in aspiration. It could cause complications if surgery is needed.

The signs and symptoms of shock are

- Altered mental status: anxiety and restlessness
- Pale, cold, and clammy skin, lips, and nail beds
- Nausea and vomiting
- Rapid breathing and pulse
- Unresponsiveness when shock is severe

Care For Shock

Even if an injured victim does not have signs or symptoms of shock, first aiders should treat for shock:

1. Treat life-threatening and other severe injuries.

2. Lay the victim on his or her back (note exceptions, page 158).

3. Raise the victim's legs 8″ to 12″ if there is no suspected spinal injury **(Figure 2).** Use the recovery position for victims with altered consciousness or who have vomited. A woman in advanced pregnancy (third trimester) should be placed on her left side to avoid pressing the vena cava. Raising the legs allows the blood to drain from the legs back to the heart.

4. Prevent loss of body heat by putting blankets and coats under and over the victim.

5. A shock victim should not be given anything to eat or drink.

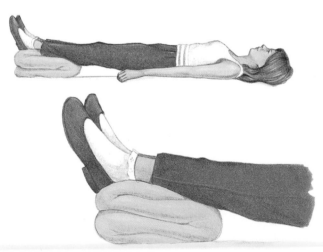

Figure 2
Elevate the legs of a shock victim 8″ to 12″ if there is no suspected spinal injury.

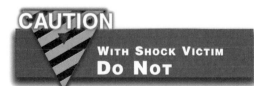

CAUTION
WITH SHOCK VICTIM
DO NOT

- place victims with altered consciousness or vomiting victims on their backs.

- move the victim if a spinal injury is suspected.

- place a woman in advanced pregnancy (third trimester) on her back.

- give the victim anything to eat or drink. It could cause nausea and vomiting, which could result in aspiration. It could also cause complications if surgery is needed.

POSITIONING THE SHOCK VICTIM

Usual shock position. Elevate the legs 8″ to 12″ (FIGURE 3A).

EXCEPTIONS:

1. **Elevate the head for stroke victim** (FIGURE 3B).

2. **Position an unresponsive, or vomiting victim on his or her left side** (FIGURE 3C) **in the recovery position.**

3. **Use a half-sitting position for those with breathing difficulties, chest injuries, or a heart attack** (FIGURE 3D).

4. **Keep the victim flat if a spinal injury is suspected or if the victim has leg fractures** (FIGURE 3E).

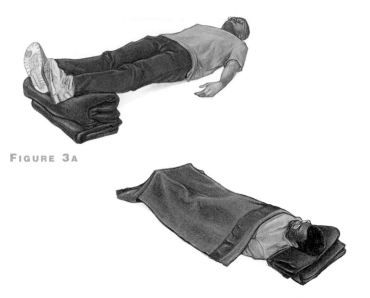

FIGURE 3A

FIGURE 3B

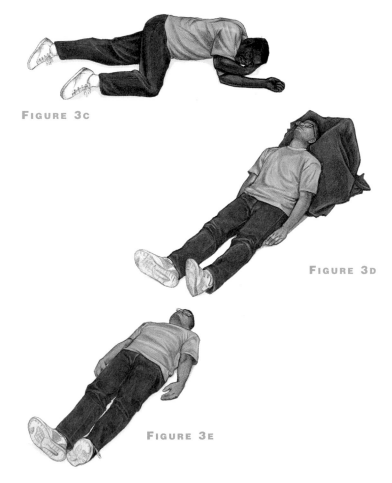

FIGURE 3C

FIGURE 3D

FIGURE 3E

SHOCK

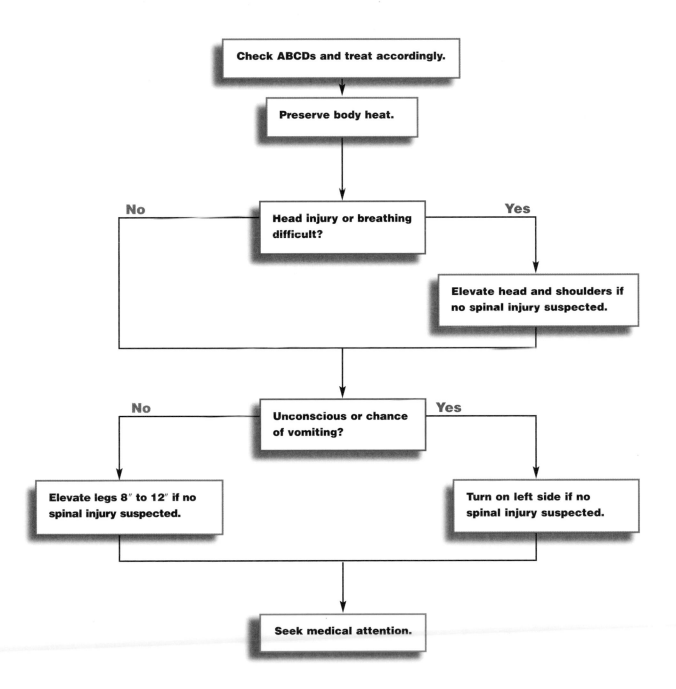

Check ABCDs and treat accordingly.

Preserve body heat.

Head injury or breathing difficult?

No   Yes

Elevate head and shoulders if no spinal injury suspected.

Unconscious or chance of vomiting?

No   Yes

Elevate legs 8″ to 12″ if no spinal injury suspected.

Turn on left side if no spinal injury suspected.

Seek medical attention.

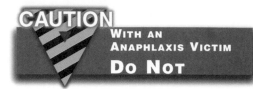

WITH AN ANAPHLAXIS VICTIM

DO NOT

- mistake anaphylaxis for other reactions such as hyperventilation, anxiety attacks, alcohol intoxication, or low blood sugar.

CAUSES OF ANAPHYLAXIS

Anaphylaxis is an abnormal response to an allergen that causes symptoms in people with a hypersensitivity. Well-known causes of anaphylaxis include

- **Medications (penicillin and related drugs, aspirin, sulfa drugs)**
- **Food and food additives (shellfish, nuts, eggs, monosodium glutamate, nitrates, nitrites)**
- **Insect stings (honeybee, yellow jacket, wasp, hornet, fire ant)**
- **Plant pollen**
- **Radiographic dyes**

fyi

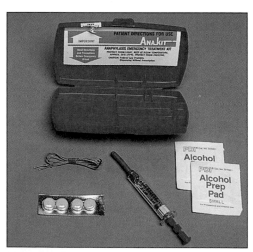

FIGURE 4
Physician-prescribed epinephrine kit.

ANAPHYLAXIS

A powerful reaction to substances eaten or injected can occur within minutes or even seconds. **This reaction, called anaphylaxis, can cause death if it is not treated immediately.** Anaphylaxis typically comes on within minutes of exposure to the offending substance, peaks in 15 to 30 minutes, and is over within hours.

The signs and symptoms of anaphylaxis include

- Sneezing, coughing, wheezing
- Shortness of breath
- Tightness and swelling in the throat
- Tightness in the chest
- Increased pulse rate
- Swelling of the mucous membranes (tongue, mouth, nose)
- Blueness around lips and mouth
- Dizziness
- Nausea and vomiting

Care for Anaphylaxis

1. Check the ABCs.
2. Seek immediate medical attention.
3. If the victim's own physician-prescribed epinephrine is available, help the victim use it (**FIGURES 4 AND 5**).

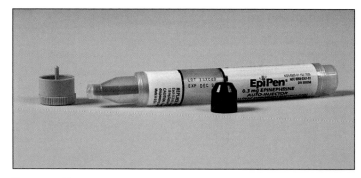

FIGURE 5
Physician-prescribed epinephrine autoinjector.

ANAPHYLAXIS

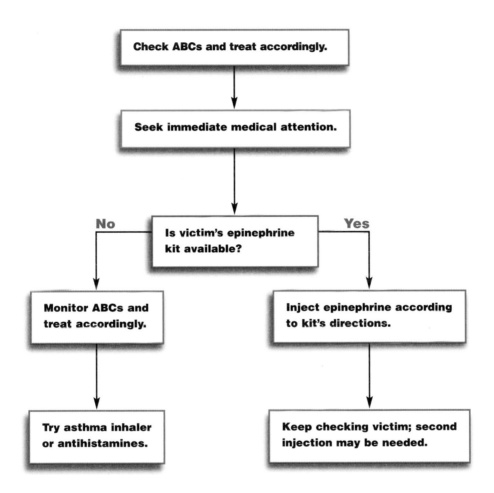

Check ABCs and treat accordingly.

↓

Seek immediate medical attention.

↓

No — Is victim's epinephrine kit available? — **Yes**

Monitor ABCs and treat accordingly.

Inject epinephrine according to kit's directions.

↓

↓

Try asthma inhaler or antihistamines.

Keep checking victim; second injection may be needed.

SUMMARY

Injuries frequently result in external or internal bleeding, which may be minor and easily controlled, or severe and life threatening. Uncontrolled bleeding, along with other causes, may result in shock.

Serious external bleeding needs to be controlled as quickly as possible. Put on medical exam gloves and cover the wound with sterile gauze or clean cloth, and then apply direct pressure on the wound. Add more dressings as needed and continue the pressure. Use a pressure bandage to hold the dressings in place. Seek immediate medical attention for serious bleeding.

Internal bleeding may be difficult to detect but can be life threatening. The victim might have bruises or an abdomen that is painful, tender, and rigid. Monitor the ABCDs, roll the victim onto his or her side if vomiting occurs, and treat the victim for shock.

Shock is a failure of the circulatory system that may result from bleeding, injury, or illness. Treat any life-threatening injuries, lay the victim on his or her back, raise the victim's legs, and prevent loss of body heat. Call EMS.

Anaphylaxis, a severe allergic reaction, occurs soon after exposure to the allergen. Check the ABCs and seek immediate medical attention. Help the victim with their own physician-prescribed epinephrine.

REVIEW QUESTIONS

Bleeding

Directions: Circle Yes if you agree with the statement, and circle No if you disagree.

Yes   No   1. Most cases of bleeding require more than direct pressure for it to stop.

Yes   No   2. Remove and replace blood-soaked dressings.

Yes   No   3. Elevating an arm or leg alone will not control bleeding and must be used in combination with direct pressure over the wound.

Yes   No   4. If direct pressure and elevation fail to control bleeding, the next step would be to use a tourniquet.

Yes   No   5. Evaluate the legs of all shock victims.

Scenario 1. **A 25-year-old construction worker has been badly cut on his thigh by a circular power saw. Blood is flowing heavily. The cut is about 6″ to 8″ long. What should you do?**

_____

_____

_____

Shock

Yes	**No**	1. Most severely injured victims should have their legs raised.
Yes	**No**	2. Give the victim something to drink.
Yes	**No**	3. Prevent loss of body heat by putting blankets under and over the victim.
Yes	**No**	4. A shock victim with head injuries should be placed on his or her side.
Yes	**No**	5. A shock victim with breathing difficulty or chest injury should be placed on his or her back with the legs raised.

Scenario 2. After you have controlled a victim's bleeding, the victim appears to be pale and is anxious and restless. What should you do?

_____

_____

_____

Anaphylaxis

Yes	**No**	1. Anaphylaxis is another form of fainting.
Yes	**No**	2. Anaphylaxis can kill.
Yes	**No**	3. Ask the victim whether he or she has doctor-prescribed epinephrine.

Scenario 3. Your neighbor comes running to your house, panicky. She says that her husband is acting strangely and is reacting to aspirin, to which he is allergic. You run with her back to her house and find the husband complaining of throat and chest tightness. You notice blueness around his lips and mouth. What should you do?

_____

_____

_____

HOW DID YOU DO?

Bleeding
1. No; 2. No; 3. Yes; 4. No; 5. No
Shock
1. Yes; 2. No; 3. Yes; 4. No; 5. No
Anaphylaxis
1. No; 2. Yes; 3. Yes

WOUNDS

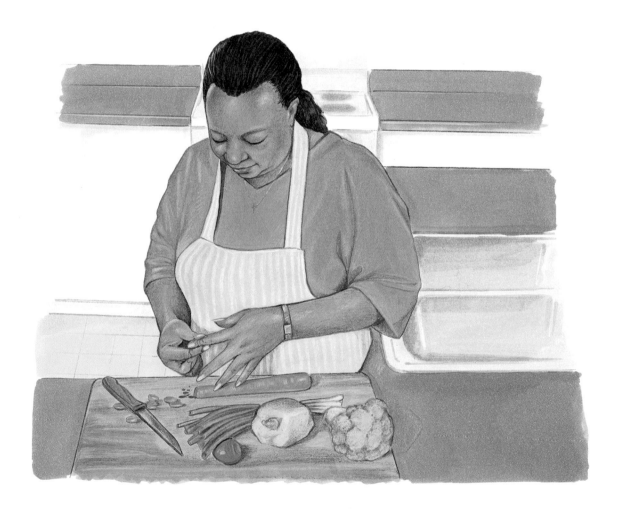

CONTENTS

11

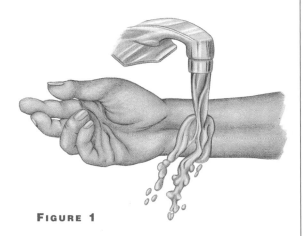

FIGURE 1

LEARNING OBJECTIVES

After reading this chapter, you should be able to

1. Describe the various types of open wounds

2. Describe how to care for an open wound

3. Describe the importance of a tetanus vaccination

4. Describe how to care for an amputation

5. Describe how to care for an impaled object

6. Describe how to care for a closed wound

7. Describe how to care for blood under a nail and how to remove a tight ring on a finger

8. Give guidelines for seeking medical attention for wounds

OPEN WOUNDS

An open wound is a break in the skin's surface in which there is external bleeding. **Victims of open wounds are susceptible to blood loss and infection.**

Cleaning a Wound

A victim's wound should be cleaned to help prevent infection. Wound cleaning might restart bleeding, but it should be done anyway for shallow wounds. It is not necessary to clean deep wounds requiring professional medical care. These wounds will be cleaned thoroughly before sutures (stitches) are used to close the wound:

1. Scrub your hands vigorously with soap and water. Then, if they are available, put on medical exam gloves.

2. Expose the wound by removing or cutting the clothing to see where the blood is coming from.

3. Clean the wound.

   For a shallow wound:

   • Wash inside the wound with soap and water.

   • Irrigate the wound with water (use water that is clean enough to drink). Run the water directly into the wound and allow it to run out. Irrigation with water needs pressure for adequate tissue cleansing. Water from a faucet generally provides the pressure and the amount needed **(FIGURE 1)**. Pouring the water or using a bulb syringe is not forceful enough.

   For a wound with a high risk for infection (eg, an animal bite, a very dirty or ragged wound, a puncture), seek medical attention for wound cleaning unless you are in a remote

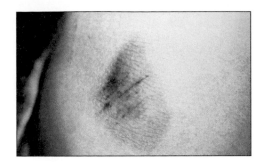

FIGURE 2
Abrasion.

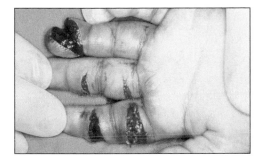

FIGURE 3
Laceration.

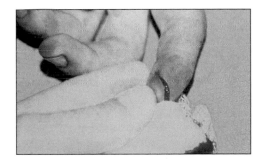

FIGURE 4
Incision.

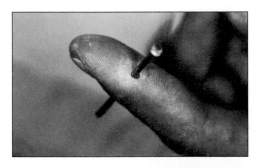

FIGURE 5
Puncture.

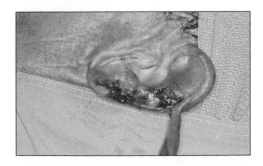

FIGURE 6
Avulsion.

FOUNDATION FACTS: TYPES OF WOUNDS

There are several types of open wounds. With an abrasion, the top layer of skin is removed, with little or no blood loss. Abrasions tend to be painful, because the nerve endings often are abraded along with the skin (FIGURE 2). Ground-in debris may be present. This type of wound can be serious if it covers a large area or if foreign matter becomes embedded in it. Other names for an abrasion are "scrape," "road rash," and "rug burn."

A laceration is cut skin with jagged, irregular edges (FIGURE 3). This type of wound is usually caused by a forceful tearing away of skin tissue.

Incisions tend to be smooth edged, resembling a surgical cut or a paper cut (FIGURE 4). The amount of bleeding depends on the depth, location, and size of the wound.

Punctures are usually deep, narrow wounds in the skin and underlying organs (FIGURE 5), such as a stab wound from a nail or a knife. The entrance is usually small, and the risk of infection is high. The object that caused the injury may remain impaled in the wound.

With an avulsion, a flap of skin is torn loose and is either hanging from the body or completely removed (FIGURE 6). This type of wound can bleed heavily. If the flap is still attached and folded back, lay it flat and realign it into its normal position. Avulsions most often involve ears, fingers, and hands.

An amputation involves the cutting or tearing off of a body part, such as a finger, toe, hand, foot, arm, or leg.

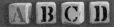

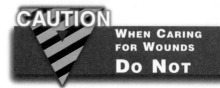

CAUTION

WHEN CARING FOR WOUNDS DO NOT

- **clean large, extremely dirty, or life-threatening wounds. Let hospital emergency department personnel do the cleaning.**
- **scrub a wound. This can bruise the tissue.**
- **irrigate a wound with full-strength iodine preparations (eg, Betadine™ 10%) or iso-propyl alcohol (70%). They kill body cells as well as bacteria and are painful. Also, some people are allergic to iodine.**
- **use hydrogen peroxide. It does not kill bacteria, and it adversely affects capillary blood flow and wound healing.**
- **use antibiotic ointment on wounds that require sutures or on puncture wounds (the ointment may prevent drainage).**
- **soak a wound to clean it.**
- **close the wound with tape (eg, butterfly tape, Steri-strips™). Infection is more likely when bacteria are trapped in the wound.**
- **breathe on a wound or the dressing.**

setting (more than 1 hour from medical attention). In this case, clean the wound as best you can.

4. With sterile tweezers, remove small objects that were not flushed out by irrigation. A dirty abrasion or other wound that is not cleaned will leave a "tattoo" on the victim's skin.

5. Cover the wound with a sterile and, if possible, nonstick dressing. Keep the dressing clean and dry. To keep the dressing in place on an arm or leg, use a self-adhering roller bandage or tape; on other parts of the body, tape the four sides of the dressing onto the skin. For a shallow wound, use an antibiotic ointment.

6. Change the dressing daily, or more often if it gets wet or dirty.

Covering a Wound

For a small wound that does not require sutures

1. Cover it with a thin layer of antibiotic ointment (eg, Neosporin™ or Polysporin™). Such ointments can kill a great many bacteria and rarely cause allergic reactions. They are available without prescription.

2. Cover the wound with a sterile dressing. Do not close the wound with tape (butterfly bandages). Bacteria may remain, leading to a greater chance of infection than if the wound were left open and covered by a sterile dressing. Closing a wound should be left to a physician.

3. If a wound bleeds after a dressing has been applied and the dressing becomes stuck, leave it on as long as the wound is healing. Pulling the scab loose to change the dressing retards healing and increases the chance of infection. If a dressing that is sticking must be removed, soak it in warm water to help soften the scab and make removal easier.

Wound Infection

Any wound, large or small, can become infected. Once an infection begins, damage can be extensive, so prevention is the best way to avoid the problem. A wound should be cleaned by using the procedures described above.

It is important to know how to recognize and treat an infected wound. The signs and symptoms of infection include

- Swelling and redness around the wound
- A sensation of warmth
- Throbbing pain
- Pus discharge
- Fever
- Swelling of the lymph nodes

If one or more red streaks appear, leading from the wound toward the heart, this is a serious sign that the infection is spreading and could cause death. If chills and fever develop, the infection has reached the circulatory system (known as blood poisoning). Seek medical attention immediately.

Tetanus

The tetanus bacterium by itself does not cause tetanus. But when it enters a wound that contains little oxygen, such as a puncture wound, the bacterium can produce a powerful poison. This toxin travels through the nervous system to the brain and the spinal cord. It then causes contractions of certain muscle groups (particularly in the jaw). There is no known antidote to the toxin once it enters the nervous system.

A vaccination can completely prevent tetanus. Everyone needs an initial series of vaccinations to prepare the immune system to defend against the toxin. Then a booster shot once every 5 to 10 years is sufficient to maintain immunity.

Guidelines for Tetanus Immunization Boosters

Anyone with a wound who has never been immunized against tetanus should be given a tetanus vaccine and booster immediately.

- A victim who was once immunized but has not received a tetanus booster within the last 10 years should receive a booster.
- A victim with a dirty wound who has not had a booster for over 5 years should receive a booster.
- Tetanus immunization shots must be given within 72 hours of the injury to be effective.

AMPUTATIONS

If a body part is amputated, immediate action is needed for reattachment. Amputated body parts that are left uncooled for more than 6 hours have little chance of survival. Muscles without blood lose viability within 4 to 6 hours. Rapid first aid for an amputation is critical.

Care for Amputations

1. Control the bleeding with direct pressure and elevate the extremity. Apply a dry dressing or bulky cloths. Be sure to protect yourself against disease. Tourniquets are rarely needed and, if used, will destroy tissue, blood vessels, and nerves that are necessary for replantation.

Tetanus immunization shots must be given within 72 hours of the injury to be effective.

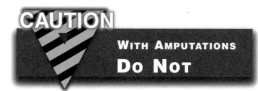

CAUTION

WITH AMPUTATIONS
DO NOT

- try to decide whether a body part is salvageable or too small to save. Leave the decision to a physician.
- wrap an amputated part in a wet dressing or cloth. Using a wet wrap on the part can cause waterlogging and tissue softening, which will make reattachment more difficult.
- bury an amputated part in ice, or place it directly on ice. Reattaching frostbitten parts is usually unsuccessful.
- use dry ice.
- cut a skin "bridge," a tendon, or other structure that is connecting a partially attached part to the rest of the body. Instead, reposition the part in its normal position, wrap the part in a dry sterile dressing or clean cloth, and place an ice pack on it.

2. Treat the victim for shock.

3. Recover the amputated part and, whenever possible, take it with the victim. However, in multicasualty cases, in reduced lighting conditions, or when untrained people transport the victim, someone may be requested to locate and take the severed body part to the hospital after the victim's departure.

4. To care for the amputated body part (FIGURE 7):

   - If possible, rinse the body part with clean water to remove any debris; do not scrub it. The amputated portion does not need to be cleaned.
   - Wrap the amputated part with dry sterile gauze or other clean cloth.
   - Put the wrapped amputated part in a plastic bag or other waterproof container.
   - Place the bag or container with the wrapped part on a bed of ice.

5. Seek medical attention immediately.

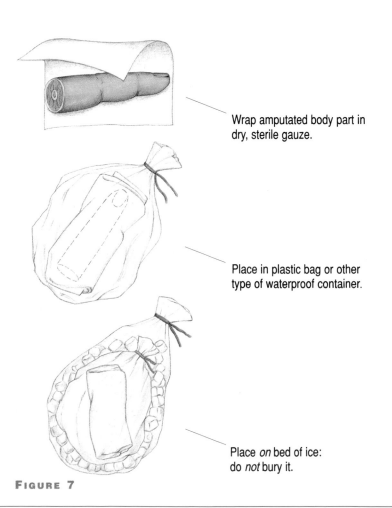

Wrap amputated body part in dry, sterile gauze.

Place in plastic bag or other type of waterproof container.

Place *on* bed of ice: do *not* bury it.

FIGURE 7

AMPUTATION

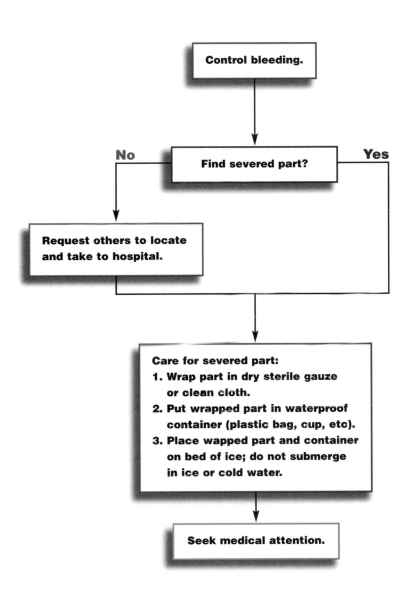

Control bleeding.

No ← **Find severed part?** → Yes

Request others to locate and take to hospital.

Care for severed part:
1. Wrap part in dry sterile gauze or clean cloth.
2. Put wrapped part in waterproof container (plastic bag, cup, etc).
3. Place wapped part and container on bed of ice; do not submerge in ice or cold water.

Seek medical attention.

Blisters are so

common that

many people

assume that they

are a fact of life.

BLISTERS

A blister is a collection of fluid in a "bubble" under the outer layer of skin. (This section applies only to friction blisters. It does not apply to blisters from burns, frostbite, drug reactions, insect or snake bites, or contact with a poisonous plant.)

Repeated rubbing of a small area of the skin will produce a blister. Blisters are so common that many people assume that they are a fact of life. But blisters are avoidable, and life for many people could be more comfortable if they knew how to treat and prevent blisters.

Rubbing—as between a sock and a foot—causes stress on the skin's surface because the supporting tissue remains stationary. The stress separates the skin into two layers, and the resulting space fills with fluid. The fluid may collect either under or within the skin's outer layer, the epidermis. Because of differences in skin, blister formation varies considerably from person to person.

When caring for a friction blister, try to (1) avoid the risk of infection, (2) minimize the victim's pain and discomfort, (3) limit the blister's development, and (4) help a fast recovery. The best care for a particular blister depends mainly on its size and location.

If an area on the skin becomes a "hot spot" (a painful, red area), tightly apply a piece of silver aluminum duct tape or cover it with a doughnut-shaped piece of moleskin secured by tape.

If a blister on a foot is closed and not very painful, a conservative approach is to tape the blister tightly with duct tape or waterproof adhesive tape. The tape must remain on the blister for several days; otherwise, tearing of the blister's roof when the tape is removed may expose unprotected skin. One limitation of this approach is that the tape may become damp and contaminated and have to be replaced, at the risk of tearing the blister roof. You could also cut a hole in a piece of moleskin to fit around the blister, making a doughnut-shaped pad, and apply it over the blister. Small blisters, especially on weight-bearing areas, generally respond better if left alone.

If a blister on the foot is open, or a very painful closed blister affects walking or running

1. Clean the area with soap and water or rubbing alcohol.

2. Drain all fluid out of the blister by making several small holes at the base of the blister with a sterilized needle. Press the fluid out. Do not remove the blister's roof unless it is torn.

3. Apply antibiotic ointment and cover it tightly with a nonstick pad or gauze pad. The pressure dressing ensures that the blister's roof sticks to the underlying skin and that the blister does not refill with fluid after it has been drained.

BLISTERS

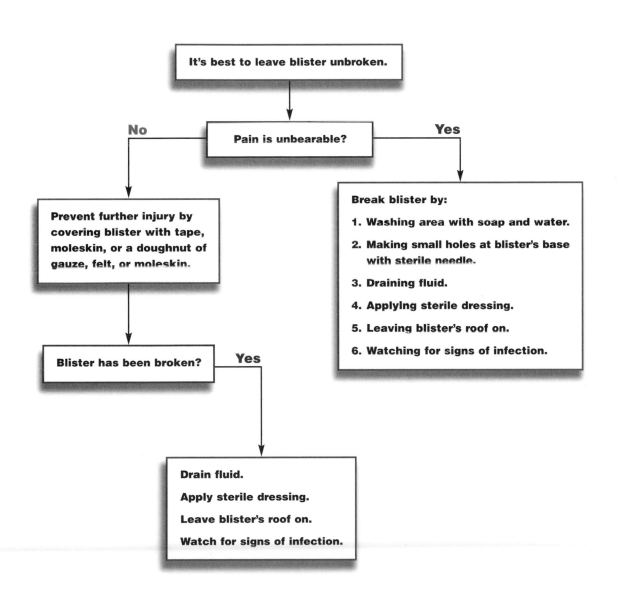

It's best to leave blister unbroken.

No   Pain is unbearable?   **Yes**

Prevent further injury by covering blister with tape, moleskin, or a doughnut of gauze, felt, or moleskin.

Break blister by:

1. Washing area with soap and water.
2. Making small holes at blister's base with sterile needle.
3. Draining fluid.
4. Applying sterile dressing.
5. Leaving blister's roof on.
6. Watching for signs of infection.

Blister has been broken?   **Yes**

Drain fluid.

Apply sterile dressing.

Leave blister's roof on.

Watch for signs of infection.

4. Duplicate the procedures described for treating a closed blister.

5. Change the dressing daily and check for signs of infection (redness and pus). Seek medical attention if infection develops.

With few exceptions, the blister's roof, which is the best and most comfortable "dressing," should be removed only when an infection is present. Once a blister has been opened, the area should be washed with soap to prevent further infection. For 10 to 14 days, or until new skin forms, a protective bandage or other cover should be used.

Impaled Objects

If an object is impaled in a wound, it should not be moved because movement could produce additional bleeding and tissue damage. Follow these steps:

1. Expose the area. Remove or cut away any clothing surrounding the injury. If clothes cover the object, leave them in place because removing them could cause the object to move.

2. Control any bleeding with direct pressure. Straddle the object with gauze. Do not press directly on the object or along the wound next to the cutting edge, especially if the object has sharp edges.

3. **Stabilize the object.** Secure a bulky dressing or clean cloth around the object.

4. Shorten the object only if necessary. In most cases, do not shorten the object by cutting or breaking it. There are times, however, when cutting off or shortening the object is needed for transportation. Be sure to stabilize the object before shortening it. Remember that the victim will feel any vibrations from the object being cut and that the injury could be worsened.

Closed Wounds

A closed wound happens when a blunt object strikes the body. The skin is not broken, but tissue and blood vessels beneath the skin's surface are crushed, causing bleeding within a confined area. Follow these guidelines for first aid:

1. Control bleeding by applying an ice pack for no more than 20 minutes.

2. Apply an elastic bandage with a gauze pad between the bandage and the skin.

3. Check for a possible fracture.

4. Elevate an injured extremity above the victim's heart level to decrease pain and swelling.

STITCHES (SUTURES)

If sutures are needed, the victim should see a physician within 6 to 8 hours of the injury. Suturing wounds allows faster healing, reduces infection, and lessens scarring.

An extremity (eg, hand or foot) wound can be sutured within 6 to 8 hours of the injury. Suturing of a head or trunk wound can wait up to 24 hours after the injury. Some wounds can be sutured 3 to 5 days after the injury.

Some wounds do not usually require sutures:

• Wounds in which the skin's cut edges tend to fall together

• Cuts less than 1″ long that are not deep

Rather than closing a gaping wound with butterfly bandages, cover the wound with sterile gauze. Closing the wound might trap bacteria inside, resulting in an infection. In most cases, a physician can be reached in time for suturing.

fyi

CRITICAL CONCEPTS: WOUNDS REQUIRING MEDICAL ATTENTION

Seek medical attention for wound victims with the following conditions:

- **Arterial bleeding**
- **Uncontrolled bleeding**
- **A deep incision, laceration, or avulsion that**
  - goes into the muscle or bone
  - is located on a body part that bends (eg, elbow or knee)
  - tends to gape widely
  - is located on the thumb or palm of the hand (nerves may be affected)
- **A large or deep puncture wound**
- **A large embedded object or a deeply embedded object of any size**
- **Foreign matter left in the wound**
- **A human or animal bite**
- **The possibility of a noticeable scar (sutured cuts usually heal with less scarring than unsutured ones)**
- **An eyelid cut (to prevent later drooping)**
- **A slit lip (easily scarred)**
- **Internal bleeding**
- **Any wound that you are not certain how to treat**
- **The victim's immunization against tetanus is not up to date**

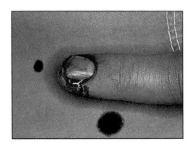

FIGURE 8
Blood under a nail.

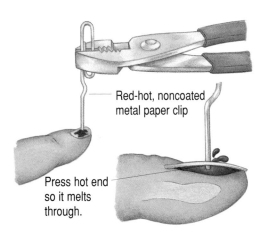

Red-hot, noncoated
metal paper clip

Press hot end
so it melts
through.

FIGURE 9
Making hole in nail to release blood.

Blood Under a Nail

When a fingernail has been crushed, blood collects under the nail **(FIGURE 8)**. This condition is usually very painful because of the pressure of the blood pressing against the nail. First aid involves removing the pressure and caring for the wound.

1. Immerse the finger in ice water or apply an ice pack with the hand elevated.

2. Relieve the pressure under the injured nail by one of the following methods:

    • Straighten the end of a metal (noncoated) paper clip or use the eye end of a sewing needle. Hold the paper clip or needle with pliers and use a match or cigarette lighter to heat it until the metal is red hot. Press the glowing end of the paper clip or needle against the nail so that it melts through **(FIGURE 9)**. Little pressure is needed. The nail has no nerves, so this treatment is painless.

    • Using a rotary action, carefully drill through the nail with the sharp point of a knife. This method may be painful.

3. Apply a dressing to absorb the draining blood and to protect the injured nail.

Ring Strangulation

Sometimes a finger is so swollen that a ring cannot be removed. Ring strangulation can be a serious problem if it cuts off circulation long enough. Try one or more of the following methods to remove a ring:

• Lubricate the finger with grease, oil, butter, petroleum jelly, or some other slippery substance, then try to remove the ring.

• Immerse the finger in cold water or apply an ice pack for several minutes to reduce the swelling.

• Massage the finger from the tip to the hand to move the swelling; lubricate the finger again and try removing the ring.

• Smoothly wind thread around the finger, starting about an inch from the ring edge and going toward the ring, with each course touching the next. Wind smoothly and tightly right up to the edge of the ring. This action will push the swelling toward the hand. Slip the end of the thread under the ring with a matchstick or toothpick, then slowly unwind the thread on the hand side of the ring. You should be able to gently twist the ring over the thread and off the finger.

- Lubricate the finger well, then pass a rubber band under the ring. Hold both ends of the rubber band and, while maintaining tension on the rubber band toward the end of the finger, pull the rubber band in a circular motion around the finger.

- Cut the narrowest part of the ring with a ring saw, jeweler's saw, ring cutter, or fine hacksaw blade. Be sure to protect the exposed portions of the finger.

- Inflate an ordinary balloon (preferably a slender, tube-shaped one) about three-fourths full. Tie the end. Insert the victim's swollen finger into the end of the balloon until the balloon evenly surrounds the entire finger. In about 15 minutes, the air pressure in the balloon should return the finger to its normal size, and the ring can be removed.

- Liberally spray window or glass cleaner onto the finger, then try to slide the ring off.

....

Open wounds

require care to

control bleeding

and protect

the wound

from infection.

....

SUMMARY

Open wounds require care to control bleeding and protect the wound from infection. Wear gloves and control bleeding first with direct pressure. Clean the wound with running water and remove any small objects from the wound. Cover the wound with a sterile, nonstick dressing that is bandaged in place.

For a small wound that will not receive medical attention, use an antibiotic ointment and cover the wound with a sterile dressing. Watch for the signs of infection and seek medical attention immediately if these signs occur. A tetanus booster may be needed.

For an amputated body part, in addition to caring for the victim, rinse the amputated part, wrap it in plastic and put it on ice, and seek medical attention immediately.

For an impaled object in a wound, do not remove the object but stabilize it with dressings around it.

For a closed wound, use an ice pack to help control bleeding and then apply an elastic bandage. Check for a fracture, and elevate an injured extremity above the heart level to decrease pain and swelling.

Wounds that require medical attention or sutures include those with arterial bleeding, uncontrolled bleeding, a deep or wide wound, an impaled object, a bite, a wound to the eyelid or lip, or any wound you are uncertain how to treat.

REVIEW QUESTIONS

Wound Care

Directions: Circle Yes if you agree with the statement, and circle No if you disagree.

Yes   No   1. Wash shallow wounds with soapy water.

Yes   No   2. Irrigating a wound with water requires pressure.

Yes   No   3. Wounds with a high risk for infection (eg, animal bites, dirty wounds) require medical attention for proper wound cleaning.

Yes   No   4. Antibiotic ointment can be applied to any wound.

Yes   No   5. Hydrogen peroxide works well on wounds.

Scenario 1. While using a knife to open a cardboard box, Nancy, a 23-year-old, lost her grip on the knife and received a shallow incision wound on her hand. What should you do?

_____

_____

_____

Scenario 2. A friend falls and skins his knee on an asphalt road that has many small rocks and dirt on it. What should you do?

_____

_____

_____

Amputations

Yes   No   1. Recover any amputated part, regardless of size, and take it with the victim to the nearest hospital.

Yes   No   2. Cut off a partially attached part.

Yes   No   3. Wrap an amputated part in a dry sterile gauze dressing, enclose it in something waterproof, and keep it cool.

Yes   No   4. Keep an amputated part packed (buried) in ice.

Yes   No   5. Do NOT let an amputated part become "waterlogged," since that would make reattachment more difficult.

Scenario 3. Matt is mowing long, wet grass, which begins to back up at his mower's discharge opening. He reaches into the discharge chute to try to brush away a clump of grass, and his fingers are struck by the mower's blade. Two fingers are cut off. You find him sitting on the ground, firmly holding what remains of his fingers. What should you do?

_____

_____

_____

Scenario 4. You respond to an injured worker calling for help who has cut his thumb off with a circular power saw. What should you do?

_____

_____

_____

Impaled Objects

Yes   No   1. Removing an impaled object could cause more bleeding.

Yes   No   2. Prevent an impaled object from moving by placing bulky padding around the object.

Scenario 5. At a construction site, a 38-year-old worker drove a large nail through her left hand with a nail gun. What should you do?

_____

_____

_____

Scenario 6. While building a fence, a worker steps on a 16-penny nail. It goes through his boot's sole and into the foot. What should you do?

_____

_____

_____

Scenario 7. While jogging on the shoulder of a street, a jogger trips and falls with her hands out. A piece of glass goes into her hand. What should you do?

_____

_____

_____

Blisters

Scenario 8. While you are on a 5-mile hike, wearing a new pair of boots, a blister appears on your foot. It is painful enough to prevent you from continuing. What should you do?

_____

_____

_____

How did you do?

Wound Care

1. Yes; 2. Yes; 3. Yes; 4. No; 5. No

Amputations

1. Yes; 2. No; 3. Yes; 4. No; 5. Yes

Impaled Objects

1. Yes; 2. Yes

BURNS

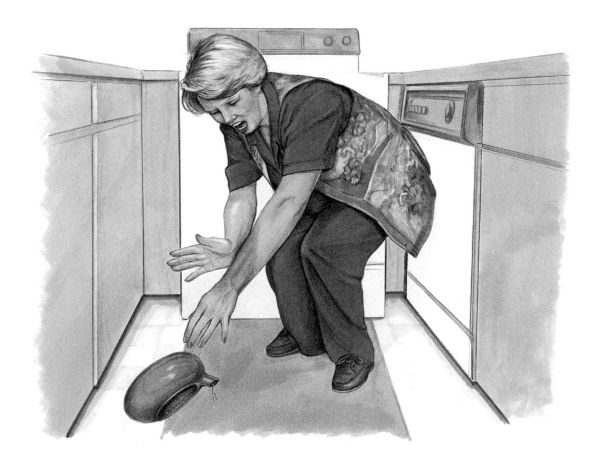

CONTENTS

12

LEARNING OBJECTIVES

After reading this chapter, you should be able to

1. Describe the characteristics of first-, second-, and third-degree burns

2. Calculate the extent of burns using the Rule of Nines and the Rule of Palm

3. Explain how to assess the severity of burns and describe appropriate burn care

4. Describe a chemical burn and its appropriate care

5. Describe what to do for an electrocution

Burn injuries can be classified as thermal (heat), chemical, or electrical:

- *Thermal burns.* Not all thermal burns are caused by flames. Contact with hot objects, flammable vapor that burns in a flash or an explosion, and steam or hot liquid are other common causes of burns.

- *Chemical burns.* A wide range of chemical agents can cause tissue damage and death on contact with the skin. The amount of tissue damage depends on the duration of contact, the skin thickness in the area of exposure, and the strength of the chemical agent. Chemicals will continue to cause tissue destruction until the chemical agent is removed. Three types of chemicals — acids, alkalis, and organic compounds — are responsible for most chemical burns.

- *Electrical burns.* The injury severity from exposure to electrical current depends on the type of current (direct or alternating), the voltage, the area of the body exposed, and the duration of contact.

Respiratory damage may result from breathing heat or the products of combustion, from being burned by a flame while in a closed space, or from being in an explosion. Swelling occurs in 2 to 24 hours, restricting or even completely shutting off the airway, so air cannot reach the lungs. All respiratory injuries must receive medical care.

FOUNDATION FACTS: DEGREE OF BURN

Historically, burns have been described as first-degree, second-degree, and third-degree injuries. Burn-care professionals often use the terms superficial, partial thickness, and full thickness because they are more descriptive of the tissue damage.

- First-degree (superficial) burns affect the skin's outer layer (epidermis) (FIGURE 1). Characteristics include redness, mild swelling, tenderness, and pain. Healing occurs without scarring, usually within a week. The outer edges of deeper burns often are first-degree burns.

- Second-degree (partial-thickness) burns extend through the entire outer layer and into the inner skin layer (FIGURE 2). Blisters, swelling, weeping of fluids, and severe pain characterize these burns, which occur because the capillary blood vessels in the dermis are damaged and give up fluid into surrounding tissues. Intact blisters provide a sterile waterproof covering. Once a blister breaks, a weeping wound results and the risk of infection increases.

- Third-degree (full-thickness) burns are severe burns that penetrate all the skin layers, into the underlying fat and muscle (FIGURE 3). The skin looks leathery, waxy, or pearly gray and is sometimes charred. There is a dry appearance, because capillary blood vessels have been destroyed and no more fluid is brought to the area. The skin does not blanch after being pressed because the area is dead. The victim feels no pain from a third-degree burn because the nerve endings have been damaged or destroyed. Any pain that is felt is from surrounding burns of lesser degrees. A third-degree burn requires medical care, which involves removal of the dead tissue and often a skin graft to heal properly.

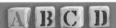

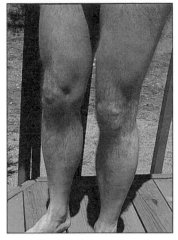

FIGURE 1

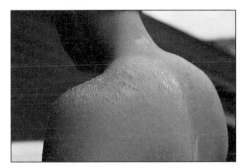

FIGURE 2

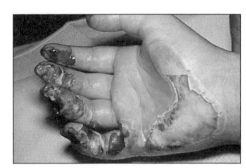

FIGURE 3

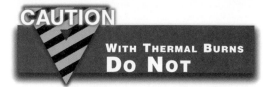

WITH THERMAL BURNS
DO NOT

- remove clothing that is stuck to the skin. Cut around the areas where clothing sticks to the skin.
- pull on stuck clothing because pulling will further damage the skin.
- forget to remove jewelry as soon as possible because swelling could make jewelry difficult to remove later.
- apply cold to more than 20% of an adult's body surface (10% for children) because wide-spread cooling can cause hypothermia. Burn victims lose large amounts of heat and water.
- leave wet packs on wounds for long periods.
- use an ice pack unless it is the only source of cold. If you must use one, apply it for only 10 to 15 minutes, since frostbite and hypothermia can develop.
- apply salve, ointment, grease, butter, cream, spray, home remedy, or any other coating on a burn until it has been cooled. Such coatings are unsterile and can lead to infection. They also can seal in heat, causing further damage.

THERMAL BURNS

Give the following care for all thermal burns. See the following sections for specific burn care for first-, second-, and third-degree burns.

1. Stop the burning! Burns can continue to injure tissue for a surprisingly long time. If clothing has ignited, have the victim roll on the ground using the "stop, drop, and roll" method. Smother the flames with a blanket or douse the victim with water. Stop a person whose clothes are on fire from running, which only fans the flames. A victim should not remain standing, because he or she is more apt to inhale flames. Once the fire is extinguished, immediately remove all hot or smoldering clothing because the burning may continue if the clothing is left on.

2. Check the ABCs.

3. Determine the depth of the burn. It is difficult to tell a burn's depth because the destruction varies within the same burn. Even experienced physicians will not know the depth for several days after the burn. However, making an assessment of burn depth will help you to decide whether to seek medical care for the victim.

4. Determine the extent of the burn. This means estimating how much body surface area the burn covers. A rough guide known as the *Rule of Nines* assigns a percentage value to each part of an adult's body (FIGURE 4). The entire head is 9%, one complete arm is 9%, the front torso is 18%, the complete back is 18%, and each leg is 18%. The Rule of Nines must be modified to take into account the different proportions of a small child. In small children and infants, the head accounts for 18% and each leg is 14%.

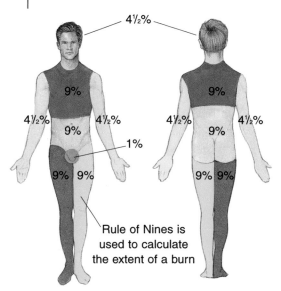

Rule of Nines is used to calculate the extent of a burn

FIGURE 4

For small or scattered burns, use the *Rule of the Palm*. The victim's hand, excluding the fingers and the thumb, represents about 1% of his or her total body surface. For a very large burn, estimate the unburned area in number of hands and subtract from 100%.

5. Determine what parts of the body are burned. Burns on the face, hands, feet, and genitals are more severe than burns on other body parts. A circumferential burn (one that goes around a finger, toe, arm, leg, neck, or chest) is considered more severe than a noncircumferential one because of the possible constriction and tourniquet effect on circulation and, in some cases, breathing. All these burns require medical care.

6. Determine whether other injuries or preexisting medical problems exist and whether the victim is an older adult (over 55) or very young (under 5). A medical problem or belonging to one of those age groups increases a burn's severity.

7. Determine the burn's severity. This forms the basis for how to treat the burned victim. After you have evaluated the burn according to Steps 3 through 6, use the American Burn Association (ABA) guidelines to determine the burn's severity. Most burns are minor, occur at home, and can be managed outside a medical setting. Seek medical attention for all moderate and critical burns, as classified by the ABA, or if any of the following conditions apply:

- The victim is under 5 or over 55 years of age
- The victim has difficulty breathing
- Other injuries exist
- An electrical injury exists
- The face, hands, feet, or genitals are burned
- Child abuse is suspected
- The surface area of a second-degree burn is greater than 15% of the body surface area
- The burn is third degree

Burn Severity*
Minor Burns
- First-degree burn covering <50% BSA**
- Second-degree burn covering <15% BSA in adults
- Second-degree burn covering <10% BSA in children or older adults
- Third-degree burn covering <2% BSA

*Source: Adapted with permission from the American Burn Association categorization.

**BSA = body surface area.

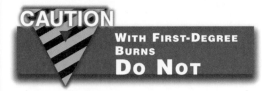

WITH FIRST-DEGREE BURNS DO NOT

- use a dressing. Most first-degree burns do not need a dressing.
- use anesthetic sprays because they may sensitize the skin to "-caine" anesthetics.

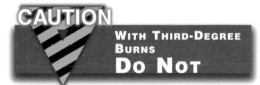

WITH THIRD-DEGREE BURNS DO NOT

- apply salve, ointment, grease, butter, cream, spray, a home remedy, or any other coating on a burn. Such coatings are unsterile and may lead to infection. They can also seal in the heat, causing further damage. For moderate and severe burns, a physician will have to scrape off the coating, causing the victim unnecessary additional pain.

Moderate Burns

- First-degree burn covering >50% BSA
- Second-degree burn covering 15%-30% BSA in adults
- Second-degree burn covering 10%-20% BSA in children or older adults
- Third-degree burn covering <10% BSA

Critical Burns

- Second-degree burn covering >30% BSA in adults
- Second-degree burn covering >20% BSA in children or older adults
- Third-degree burn covering >10% BSA
- Burns of hands, face, eyes, feet, or genitalia; also most inhalation injuries, electrical injuries, and burns accompanied by major trauma or significant preexisting conditions

BURN CARE

Burn care aims to reduce pain, protect against infection, and prevent evaporation.

Care for First-Degree Burns

1. Relieve pain by immersing the burned area in cold tap water or by applying a wet, cold cloth (FIGURE 5). Apply cold until the part is pain free both in and out of the water (usually 15 to 30 minutes). Cold also stops the burn's progression into deeper tissue. If cold water is unavailable, use any cold, drinkable liquid to reduce the burned skin's temperature.

2. Relieve pain and inflammation with aspirin (adults only) or ibuprofen. Acetaminophen relieves pain but not inflammation.

Care for Second-Degree Burns

1. Seek medical attention for moderate burns covering 15% to 20% of the body surface area in adults or 10% to 20% in children or elderly victims.

2. Relieve pain by immersing the burned area in cold tap water or by applying a wet, cold cloth. Apply cold until the part is pain free both in and out of the water (usually 15 to 30 minutes). Cold also stops the burn's progression into deeper tissue.

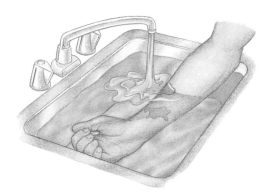

FIGURE 5

3. Relieve pain and inflammation with aspirin (adults only) or ibuprofen. Acetaminophen relieves pain but not inflammation. Keep a burned extremity elevated to reduce gravity-induced swelling.

4. Cover the burn with a dry, nonsticking, clean dressing or a clean cloth. Covering the burn reduces the amount of pain by keeping air from reaching the exposed nerve endings. The main purpose of a dressing over a burn is to keep the burn clean, prevent evaporative loss, and reduce the pain.

Care for Third-Degree Burns

It is usually not necessary to apply cold to third-degree burns, since pain is absent. Any pain that is felt with a third-degree burn comes from accompanying first- and second-degree burns, for which cold applications can be helpful.

1. Seek medical attention immediately.

2. Cover the burn with a dry, nonsticking, clean dressing or a clean cloth.

3. Treat the victim for shock by elevating the legs and keeping the victim warm with a clean sheet or blanket.

Later Burn Care

Follow a physician's recommendations for later burn care. The following guidelines may apply:

• Elevate the area if possible for the first 24 hours

• Give pain medication if needed

• Change dressings once or twice a day or as the doctor instructed

• Report any signs of infection to a doctor: redness, pain, tenderness, swelling, pus, or fever

• Keep the area and dressing clean and dry

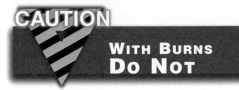

CAUTION
WITH BURNS DO NOT

- cool more than 20% of an adult's body surface area (10% for a child) except to extinguish flames.

- break any blisters. Intact blisters serve as excellent burn dressings.

- apply salve, ointment, grease, butter, cream, spray, a home remedy, or any other coating on a burn until it has cooled. Such coatings are unsterile and may lead to infection. They can also seal in heat, causing further damage. For moderate and severe burns, a physician will have to scrape off the coating, causing the victim unnecessary additional pain.

- place a moist dressing over a burn, since it will dry out quickly. A wet dressing over a large area can induce hypothermia.

- use plastic as a dressing (its only advantage is that it will not stick to the burn), since it will trap moisture and provide a good place for bacteria to grow.

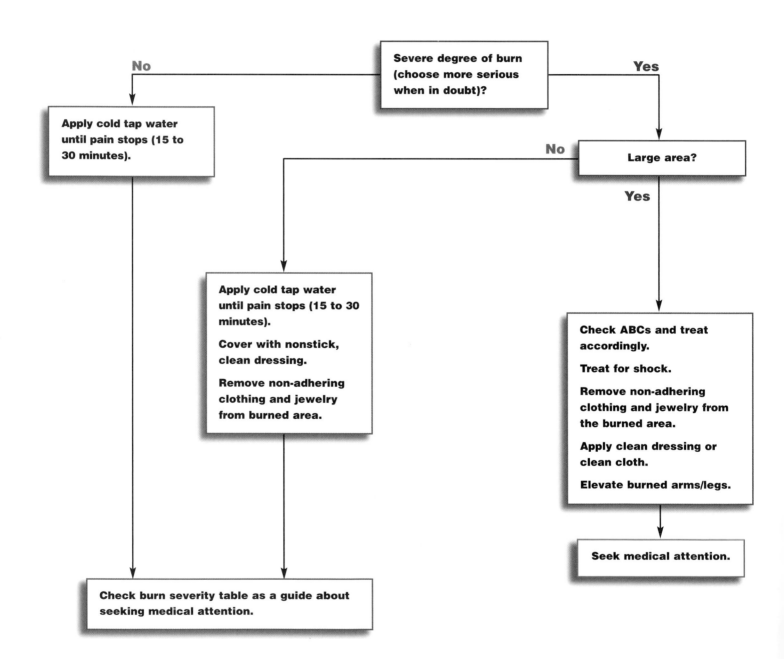

Severe degree of burn (choose more serious when in doubt)?

No → **Apply cold tap water until pain stops (15 to 30 minutes).**

Yes → **Large area?**

No → **Apply cold tap water until pain stops (15 to 30 minutes).**

Cover with nonstick, clean dressing.

Remove non-adhering clothing and jewelry from burned area.

Yes → **Check ABCs and treat accordingly.**

Treat for shock.

Remove non-adhering clothing and jewelry from the burned area.

Apply clean dressing or clean cloth.

Elevate burned arms/legs.

Seek medical attention.

Check burn severity table as a guide about seeking medical attention.

To change dressings

1. Wash your hands.

2. If the old dressing sticks when removed, soak it off with cool, clean water.

3. Wash the area gently with mild soap and water. Do not break blisters.

4. Pat the area dry with a clean cloth.

5. Apply a thin layer of antibiotic (bacitracin) ointment to the burn.

6. Apply a nonsticking sterile dressing.

CHEMICAL BURNS

A chemical burn is the result of a caustic or corrosive substance touching the skin (FIGURE 6). Since chemicals continue to "burn" as long as they are in contact with the skin, they should be removed from the victim as rapidly as possible.

First aid is the same for all chemical burns, except a few specific ones for which a chemical neutralizer has to be used. Alkalies (eg, drain cleaners) cause more serious burns than acids (eg, battery acid) because they penetrate deeper and remain active longer. Organic compounds (eg, petroleum products) are also capable of burning.

Care for a Chemical Burn

1. Immediately remove the chemical by flushing with water (FIGURE 7). If available, use a hose or a shower. Brush dry powder chemicals from the skin before flushing, unless large amounts of water are immediately available. Water may activate a dry chemical and cause more damage to the skin. Take precautions to protect yourself from exposure to the chemical.

2. Remove the victim's contaminated clothing while flushing with water. Clothing can hold chemicals, allowing them to continue to burn as long as they are in contact with the skin.

3. Flush for 20 minutes or longer. Let the victim wash with a mild soap before a final rinse. Dilution with large amounts of water decreases the chemical concentration and washes it away.

4. Cover the burned area with a dry, sterile dressing or, for large areas, a clean pillowcase.

5. If the chemical is in an eye, flood it for at least 20 minutes, using low pressure.

6. Seek medical attention immediately for all chemical burns.

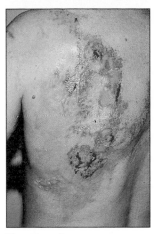

FIGURE 6

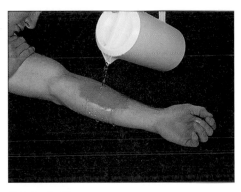

FIGURE 7

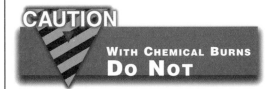

CAUTION

WITH CHEMICAL BURNS
DO NOT

- waste time! A chemical burn is an emergency.

- apply water under high pressure. It will drive the chemical deeper into the tissue.

- try to neutralize a chemical even if you know which chemical is involved. Heat may be produced, resulting in more damage. Some product labels for neutralizing may be wrong. Save the container or the label for the chemical's name.

CHEMICAL BURNS

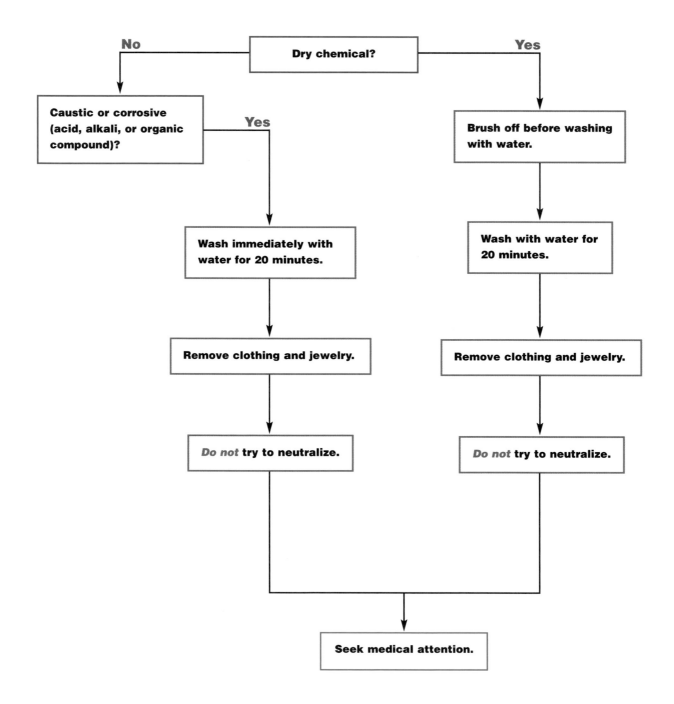

Dry chemical?

No ← → **Yes**

Caustic or corrosive (acid, alkali, or organic compound)?

Yes

Wash immediately with water for 20 minutes.

Remove clothing and jewelry.

Do not **try to neutralize.**

Brush off before washing with water.

Wash with water for 20 minutes.

Remove clothing and jewelry.

Do not **try to neutralize.**

Seek medical attention.

ELECTROCUTION

Even a mild electrical shock can cause serious internal injuries. A current of 1000 volts or more is considered high voltage, but even the 110 volts found in ordinary household current can be deadly.

There are three types of electrical injuries: thermal (flame), arc (flash), and true electrical injury (contact). A thermal burn (flame) results when clothing or objects that are in direct contact with the skin are ignited by an electrical current (FIGURES 8 AND 9). These injuries are caused by the flames produced by the electrical current and not by the passage of the electrical current or arc.

An arc burn (flash) occurs from electricity jumping, or arcing, from one spot to another and not from the passage of an electrical current through the body. Although the duration of the flash may be brief, it usually causes extensive superficial injuries.

A true electrical injury (contact) happens when an electric current has truly passed through the body. This type of injury is characterized by an entrance wound and an exit wound. The important factor with this type of injury is that the surface injury may be just the tip of the iceberg. High-voltage electrical currents passing through the body may disrupt the normal heart rhythm and cause cardiac arrest, burns, and other injuries.

During an electric shock, electricity enters the body at the point of contact and travels along the path of least resistance (nerves and blood vessels). The major damage occurs inside the body, and the outside burn might appear small. Usually, the electricity exits where the body is touching a surface or is in contact with a ground (eg, a metal object). Sometimes, a victim has more than one exit site.

Care for Electrocution

1. Make sure the area is safe. Unplug, disconnect, or turn off the power. If that is impossible, call the power company or EMS for help.

2. Check the ABCDs.

3. If the victim fell, check for a spinal injury.

4. Treat the victim for shock by elevating the legs 8″ to 12″ if no spinal injury is suspected and prevent heat loss by covering the victim with a coat or blanket.

5. Seek medical attention immediately. The ABA recommends that electrical injuries be treated in a burn center.

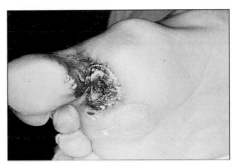

FIGURE 8

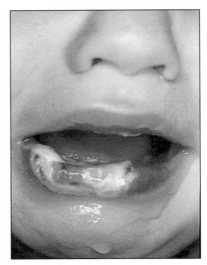

FIGURE 9

ELECTROCUTION

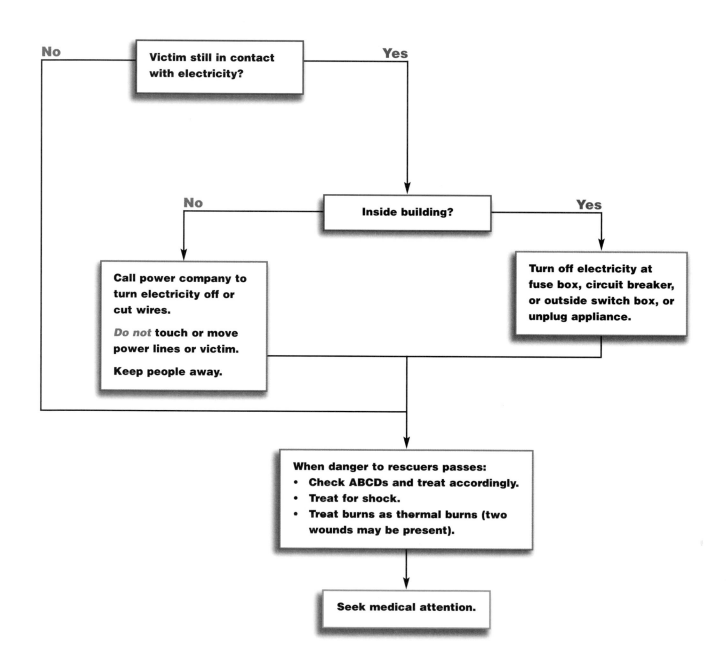

Victim still in contact with electricity?
No — Yes

Inside building?
No — Yes

Call power company to turn electricity off or cut wires.

Do not **touch or move power lines or victim.**

Keep people away.

Turn off electricity at fuse box, circuit breaker, or outside switch box, or unplug appliance.

When danger to rescuers passes:
- **Check ABCDs and treat accordingly.**
- **Treat for shock.**
- **Treat burns as thermal burns (two wounds may be present).**

Seek medical attention.

Contact With a Power Line (Outdoors)

If the electric shock is from contact with a downed power line, the power must be turned off before a rescuer approaches anyone who may be in contact with the wire.

If, as you approach a victim, you feel a tingling sensation in your legs and lower body, stop. The sensation signals that you are on energized ground and that an electrical current is entering through one foot, passing through your lower body, and leaving through the other foot. Raise one foot off the ground, turn around, and hop to a safe place.

If you can safely reach the victim, do not attempt to move any wires, even with wooden poles, tools with wood handles, or tree branches. Do not use objects with a high moisture content and certainly do not use metal objects. The recommendation for not using wood-handled rakes, brooms, or shovels is that if the voltage is high enough (you seldom will know how much voltage is involved), those objects can conduct electricity and the rescuer will be electrocuted. Do not attempt to move downed wires at all unless you are trained and are equipped with tools able to handle the high voltage.

Wait until trained personnel with the proper equipment can cut the wires or disconnect them. Prevent bystanders from entering the danger area.

Contact Inside Buildings

Most electrical burns that occur indoors are caused by faulty electrical equipment or careless use of electrical appliances. Turn off the electricity at the circuit breaker, fuse box, or outside switch box or unplug the appliance if the plug is undamaged. Do not touch the appliance or the victim until the current is off.

Care for Electrical Burns

Once there is no danger to rescuers, give this first aid:

1. Check the ABCDs and treat accordingly.

2. Check the victim for multiple burns and treat for shock by elevating the legs 8″ to 12″ and keeping the victim warm. Most electrical burns are third-degree burns, so cover them with a sterile dressing and elevate affected parts if possible.

3. Seek medical attention immediately.

A true electrical injury (contact) happens when an electric current has truly passed through the body.

SUMMARY

Burns may result from heat, chemical contact, or electricity and may be mild to life threatening. Traditionally, burns are classified as first-, second-, or third-degree, depending on their depth in or through the skin. Burns can also be classified as minor, moderate, or critical, depending on what parts of the body are affected as well as the percentage of the total body area that is burned.

The care of thermal burns depends on both the depth and extent of the burn. The general principles of care include the following:

- Stop the burning and cool the burn area
- Check the ABCs
- Determine the burn depth and extent and the body areas affected
- Determine whether other injuries or illnesses are present
- Determine the severity of the burn
- Seek immediate medical attention for moderate and critical burns

The specific care for burns depends on the degree (depth and size). Third-degree burns should be covered with a sterile dressing, and the victim should be treated for shock.

Chemical burns require immediate removal of the chemical and extensive flushing with water. The area should be covered with a dry, sterile dressing, and medical attention should be sought.

Electrical shock can cause a thermal burn, arc burn, or contact electrical injury in which the electricity causes an entrance and exit wound, and may cause extensive damage inside the body. Seek medical attention immediately. The victim might need treatment for shock. Avoid contact with power lines or electrical appliances or other sources of electricity at the scene.

REVIEW QUESTIONS

Thermal (Heat) Burns

Directions: Circle Yes if you agree with the statement, and circle No if you disagree.

Yes   No   1. Relieve pain and tissue damage from a burn by holding the part in a sink filled with running cold water.

Yes   No   2. Pain and inflammation can be relieved with aspirin (adults only) or ibuprofen in those who can tolerate these over-the-counter medications.

Yes   No   3. Later, a layer of antibiotic ointment or aloe vera gel can be applied on first- and second-degree burns.

Yes   No   4. Butter can be effective on first- and second-degree burns.

Scenario 1. A woman is boiling water in the office kitchen. She reaches across the stove for a cup. The sleeve of her blouse touches the flame of the gas burner and ignites, sending fire racing up her arm. Her screams bring you and others racing into the kitchen. She has second-degree burns on about 7% of her body. What should you do?

_____

_____

_____

Scenario 2. A fire breaks out in your company's storeroom. Two workers put the fire out with fire extinguishers. One of the workers complains of severe pain to both arms. You can see that these areas appear red and blisters have started to form. What should you do?

_____

_____

_____

Chemical Burns

Yes   No   1. When washing chemicals off the body, flush with water for at least five minutes.

Yes   No   2. When washing chemicals off the body, use high pressure water.

Yes   No   3. Do not try to neutralize a chemical because more damage may result.

Yes   No   4. Brush dry powder chemicals from the skin before flushing unless large amounts of water are immediately available.

Scenario 3. A 28-year-old man is using a caustic drain cleaner to unclog a bathroom sink. Fifteen minutes after applying the chemical, he runs water into the sink, but the drain remains clogged. Then, contrary to the instructions on the drain cleaner package, he attempts to use a plunger to clear the drain, and the solution in the sink splashes on his arm. What should you do?

_____

_____

_____

Scenario 4. You are helping a fellow worker replace a battery when it explodes in his face, showering him with battery acid. You see that the acid is already causing second-degree burns to his face and arms. What should you do?

_____

_____

_____

Electrocution

Yes   No   1. If a victim is in contact with an outdoor electrical wire, try to move it with a wooden pole or handle.

Yes   No   2. For a victim who is inside a building, turn off the electricity at the fuse box, circuit-breaker, or outside switch box, or unplug the appliance.

Scenario 5. Kelly is trimming hedges using an old electric hedge trimmer, which is falling apart, but works. Because the three-pronged grounding plug is a little wobbly, she has connected it to a two-pronged adapter, plugged the adapter into an outlet, and started to work on hedges growing along a metal chain-link fence. Things are going well until she reaches for the fence for support, and a powerful electric current shoots through her body, causing her to fall over. When you arrive, she is unresponsive. What do you do?

_____

_____

_____

Scenario 6. You come into the office and see the custodian lying in the room next to an old, frayed electrical wire. His face is pale white with blue coloring underneath the eyes and around the lips. What do you do?

_____

_____

_____

How did you do?

Thermal (Heat) Burns

1. Yes; **2.** Yes; **3.** Yes; **4.** No

Chemical Burns

1. No; **2.** No; **3.** Yes; **4.** Yes

Electrocution

1. No; **2.** Yes

DRESSINGS AND BANDAGES

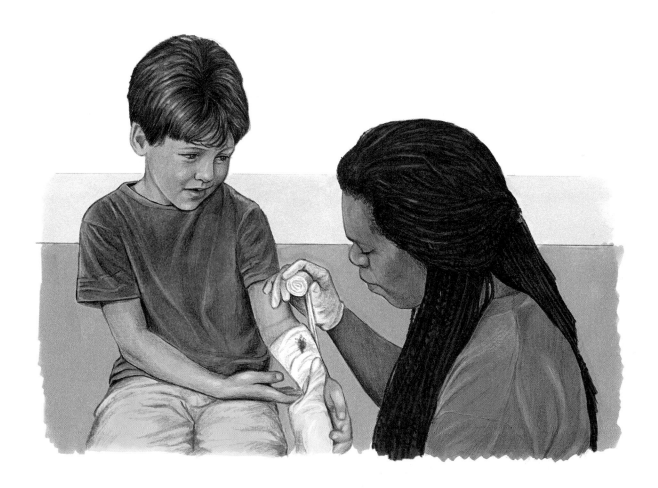

CONTENTS

13

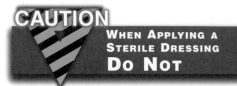

CAUTION

**WHEN APPLYING A
STERILE DRESSING
DO NOT**

- touch any part of the wound or any part of the dressing that will be in contact with the wound.
- cough, breathe, or talk over the wound or dressing.

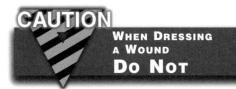

CAUTION

**WHEN DRESSING
A WOUND
DO NOT**

- use fluffy cotton or cotton balls as a dressing. Cotton fibers can get in the wound and be difficult to remove.
- remove a blood-soaked dressing until the bleeding stops.
- pull off a dressing stuck to a wound. If it needs to be removed, soak it off in warm water.

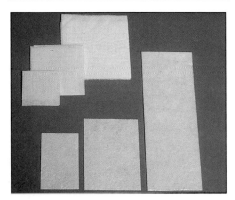

FIGURE 1

LEARNING OBJECTIVES

After reading this chapter, you should be able to

1. Describe the purposes of a dressing
2. Identify various types of dressings
3. Describe the uses of a bandage
4. Identify various types of bandages
5. Demonstrate how to apply a roller bandage to a hand, elbow or knee, and ankle

DRESSINGS

A dressing covers an open wound, and touches the wound. Whenever possible, a dressing should be

- Sterile (if a sterile dressing is not available, use a clean cloth such as a handkerchief, washcloth, or towel)
- Larger than the wound
- Thick, soft, and compressible so that pressure is evenly distributed over the wound
- Lint free

The purposes of a dressing are to

- Control bleeding
- Prevent infection and contamination
- Absorb blood and wound drainage
- Protect the wound from further injury

Applying a Sterile Dressing

1. Wear medical exam gloves whenever possible.
2. Use a dressing that is large enough to extend beyond the wound's edges. Hold the dressing by a corner. Place the dressing directly over the wound. Do not slide it on.
3. Cover the dressing with one of the types of bandages.

Types of Dressings

- *Gauze pads* are used for small wounds (**FIGURE 1**). They come in separately wrapped packages of various sizes (eg, 2″ by 2″, 4″ by 4″) and are sterile unless the package is open. Some gauze pads have a special coating to keep them from sticking to the wound and are especially helpful for dressing burns or wounds secreting fluids.
- *Adhesive strips* (eg, Band-Aids™) are used for small cuts and abrasions and are a combination of both a sterile dressing and a bandage (**FIGURE 2**).

- *Trauma dressings* are made of large, thick, absorbent, sterile materials (**FIGURE 3**). Individually wrapped sanitary napkins can serve because of their bulk and absorbency, but they usually are not sterile.

BANDAGES

Bandages are used to

- Hold a dressing in place over an open wound
- Apply direct pressure over a dressing to control bleeding
- Prevent or reduce swelling
- Provide support and stability for an extremity or joint

A bandage should be clean but need not be sterile. Following are signs that a bandage is too tight:

- Blue tinge of the fingernails or toenails
- Blue or pale skin color
- Tingling or loss of sensation
- Coldness of the extremity
- Inability to move the fingers or toes

Types of Bandages

There are four basic types of bandages.

1. *Roller bandages* come in various widths, lengths, and types of material. For best results, use different widths for different body areas.
   - 1″ width for fingers
   - 2″ width for wrists, hands, and feet
   - 3″ width for elbows and arms
   - 4″ or 6″ width for ankles, knees, and legs
   - *Self-adhering, conforming bandages* come as rolls of slightly elastic, gauzelike material in various widths (**FIGURE 4**). Their self-adherent quality makes them easy to use.
   - *Gauze rollers* are cotton, rigid, and nonelastic. They come in various widths (1″, 2″, and 3″) and usually are 10 yards long.
   - *Elastic roller bandages* are used for compression on sprains, strains, and contusions and come in various widths (**FIGURE 5**). Elastic bandages are not usually applied over dressings covering a wound.

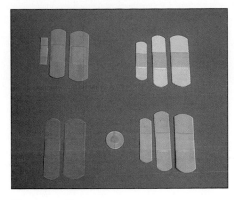

FIGURE 2

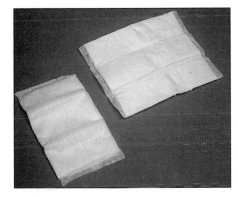

FIGURE 3

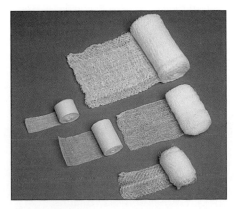

FIGURE 4

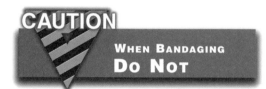

FIGURE 5

If commercial roller bandages are unavailable, you can improvise bandages from neckties or strips of cloth torn from a sheet or other similar material.

2. *Triangular bandages* are available commercially or can be made from a 36″ to 40″ square of preshrunk cotton muslin material that is cut diagonally from corner to corner to produce two triangular pieces of cloth. The longest side is called the base; the corner directly across from the base is the point; the other two corners are called ends. A triangular bandage may be applied in two ways:

   - Fully opened (not folded). Best used for an arm sling. When used to hold dressings in place, fully opened triangular bandages do not apply sufficient pressure on the wound.

   - As a cravat (folded triangular). The point is folded to the center of the base and folded in half again from the top to the base to form a cravat. It is used to hold splints in place, to apply pressure evenly over a dressing, or as a swathe (binder) around the victim's body to stabilize an injured arm in an arm sling.

3. *Adhesive tape* comes in rolls and in a variety of widths. It is often used to secure roller bandages and small dressings in place. For victims who are allergic to adhesive tape, use paper tape or special dermatologic tape.

4. *Adhesive strips* are used for small cuts and abrasions and are a combination of a dressing and a bandage.

Applying a Roller Bandage

Roller bandages are common in first aid kits. Because they are self-adhering and conform well to various body parts, they eliminate the need for complicated bandaging techniques.

Apply the bandage directly over a sterile dressing on the wound. Avoid making it so tight that it reduces circulation, or too loose so that it allows the dressing to slip. When using a roller bandage, start below the wound and work upward. Unless they are injured, leave fingers or toes exposed so that they can be checked to ensure that circulation is not affected by the bandage. See the Skill Scan on pages 206-207 for methods of applying a roller bandage for a hand, elbow, knee, or ankle.

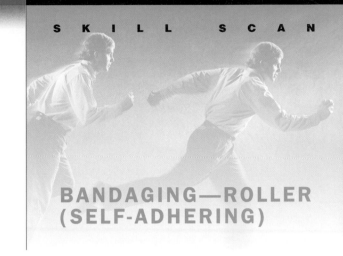

BANDAGING—ROLLER (SELF-ADHERING)

ROLLER BANDAGE FOR HAND: METHOD 1

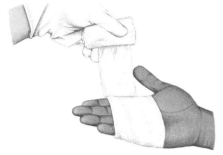

FIGURE 6A

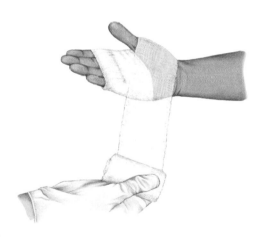

FIGURE 6B

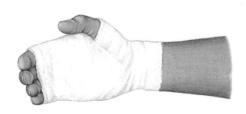

FIGURE 6C

ROLLER BANDAGE FOR HAND: METHOD 2

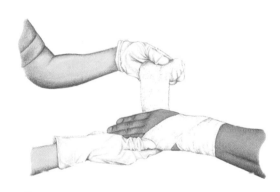

FIGURE 6D

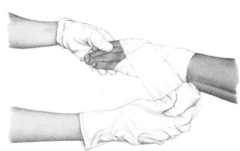

FIGURE 6E

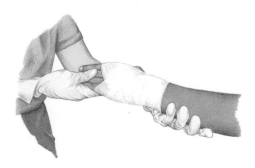

FIGURE 6F

BANDAGING—ROLLER (SELF-ADHERING)

ROLLER BANDAGE FOR ELBOW (OR KNEE)

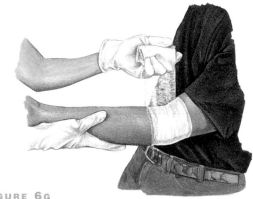

FIGURE 6G

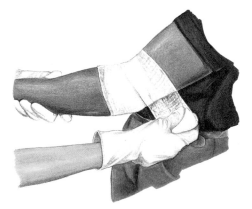

FIGURE 6H

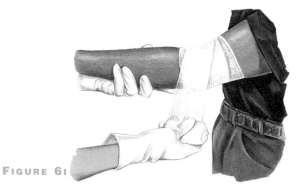

FIGURE 6I

ROLLER BANDAGE FOR ANKLE

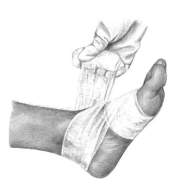

FIGURE 6J

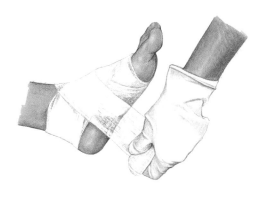

FIGURE 6K

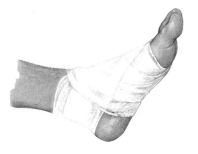

FIGURE 6L

SUMMARY

Dressings are applied over open wounds to help control bleeding, prevent infection, absorb blood and drainage, and protect the wound. Commercially available dressings include gauze pads, adhesive strips, and trauma dressings. Dressings are held in place by bandages.

Bandages are also used to apply direct pressure to control bleeding, to prevent or reduce swelling, and to support an extremity or joint. Types of bandages include

- Roller bandages (self-adhesive, conforming bandages; gauze roller bandages; elastic roller bandages)

- Triangular bandages

- Adhesive tape

- Adhesive strips

When applying a bandage, make certain that it covers the dressing and is secure, but not too tight that it interrupts circulation.

HEAD AND SPINAL INJURIES

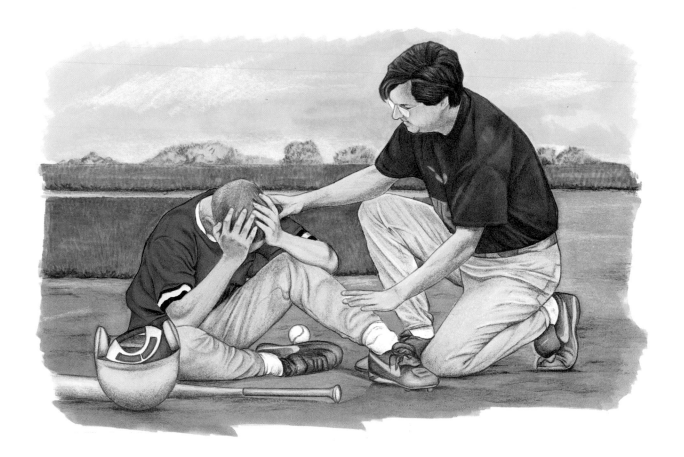

CONTENTS

14

LEARNING OBJECTIVES

After reading this chapter, you should be able to

1. Describe how to care for scalp wounds, skull fractures, eye injuries, nose injuries, and dental injuries
2. Check a responsive and an unresponsive victim with a suspected spinal injury
3. Immobilize a victim with a suspected spinal injury

HEAD INJURIES

Scalp Wounds

A bleeding scalp wound does not affect the blood supply to the brain. Look into the wound for exposed skull bone or brain tissue and indentation of the skull. Suspect a spinal injury. Give the following care:

Care for Scalp Wounds

1. Control bleeding by gently applying direct pressure with a dry sterile dressing. If the dressing becomes blood soaked, do not remove it. Add another dressing on top of the first one.
2. **If you suspect a skull fracture, apply pressure around the edges of the wound** and over a broad area rather than on the center of the wound. Use a doughnut (ring) pad around the area.
3. Keep the head and shoulders slightly elevated to help control bleeding if no spinal injury is suspected.

Skull Fracture

It is very difficult to determine a skull fracture except by X-ray, unless the skull deformity is severe. The signs and symptoms of a skull fracture include the following:

- Pain at the point of injury
- Deformity of the skull
- Bleeding from the ears or nose
- Leakage of clear, pink, watery fluid known as cerebrospinal fluid (CSF) from an ear or the nose. A drop of CSF fluid on a gauze pad, handkerchief, or other cloth will form a pink ring resembling a target around a slightly blood-tinged center; this is called the "halo sign" or "ring sign."
- Discoloration around the eyes ("raccoon eyes") appearing several hours after the injury
- Discoloration behind an ear (known as "Battle's sign"), appearing several hours after the injury

CAUTION

WITH A SCALP INJURY DO NOT

- remove an embedded object. Instead, stabilize it in place with bulky dressings. If a skull fracture is suspected, do not clean a scalp wound or irrigate it, since the fluid can carry debris and bacteria into the brain.

- Unequal-sized pupils

- Profuse scalp bleeding if the skin is broken. A scalp wound may expose the skull or brain tissue.

- Penetrating wound (eg, from a bullet) or impaled object

Care for a Skull Fracture

1. Monitor the ABCDs.

2. Cover wounds with a sterile dressing.

3. Immobilize the victim's neck against movement.

4. Apply pressure around the edges of the wound, not directly on it.

Brain Injuries

When the head is struck with force, the brain bounces against the inside of the skull. Like other body tissue, the brain will swell when injured. Unlike other tissue, the brain is confined in the skull where there is little space for swelling. Swelling of brain tissue or accumulating of blood inside the skull therefore compresses the brain and increases the pressure inside the skull, interfering with brain functioning.

Assessment is directed at determining whether injured brain tissue is swelling. The following signs and symptoms, which may go unnoticed for the first 6 to 18 hours after the injury, indicate brain swelling:

- Altered level of responsiveness. Loss of responsiveness may be short or may persist for hours or days. The victim may alternate between periods of responsiveness and unresponsiveness or be responsive but disoriented, confused, and incoherent.

- Memory loss

- Vomiting and nausea

- Headache

- Vision disturbance. The victim sees "double," or the eyes fail to move together.

- Unequal-sized pupils

- Weakness, loss of balance, or paralysis

- Seizures

- Blood or CSF leaking from ears or nose

- Combativeness. The victim may strike out randomly and with surprising strength at the nearest person.

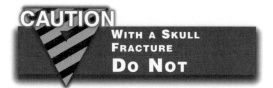

CAUTION

WITH A SKULL FRACTURE

DO NOT

- stop the flow of blood or CSF from an ear or nose. Blocking the flow could increase pressure within the skull.

- remove an impaled object from the head. Instead, stabilize it in place with bulky dressings.

- clean an open skull fracture. Infection of the brain could result.

With a responsive victim, ask what day it is, where he or she is, and his or her name. If the victim cannot answer those questions, there may be a significant problem.

Care for Brain Injuries

1. Seek immediate medical attention for all brain-injury victims.

2. Suspect a spinal injury in an unresponsive victim until proven otherwise. (See page 223 on how to immobilize the victim's head and neck.)

3. Monitor the ABCDs.

4. Control scalp bleeding by covering wounds with sterile dressings as a barrier against infection. If you suspect a skull fracture, apply pressure around the wound edges, not directly on the wound. Do not try to clean a scalp wound of a suspected skull fracture. Stabilize impaled objects in place. Do not try to stop blood or CSF draining from the ears or nose. Blocking either flow could increase pressure within the skull.

5. Brain-injury victims tend to vomit. Rolling the victim onto his or her side while stabilizing the neck against movement will help to drain vomit while keeping the airway open.

6. Minimize movement of the victim since a spinal injury could exist. If the victim is unconscious, roll the victim onto his or her side.

7. The victim's level of responsiveness or mental status is one of the best indicators of neurologic function. Observations over the first 24 hours may reveal problems. Use the mnemonic "AVPU" to assess and describe a victim's mental status, especially with small children who don't talk.

Head Injury Follow-Up

If any of the following signs appears within 48 hours of a head injury, seek medical attention:

- *Headache*. Expect a headache. If it lasts more than one or two days or increases in severity, however, seek medical advice.

- *Nausea, vomiting*. If nausea lasts more than 2 hours, seek medical advice. Vomiting once or twice, especially in children, may be expected after a head injury. Vomiting does not reveal anything about the severity of the injury. However, if vomiting begins again hours after one or two episodes have ceased, consult a doctor.

- *Drowsiness*. Allow a victim to sleep, but wake the victim at least every 2 hours to check the state of consciousness and

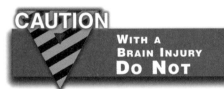

CAUTION

WITH A
BRAIN INJURY
DO NOT

- stop the flow of blood or CSF from the ears or nose. Blocking either flow could increase pressure inside the skull.

- elevate the legs. There may also be a spinal injury.

- clean an open skull injury. This could result in infection.

FLOW CHART

HEAD INJURIES

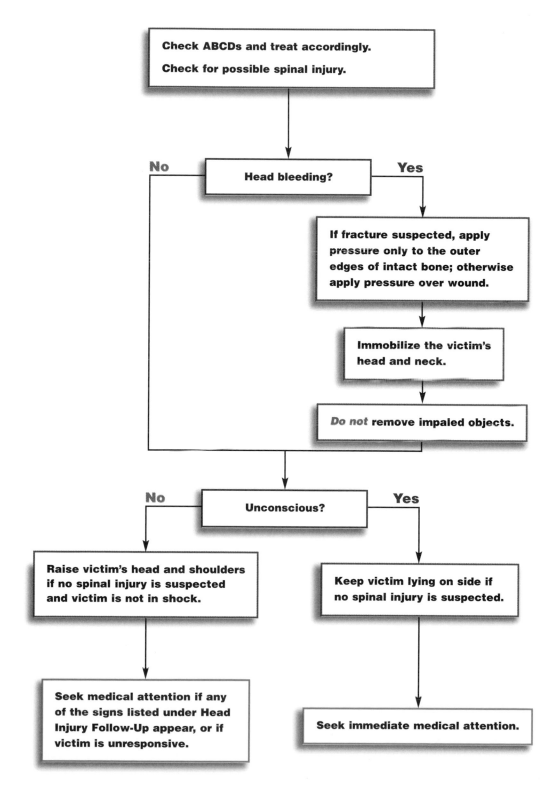

Check ABCDs and treat accordingly.

Check for possible spinal injury.

Head bleeding?

No · Yes

If fracture suspected, apply pressure only to the outer edges of intact bone; otherwise apply pressure over wound.

Immobilize the victim's head and neck.

Do not remove impaled objects.

Unconscious?

No · Yes

Raise victim's head and shoulders if no spinal injury is suspected and victim is not in shock.

Keep victim lying on side if no spinal injury is suspected.

Seek medical attention if any of the signs listed under Head Injury Follow-Up appear, or if victim is unresponsive.

Seek immediate medical attention.

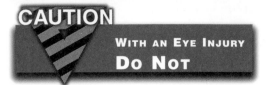

CAUTION

WITH AN EYE INJURY
DO NOT

- assume that any eye injury is innocent. When in doubt, seek medical attention immediately.

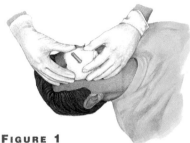

FIGURE 1
Bulky gauze stabilizes object impaled in eye.

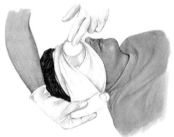

FIGURE 2
Paper cup used to prevent object from moving.

Bandaging holds cup in place.

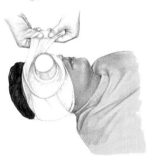

CAUTION

WITH A PENETRATING EYE INJURY
DO NOT

- remove an object stuck in the eye or try to wash out an object with water.
- exert pressure on an injured eyeball or a penetrating object.

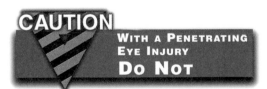

sense of orientation by asking his or her name, and an information-processing question (eg, recite months of the year backwards). If the victim cannot answer correctly or appears confused or disoriented, call a physician.

- *Vision problems.* If the victim "sees double," if the eyes fail to move together, or if one pupil appears to be larger than the other, seek medical advice.

- *Mobility.* If the victim cannot use his or her arms or legs as well as previously or is unsteady in walking, seek medical care.

- *Speech.* If the victim has slurred speech or is unable to talk, consult a doctor.

- *Seizures or convulsions.* If the victim has a violent involuntary contraction (spasm) or series of contractions of the skeletal muscles, seek medical assistance.

EYE INJURIES

Care for Penetrating Eye Injuries

Penetrating eye injuries are severe injuries that result when a sharp object, such as a knife or a needle, penetrates the eye and then is withdrawn or when pieces from a tool enter the eye and lodge there as foreign bodies.

1. Seek immediate medical attention. Any penetrating eye injury should be managed in the hospital.

2. Protect the injured eye with a paper cup, cardboard folded into a cone, or a doughnut-shaped pad made from a roller gauze bandage or a cravat bandage to prevent the object from being driven deeper into the eye **(FIGURE 1)**.

3. Cover the undamaged eye to stop movement of the damaged eye (known as sympathetic eye movement).

4. Bandage the protective cup or pad in place **(FIGURE 2)**.

EYE INJURIES

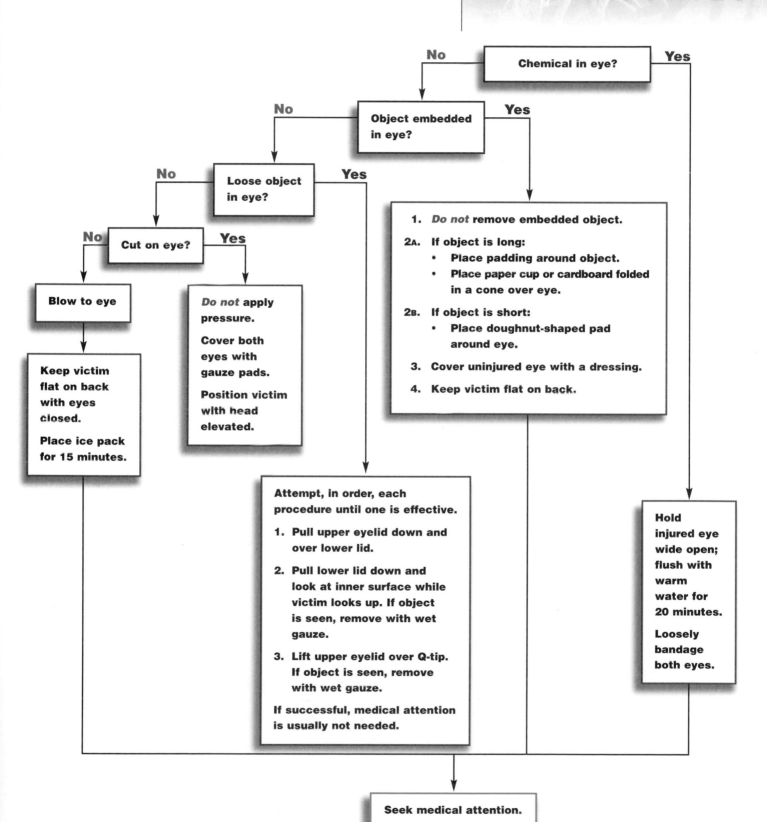

No ← **Chemical in eye?** → **Yes**

No ← **Object embedded in eye?** → **Yes**

No ← **Loose object in eye?** → **Yes**

No ← **Cut on eye?** → **Yes**

Blow to eye

Keep victim flat on back with eyes closed.

Place ice pack for 15 minutes.

Do not **apply pressure.**

Cover both eyes with gauze pads.

Position victim with head elevated.

1. *Do not* remove embedded object.

2A. If object is long:
   • Place padding around object.
   • Place paper cup or cardboard folded in a cone over eye.

2B. If object is short:
   • Place doughnut-shaped pad around eye.

3. Cover uninjured eye with a dressing.

4. Keep victim flat on back.

Attempt, in order, each procedure until one is effective.

1. Pull upper eyelid down and over lower lid.

2. Pull lower lid down and look at inner surface while victim looks up. If object is seen, remove with wet gauze.

3. Lift upper eyelid over Q-tip. If object is seen, remove with wet gauze.

If successful, medical attention is usually not needed.

Hold injured eye wide open; flush with warm water for 20 minutes.

Loosely bandage both eyes.

Seek medical attention.

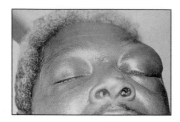

FIGURE 3

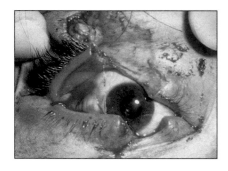

FIGURE 4

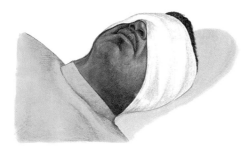

FIGURE 5

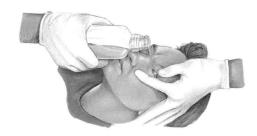

FIGURE 6
Flush eye for chemical burn.

Care for Blows to the Eye

Blows to the eye can be minor or sight threatening (**FIGURE 3**):

1. Apply an ice pack immediately for about 15 minutes to reduce pain and swelling. Do not exert any pressure on the eye.

2. Seek medical attention immediately in cases of pain, reduced vision, or discoloration (a black eye).

Care for Cuts of the Eye and Lid

For first aid for a cut of the eye or lid (**FIGURE 4**):

1. Bandage both eyes lightly (**FIGURE 5**).

2. Seek medical attention immediately.

Care for Chemical Burns of the Eye

Chemical burns of the eyes are extremely sight threatening. First aid may determine the fate of the eye and vision.

Alkalies cause more damage than acids do because alkalies penetrate deeper and continue to burn longer. Common alkalies include drain cleaners, cleaning agents, ammonia, cement, plaster, and caustic soda. Common acids include hydrochloric acid, nitric acid, sulfuric (battery) acid, and acetic acid.

Because damage can happen in 1 to 5 minutes, the chemical must be removed immediately:

1. Use your fingers to keep the eye open as wide as possible.

2. Flush the eye with water immediately. If possible, use warm water. If water is not available, use any nonirritating liquid.

   • Hold the victim's head under a faucet or pour water into the eye from any clean container for at least 20 minutes, continuously and gently. It is not possible to use too much water on these injuries.

   • Irrigate from the nose side of the eye toward the outside to avoid flushing material into the other eye (**FIGURE 6**).

   • Tell the victim to roll the eyeball as much as possible to help wash out the eye.

3. Loosely bandage both eyes with cold, wet dressings.

4. Seek immediate medical attention.

Care for an Eye Knocked Out

A blow to the eye can avulse it (knock it out) from its socket:

1. Cover the eye loosely with a sterile dressing that has been moistened with clean water. Do not try to push the eyeball back into the socket.

2. Protect the injured eye with a paper cup, cardboard folded into a cone, or a doughnut-shaped pad made from a roller gauze bandage or a cravat bandage.

3. Cover the undamaged eye with a patch to stop movement of the damaged eye (known as sympathetic eye movement).

4. Seek medical attention immediately.

Care for Foreign Objects in Eye

To remove a foreign object in the eye, try one or more of the following, starting with number 1:

1. Lift the upper lid over the lower lid, allowing the lashes to brush the object off the inside of the upper lid. Have the victim blink a few times and let the eye move the object out. If the object remains, keep the eye closed.

2. Try flushing the object out by rinsing the eye gently with warm water. Hold the eyelid open and tell the victim to move the eye as it is rinsed.

3. Examine the lower lid by pulling it down gently. If you can see the object, remove it with a moistened sterile gauze or clean cloth (FIGURE 7).

4. Many foreign bodies lodge under the upper eyelid, requiring some expertise in everting the lid and removing the object. Examine the upper lid by grasping the lashes of the upper lid, placing a matchstick or cotton-tipped swab across the upper lid, and rolling the lid upward over the stick or swab (FIGURES 8A AND 8B). If you can see the object, remove it with a moistened sterile gauze or clean cloth.

Care for Eye Burns From Light

Burns can result if a person looks at a source of ultraviolet light (eg, sunlight, arc welding, bright snow, tanning lamps). Severe pain happens 1 to 6 hours after exposure. To care for eye burns from light, do the following:

1. Cover both eyes with cold, wet packs. Tell the victim not to rub his or her eyes.

2. Have the victim rest in a darkened room. Do not allow light to reach the victim's eyes.

3. Give an aspirin (adults only), acetaminophen, or ibuprofen for pain, if needed.

4. Call an ophthalmologist for advice.

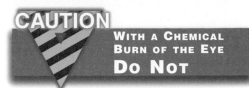

CAUTION

WITH A CHEMICAL BURN OF THE EYE DO NOT

- try to neutralize the chemical. Use water for eye irrigation.
- use an eye cup for a chemical burn.

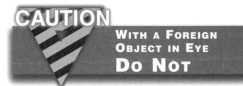

CAUTION

WITH A FOREIGN OBJECT IN EYE DO NOT

- allow the victim to rub the eye.
- try to remove an embedded foreign object.
- use dry cotton (cotton balls or cotton-tipped swabs) or instruments (eg, tweezers) on an eye.

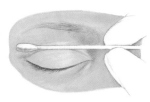

FIGURE 7
Removing an object from the eye with wet sterile gauze.

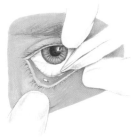

FIGURE 8A
Have the victim look down. Pull gently downward on upper eyelashes. Lay a swab or matchstick across the top of the lid.

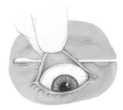

FIGURE 8B
Fold the lid over the swab or matchstick. Remove an object by gently flushing with lukewarm water or a wet sterile gauze.

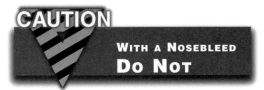

- **allow the victim to tilt the head backward.**
- **probe the nose with a cotton-tipped swab.**
- **move the victim's head and neck if a spinal injury is suspected.**

NOSE INJURIES

Care for Nosebleeds

There are two types of nosebleeds:

- Anterior (front of nose) is the most common type (90%). Blood comes out of the nose through one nostril.
- Posterior (back of nose) type involves massive bleeding backward into the mouth or down the back of the throat. A posterior nosebleed is serious and requires medical attention.

To care for an anterior nosebleed using the American Academy of Otolaryngology guidelines, do the following:

1. Pinch all the soft parts of the nose together between your thumb and two fingers.
2. Press firmly toward the face, compressing the pinched parts of the nose against the bones of the face.
3. Hold it for 5 minutes.
4. Keep the head higher than the level of the heart. Have the victim sit and lean slightly forward or lie with the head elevated.
5. Apply ice (crushed in a plastic bag or washcloth) to the nose and cheeks.

If bleeding continues:

6. Clear the nose of all blood clots by gently blowing or sniffing in.
7. Spray the nose four times on both sides with decongestant spray (such as Afrin™ or Neo-Synephrin™).
8. Pinch and press the nose toward the face again, as in Steps 1 to 3.
9. If the nosebleed continues, consult a physician.

Seek professional medical help if:

- Bleeding cannot be stopped or keeps reappearing
- Bleeding is rapid or if blood loss is large
- Weakness or fainting are present
- Bleeding begins going down the back of the throat rather than the front of the nose

Care for a Broken Nose

For a broken nose, seek medical attention and give care as for a nosebleed. Apply an ice pack to the nose for 15 minutes. Do not try to straighten a crooked nose.

NOSEBLEEDS

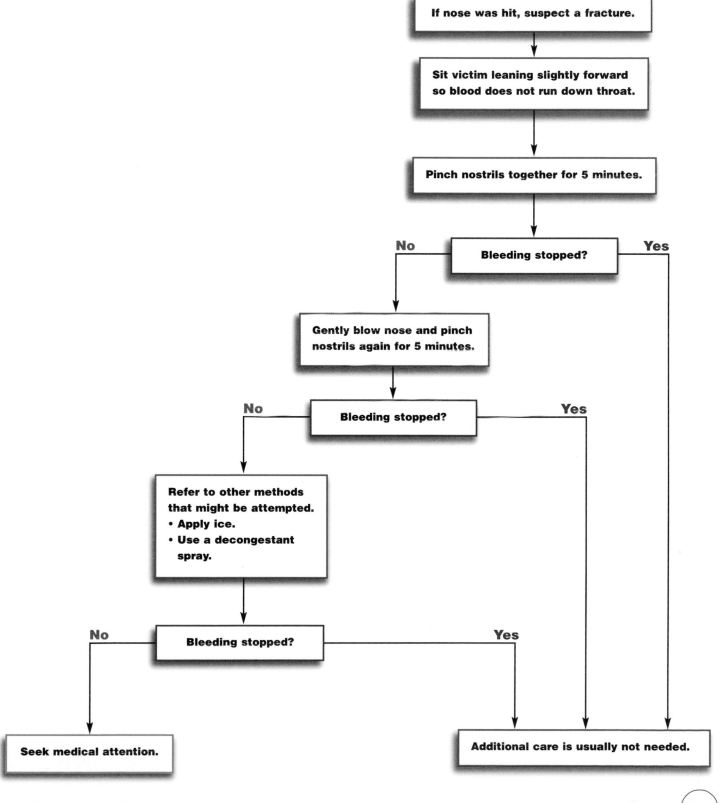

If nose was hit, suspect a fracture.

Sit victim leaning slightly forward so blood does not run down throat.

Pinch nostrils together for 5 minutes.

No ← Bleeding stopped? → **Yes**

Gently blow nose and pinch nostrils again for 5 minutes.

No ← Bleeding stopped? → **Yes**

Refer to other methods that might be attempted.
• Apply ice.
• Use a decongestant spray.

No ← Bleeding stopped? → **Yes**

Seek medical attention.

Additional care is usually not needed.

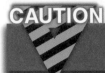

CAUTION

WITH TOOTHACHE
DO NOT

- place aspirin, acetaminophen, or ibuprofen on the aching tooth or gum tissues or allow them to dissolve in the mouth. A serious acid burn can result.
- cover a cavity with cotton if there is any pus discharge or facial swelling. See a dentist immediately.
- stick anything into the exposed cavity or into the softened exposed root.

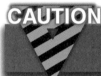

CAUTION

WITH A
KNOCKED-OUT TOOTH
DO NOT

- handle a knocked-out tooth roughly.
- put a knocked-out tooth in water, mouthwash, alcohol, or Betadine™.
- put a knocked-out tooth in skim milk, reconstituted powdered milk, or milk by-products such as yogurt.
- rinse a knocked-out tooth unless you are reinserting it in the socket.
- place a knocked-out tooth in anything that can dry or crush the outside of the tooth.
- scrub a knocked-out tooth or remove any attached tissue fragments.
- remove a partially extracted tooth. Push it back into place and seek a dentist so that the loose tooth can be stabilized.

DENTAL INJURIES

Because dental emergencies generally cause considerable pain and anxiety, managing them promptly can provide great relief to the victim.

Care for a Toothache

A diseased tooth is sensitive to heat and cold. The victim needs to see a dentist immediately. For relief of pain, follow these steps:

1. Rinse the mouth with warm water to clean it out.

2. Use dental floss to remove any food that might be trapped between the teeth.

3. If you suspect a cavity, paint the tooth by using a small cotton swab soaked in oil of cloves (eugenol) to help depress the pain. Take care to keep the oil off the gums, lips, and inside surfaces of the cheeks. If applicable, follow the same procedures as for a broken tooth.

4. Give the victim aspirin (adults only), acetaminophen, or ibuprofen to reduce pain.

5. Seek a dentist immediately.

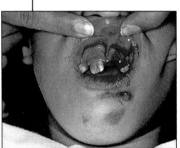

FIGURE 9

Care for a Knocked-Out Tooth

1. To care for a knocked-out tooth (FIGURE 9) have the victim rinse his or her mouth, and put a rolled gauze pad in the socket to control bleeding.

2. Find the tooth and handle it by the crown, not the root, to minimize damage to it.

3. The best place for a knocked-out tooth is its socket. A tooth often can be successfully reimplanted if it has been put back in its socket within 30 minutes after the injury.

Try to replace the tooth into the socket, using adjacent teeth as a guide. Push down on the tooth so that the top is even with the adjacent teeth. Biting down gently on gauze is helpful. When a dentist cannot be seen immediately, do not let a knocked-out tooth dry out. Keep it in the victim's saliva for short-term transport to the dentist (less than 1 hour). If available, preserve the tooth with a Save-a-Tooth™ kit. This can help to preserve the tooth for 6 to 12 hours.

Some experts recommend that the tooth be placed in the victim's mouth to keep it moist until the victim sees a dentist. Do not use this method for children or others who may swallow the tooth.

4. Take the victim and the tooth to a dentist immediately.

DENTAL INJURIES

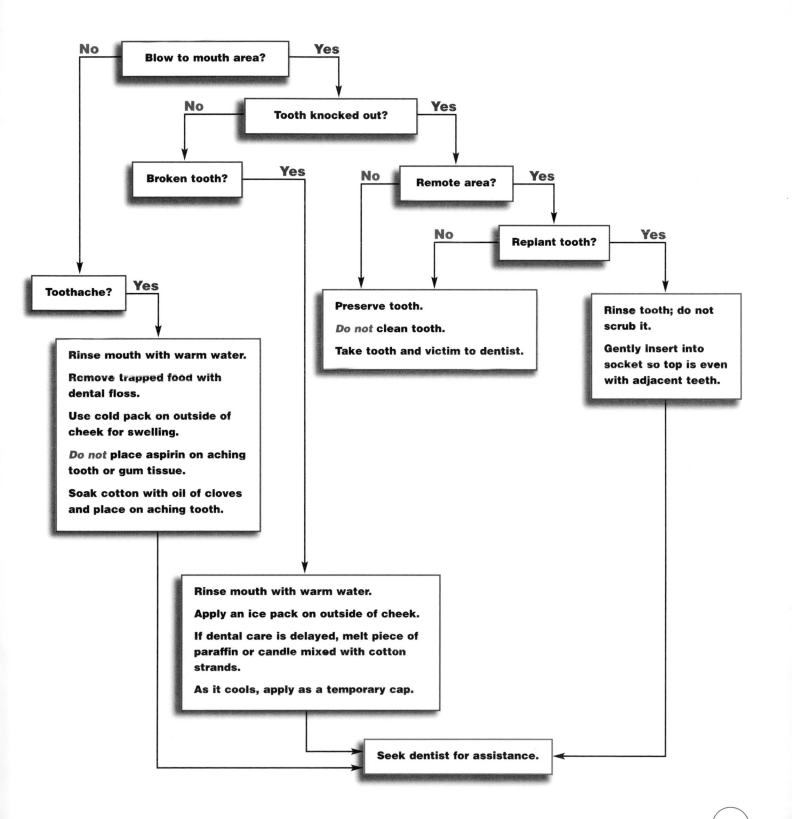

No ← **Blow to mouth area?** → **Yes**

No ← **Tooth knocked out?** → **Yes**

Broken tooth? — **Yes**

No ← **Remote area?** → **Yes**

No ← **Replant tooth?** → **Yes**

Toothache? — **Yes**

Preserve tooth.

Do not **clean tooth.**

Take tooth and victim to dentist.

Rinse tooth; do not scrub it.

Gently insert into socket so top is even with adjacent teeth.

Rinse mouth with warm water.

Remove trapped food with dental floss.

Use cold pack on outside of cheek for swelling.

Do not **place aspirin on aching tooth or gum tissue.**

Soak cotton with oil of cloves and place on aching tooth.

Rinse mouth with warm water.

Apply an ice pack on outside of cheek.

If dental care is delayed, melt piece of paraffin or candle mixed with cotton strands.

As it cools, apply as a temporary cap.

Seek dentist for assistance.

FIGURE 10

Care for a Broken Tooth

1. To care for a broken tooth **(FIGURE 10),** gently clean dirt and blood from the injured area with a sterile gauze pad or a clean cloth and warm water.

2. If you are in a remote area with no dentist nearby, you can make a temporary cap from melted candle wax or paraffin and a few strands of cotton. When the wax begins to harden but can still be molded, press a wad of it onto the tooth. Other improvisations include using ski wax or chewing gum (preferably sugarless).

3. Apply an ice pack on the face in the area of the injured tooth to decrease swelling.

4. If you suspect a jaw fracture, stabilize the jaw by wrapping a bandage under the chin and over the top of the head.

5. Seek a dentist immediately.

SPINAL INJURIES

Any time there is a head injury, there may also be a spinal injury, since the head may have been snapped suddenly in one or more directions. Following are signs and symptoms of spinal injuries:

- Painful movement of the arms or legs
- Numbness, tingling, weakness, or burning sensation in the arms or legs
- Loss of bowel or bladder control
- Paralysis of the arms or legs
- Deformity (odd-looking angle of the victim's head and neck)

To further assess the victim for a spinal injury, see the Skill Scan: "Checking for Spinal Injuries" following this section and ask a responsive victim these questions:

- Are you in pain? Neck (cervical spine) injuries radiate pain to the arms; upper-back (thoracic spine) injuries radiate pain around the ribs; lower-back injuries usually radiate pain down the legs. Often, the victim will describe the pain as "electric."
- Can you move your fingers? Moving the fingers is a sign that nerve pathways are intact. Ask the victim to grip your hand. A strong grip indicates that a spinal injury is unlikely.
- Can you move your feet? Ask the victim to press a foot against your hand. If the victim cannot perform this movement, or if the movement is extremely weak against your hand, the victim may have a spinal injury.

If the victim is unresponsive, do the following:

- Look for cuts, bruises, and deformities.

- Test responses by pinching the victim's hand (either palm or back of the hand) and bare foot (sole or top of the foot). A lack of reaction could mean spinal damage.

- Stroke the bottom of the bare foot firmly, toward the big toe with a key or similar sharp object. This is the Babinski reflex test. The normal response is the big toe goes down (except in infants). If the spinal cord is injured, an adult's or child's big toes will flex upward.

- Ask bystanders what happened. If you still are not sure about a possible spinal injury, assume that the victim has one until it is proved otherwise.

Care for Spinal Injuries

1. Check and monitor the ABCDs.

2. Immobilize the victim against any movement, using one of the following methods. Whichever method you use, tell the victim not to move:

   - Grasp the victim's clavicle and trapezius muscle (shoulder) and cradle his or her head between the inside of your forearms. Hold the victim's head and neck still until the ambulance arrives **(FIGURE 11)**.

   - Grasp the victim's head over the ears and hold the head and neck still until the ambulance arrives **(FIGURE 12)**.

   - If a long wait is anticipated or if you are tired from holding the victim's head in place, kneel with the victim's head between your knees or place objects on each side of the head to prevent it from rolling from side to side **(FIGURE 13)**.

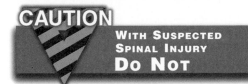

CAUTION
WITH SUSPECTED SPINAL INJURY
DO NOT

- move the victim, even if the victim is in water. Wait for EMS to arrive; EMS personnel have the proper training and equipment. Victims with suspected spinal injury require cervical collars and stabilization on a spine board. It is better to do nothing than to mishandle a victim with a spinal injury.

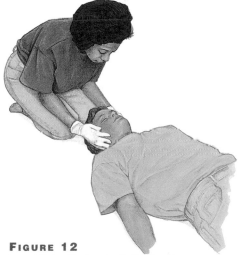

FIGURE 12
Immobilizing the head with the hands.

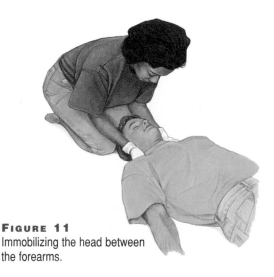

FIGURE 11
Immobilizing the head between the forearms.

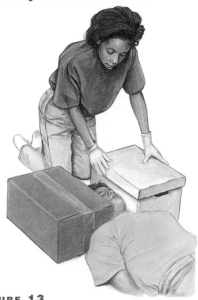

FIGURE 13
Immobilizing the head with objects.

CHECKING FOR SPINAL INJURIES

Conscious Victim: Upper Extremity Checks

1. **Victim wiggles fingers** (FIGURE 14A).
2. **Rescuer touches fingers** (FIGURE 14B).
3. **Victim squeezes rescuer's hand** (FIGURE 14C).

Conscious Victim: Lower-Extremity Checks

4. **Victim wiggles toes** (FIGURE 14D).
5. **Rescuer touches toes** (FIGURE 14E).
6. **Victim pushes foot against rescuer's hand** (FIGURE 14F). **Victim's inability to perform may mean spinal injury!**

Unconscious Victim

7. **Pinch hand** (FIGURE 14G).
8. **Pinch foot** (FIGURE 14H).

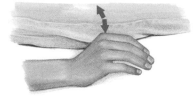

FIGURE 14A

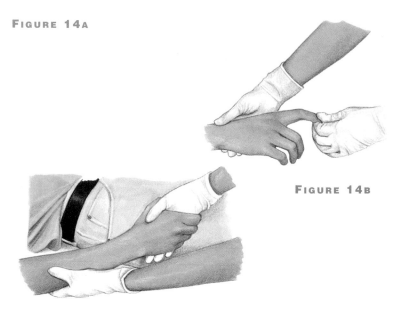

FIGURE 14B

FIGURE 14C

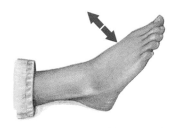

FIGURE 14D

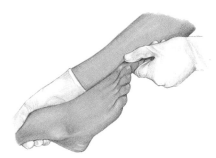

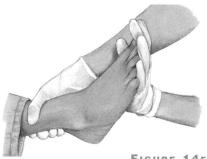

FIGURE 14F

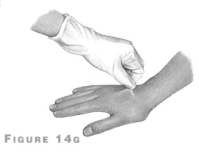

FIGURE 14E

FIGURE 14G

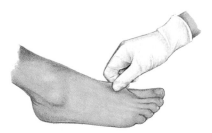

FIGURE 14H

SPINAL INJURIES

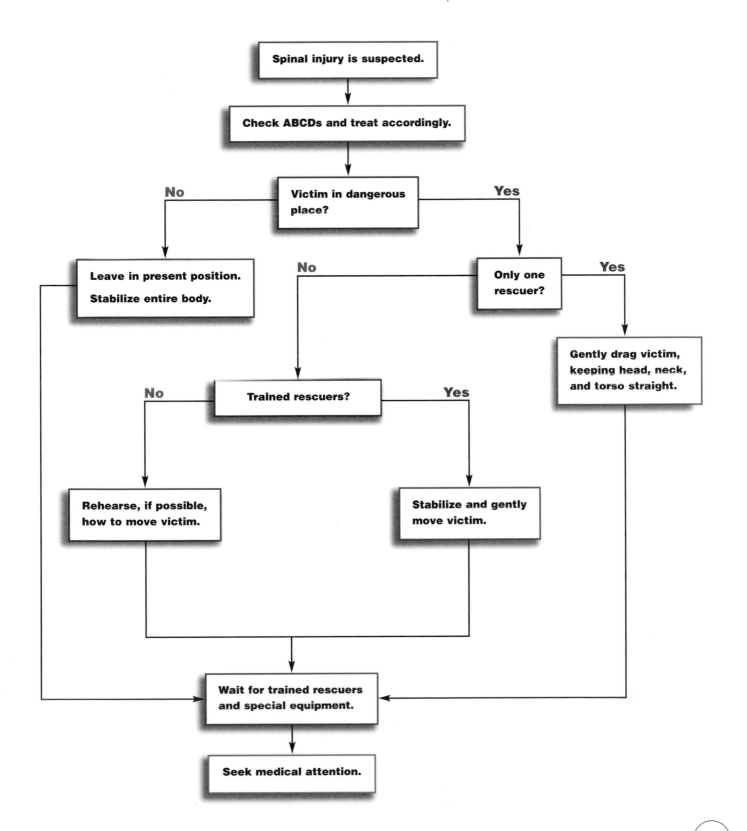

Spinal injury is suspected.

↓

Check ABCDs and treat accordingly.

↓

No ← Victim in dangerous place? → **Yes**

Leave in present position. Stabilize entire body.

No ← Only one rescuer? → **Yes**

Gently drag victim, keeping head, neck, and torso straight.

No ← Trained rescuers? → **Yes**

Rehearse, if possible, how to move victim.

Stabilize and gently move victim.

Wait for trained rescuers and special equipment.

↓

Seek medical attention.

Head and

spinal injuries

are typically

serious, and

the victim

should receive

medical attention

immediately.

SUMMARY

Head and spinal injuries are typically serious, and the victim should receive medical attention immediately.

With a possible skull fracture or brain injury, call EMS. Suspect a spinal injury also, and immobilize the victim's head and neck. Monitor the ABCDs and cover external wounds with a sterile dressing. Be prepared to move the victim into the recovery position if vomiting occurs.

Eye injuries are important because they may result in disability. Except for mild cases of a foreign body in the eye being successfully flushed out, all eye injuries should be seen by a doctor. Protect the injured eye with a loose bandage, and cover the other eye as well to prevent eye movements.

With a dental injury such as a knocked-out or broken tooth, the victim needs to see a dentist as soon as possible. Rinse the mouth with water and place a sterile gauze pad in the socket. In some cases, replace a knocked-out tooth in the socket.

If the victim has a possible spinal injury, it is important to immobilize the head, neck, and torso to prevent any movement. With the victim on his or her back, immobilize the head with your hands, forearms, or objects on both sides. Call EMS and monitor the ABCDs.

REVIEW QUESTIONS

Head Injuries

Directions: Circle Yes if you agree with the statement, and circle No if you disagree.

Yes   No   1. For a suspected skull fracture, press around the edges and not directly on the wound.

Yes   No   2. Do NOT remove impaled (embedded) objects.

Yes   No   3. Head-injured victims should be checked for a possible spinal injury.

Scenario 1. At work, you are called to help a carpenter who fell from a ladder. A bystander says that, though responsive now, the victim was previously motionless for a couple of minutes. The victim complains about a severe headache and dizziness. There is swelling on the back of his head. What should you do?

_____

_____

_____

Scenario 2. Several children are playing on a swing set. One child is hit on the forehead by another child coming back on a swing. The child is knocked several feet behind the swing set by the impact and appears dizzy, confused, and very weak. There is no bleeding. What should you do?

_____

_____

_____

Eye Injuries

Yes   No   1. After a blow to an eye, apply a cold pack for about 15 minutes.

Yes   No   2. Tears are sufficient to flush a chemical from the eye.

Yes   No   3. A clean, damp cloth can be used to remove an object from the eyeball's surface.

Scenario 3. As Sandy is attempting to jump-start the company car, a spark from the jump-cables ignites hydrogen gas that has accumulated in the battery. This causes the battery to explode. The battery cap flies off, and battery acid splashes into Sandy's eyes. What should you do?

_____

_____

_____

Scenario 4. While you and a companion are riding bicycles, an object hits your companion's eye. You have the victim open his eyes, and you see what looks like a small insect resting on the inner eyelid. What should you do?

_____

_____

_____

Dental Injuries

Yes	No	1.	Preserve a knocked-out tooth in mouthwash or rubbing alcohol.
Yes	No	2.	Scrub a knocked-out tooth before taking the victim to a dentist.
Yes	No	3.	Sometimes a knocked-out tooth should be reinserted by a first aider.

Scenario 5. Merrilyn, age 20, was struck in the mouth by a pipe that was loosely suspended from a cable. She has spit out two of her front teeth, which are lying on the ground. What should you do?

_____

_____

_____

Scenario 6. A teenager falls off a bike and breaks a piece off of two front teeth. The victim's dentist is minutes away. What should you do?

_____

_____

_____

Spinal Injuries

Yes	No	1.	Do NOT move, and stabilize against movement, a victim with a suspected spinal injury.
Yes	No	2.	Inability of fingers and/or feet to move may indicate a spinal injury.
Yes	No	3.	A head injury may be a reason to suspect a spinal injury.

Scenario 7. You hear a loud crash as a car hits a concrete median. The driver complains of numbness and loss of feeling in both legs. What should you do?

_____

_____

_____

Scenario 8. At the scene of a motorcycle accident, the victim is complaining about a loss of sensation. He can't move the toes on either foot. You found him lying on his back with no other obvious injury. What should you do?

_____

_____

_____

Nosebleeds

Scenario 9 While Jackie is turning right around the corner in an office hallway, another office worker accidentally but abruptly collides with her. The co-worker's head strikes Jackie's nose. Blood begins to flow from Jackie's nostril. What should you do?

_____

_____

_____

Scenario 10. A worker played a practical joke on another worker, who jumped and hit his nose against his elbow, causing a nosebleed. What should you do?

_____

_____

_____

HOW DID YOU DO?

Head Injuries

1. Yes; 2. Yes; 3. Yes

Eye Injuries

1. Yes; 2. No; 3. Yes

Dental Injuries

1. No; 2. No; 3. Yes

Spinal Injuries

1. Yes; 2. Yes; 3. Yes

CHEST, ABDOMINAL, AND PELVIC INJURIES

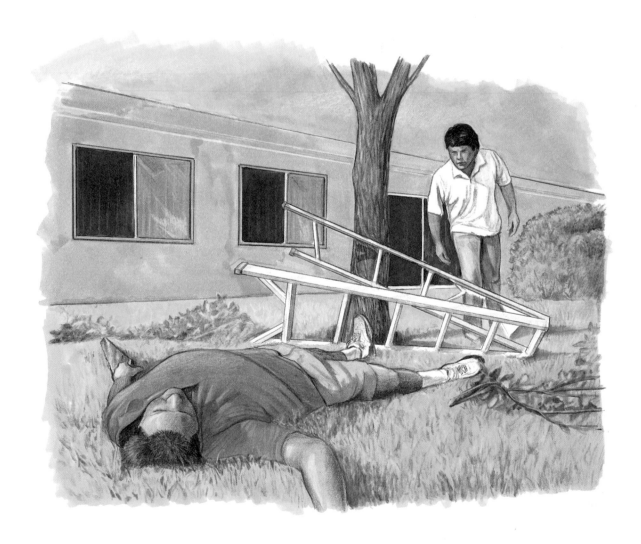

CONTENTS

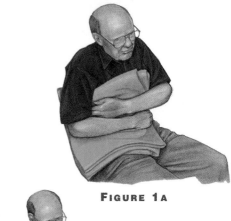

FIGURE 1A

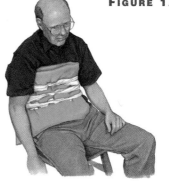

FIGURE 1B
For rib fracture, stabilize the chest with a blanket held in place (A) or loosely bandaged (B).

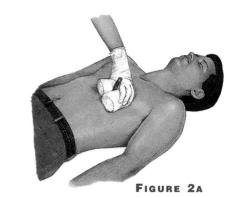

FIGURE 2A

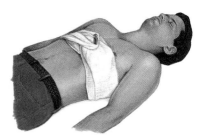

FIGURE 2B
For an impaled object in the chest, stabilize the object with bulky padding (A) and bandage to secure the object and padding (B).

LEARNING OBJECTIVES

After reading this chapter, you should be able to

1. Recognize rib fractures, impaled objects in the chest, and sucking chest wounds
2. Describe the first aid for treating chest injuries
3. Recognize blunt wounds, penetrating wounds, and protruding organs of the abdomen
4. Describe the first aid for treating abdominal injuries
5. Recognize and treat a fractured pelvis

CHEST INJURIES

All chest injury victims should have their ABCDs checked and rechecked. A responsive chest-injury victim should usually sit up or be placed with the injured side down. That position protects the uninjured side from blood inside the chest cavity and allows the lung on the uninjured side to expand.

The major symptom of a rib fracture is pain when the victim breathes, coughs, or moves. A sucking chest wound results when a chest wound allows air to pass into and out of the chest through the wound with each breath.

Care for Chest Injuries

Rib Fractures

1. Stabilize the ribs by having the victim hold a blanket or other similar soft object against the injured area **(FIGURE 1A)**. Or you can use bandages to hold the blanket in place or tie an arm over the injured area **(FIGURE 1B)**.
2. Seek medical attention.

Impaled Object in Chest

1. Stabilize the object in place with bulky dressings **(FIGURE 2A)**. Do not try to remove an impaled object. Bleeding and air in the chest cavity can result **(FIGURE 2B)**.
2. Seek medical attention.

Sucking Chest Wound

1. Have the victim take a breath and let it out; then seal the wound with anything available to stop air from entering the chest cavity. Plastic wrap or a plastic bag works well. Tape it in place with one corner untaped. That creates a flutter valve to prevent air from being trapped in the chest cavity. If plastic wrap is not available, use your gloved hand.

2. If the victim has trouble breathing or seems to be getting worse, remove the plastic cover (or your hand) to let air escape, then reapply it.

3. Seek medical attention.

ABDOMINAL INJURIES

Abdominal injuries may involve damage to internal organs. Seek medical care immediately.

Care for Abdominal Injuries

Blunt Wound

1. Place the victim on one side in a comfortable position and expect vomiting. Do not give the victim any food or drink. If you are hours from a medical facility, allow the victim to suck on a clean cloth soaked in water to relieve a dry mouth.

2. Seek medical attention.

Penetrating Wound

1. If the penetrating object is still in place, **stabilize the object and control bleeding** by using bulky dressings around it. Do not try to remove the object.

2. Seek medical attention.

Protruding Organs

1. Cover protruding organs with a sterile moist dressing or clean cloth.

2. Cover the victim lightly with a towel or blanket to maintain warmth.

3. Seek medical attention.

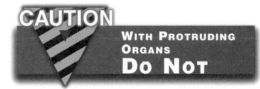

CAUTION

WITH PROTRUDING ORGANS
DO NOT

- try to reinsert protruding organs into the abdomen. You could introduce infection or damage the intestines (**FIGURE 3**).
- cover the organs tightly.
- cover the organs with any material that clings or disintegrates when wet.

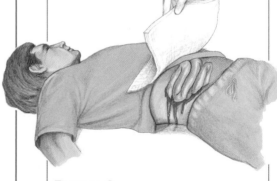

FIGURE 3
Do not reinsert protruding organs. Cover them with a moist, sterile dressing.

CHEST INJURIES

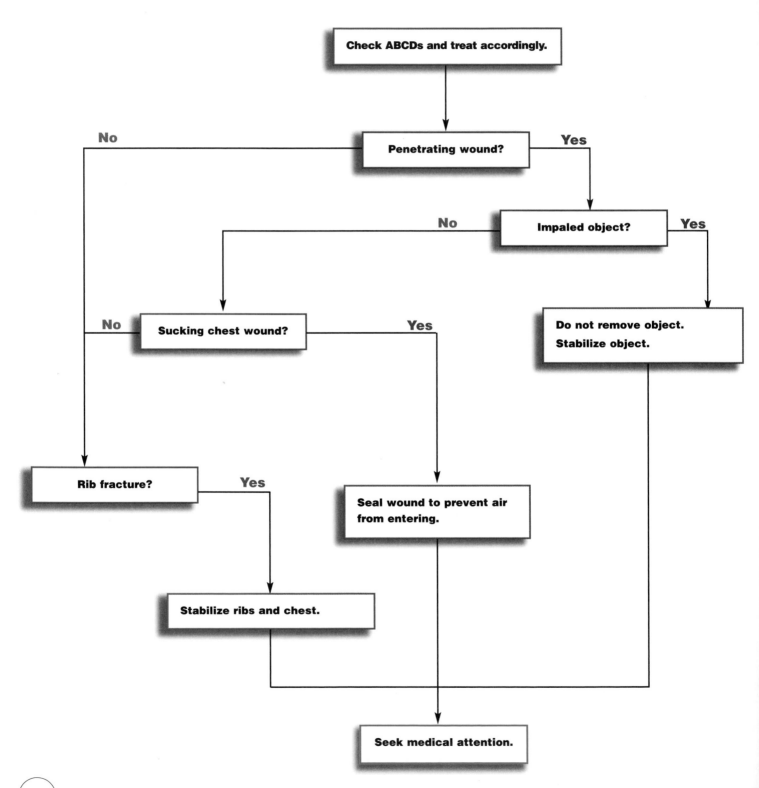

Check ABCDs and treat accordingly.

Penetrating wound?

No

Yes

Impaled object?

No

Yes

Sucking chest wound?

No

Yes

Do not remove object.
Stabilize object.

Rib fracture?

Yes

Seal wound to prevent air
from entering.

Stabilize ribs and chest.

Seek medical attention.

ABDOMINAL INJURIES

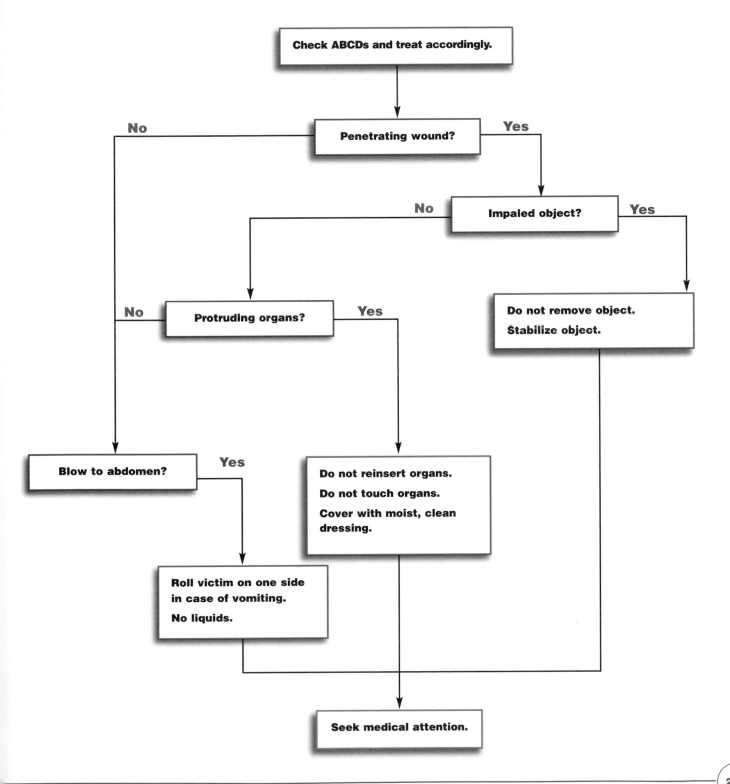

Check ABCDs and treat accordingly.

Penetrating wound?

No   Yes

Impaled object?

No   Yes

Protruding organs?

No   Yes

Do not remove object.
Stabilize object.

Blow to abdomen?   Yes

Do not reinsert organs.
Do not touch organs.
Cover with moist, clean dressing.

Roll victim on one side in case of vomiting.
No liquids.

Seek medical attention.

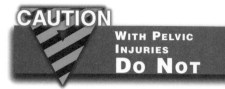

CAUTION

WITH PELVIC
INJURIES
DO NOT

- roll the victim. Additional
  internal damage could result.

- move the victim. Whenever
  possible, wait for the
  ambulance.

- apply pressure to the pelvis if
  the victim is already stating
  that it is painful.

PELVIC INJURIES

If you must move the victim, and there is concern about whether the victim's pelvis is fractured, gently press the sides of the pelvis downward and squeeze them inward at the iliac crests (upper points of the hips). A fractured pelvis will be painful. If the victim is already complaining of pain, do not apply pressure.

Care for Pelvic Injuries

1. Treat the victim for shock.

2. Place padding between the victim's thighs, then tie the victim's knees and ankles together. If the knees are bent, place padding under them for support.

3. Keep the victim on a firm surface.

4. Seek medical attention.

SUMMARY

Chest injuries include rib fractures, an impaled object in the chest, and sucking chest wounds. All are serious and require immediate medical attention. With a rib fracture, stabilize the ribs with a blanket or other bulky soft object held against the side. With an impaled object, leave the object in the chest and stabilize it with bulky dressings. With a sucking chest wound, create a flutter valve by taping plastic wrap over the wound and leaving one corner untaped to allow air out of the wound but not into it.

Abdominal injuries include blunt wounds, penetrating wounds, and protruding organs. Seek immediate medical attention for all. For a blunt wound, place the victim on one side in a comfortable position until medical assistance arrives. With an impaled object in the wound, stabilize the object with bulky dressings. If organs protrude from the wound, do not try to push the organs back into the body; cover them with a moist sterile dressing to prevent the organs from drying out. Cover the victim loosely with a towel or blanket to maintain warmth.

With a possible pelvic fracture, treat the victim for shock. Place a pad beneath the victim's thighs and tie the knees and ankles together. Keep the victim on a firm surface until the ambulance arrives.

....

All chest wounds are serious and require immediate medical attention.

....

REVIEW QUESTIONS

Chest Injuries

Directions: Circle Yes if you agree with the statement, and circle No if you disagree.

Yes   No   **1.** Stabilize a rib fracture by strapping (taping) a victim's chest as tight as possible.

Yes   No   **2.** Stabilize an impaled (embedded) object in the chest with bulky padding to prevent movement.

Yes   No   **3.** Seal off a chest wound that has air passing into and out of the chest.

Scenario 1. An iron rod breaks off and sticks into a construction worker's chest while she is tying the rods for a concrete foundation. You are called over to help with the injured worker, and you find that the iron rod has been removed. Air is passing into and out of the victim's chest with each breath she takes. What should you do?

_____

_____

_____

Scenario 2. An elderly man, shoveling snow from his driveway, slips and falls. He complains of pain when he breathes or moves. You perform a physical exam. While you are gently squeezing the sides of the chest together, he complains about the additional pain. What should you do?

_____

_____

_____

Abdominal Injuries

Yes   No   **1.** Gently push protruding organs back through the abdominal wound.

Yes   No   **2.** The dressing that is placed over protruding intestines should be kept dry.

Yes   No   **3.** Remove any penetrating object from the abdomen.

Yes   No   **4.** For a blow to the abdomen and when internal injuries are suspected, place the victim on his or her side.

Scenario 3. A 45-year-old repairman falls while carrying replacement glass for a broken window. The new glass breaks into several jagged pieces. You find him lying on his back with a blood-soaked shirt. You see a lacerated abdomen with several loops of bowel protruding through the laceration. What should you do?

_____

_____

_____

Scenario 4. A baseball runner collides with the shortstop when trying to break up a double play. The runner's shoulder hits the shortstop in the abdomen. The shortstop lies moaning on the ground and holding his abdomen. What should you do?

_____

_____

_____

Pelvic Injuries

Yes	No	**1.**	Keep the victim on a firm surface.
Yes	No	**2.**	Keep the victim's knees bent and place padding between the legs.

Scenario 5. An older secretary slips while on stairs and falls down five steps. She is at the bottom of the stairs, lying on her side. You suspect a pelvic fracture because she is complaining about severe pain in the pelvic area. What should you do?

_____

_____

_____

How did you do?

Chest Injuries
1. No; 2. Yes; 3. Yes

Abdominal Injuries
1. No; 2. No; 3. No; 4. Yes

Pelvic Injuries
1. Yes; 2. Yes

BONE, JOINT, AND MUSCLE INJURIES

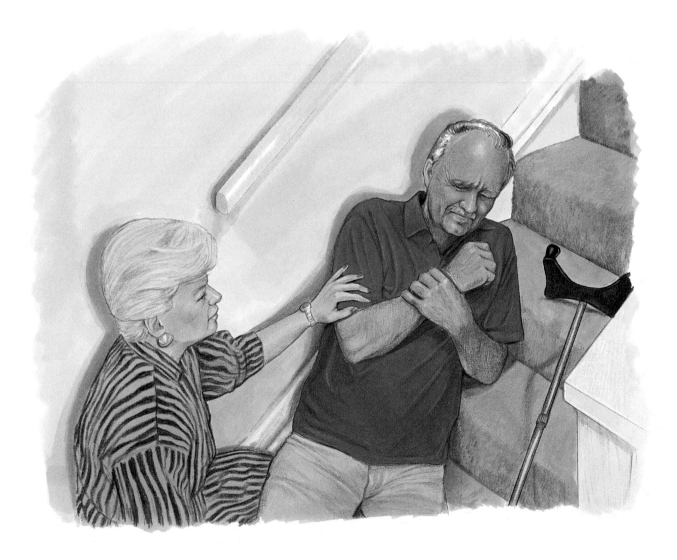

CONTENTS

16

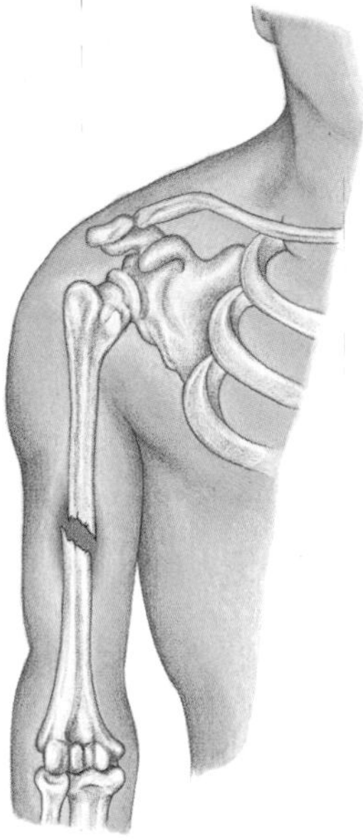

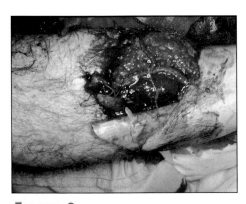

FIGURE 1A
Closed fracture.

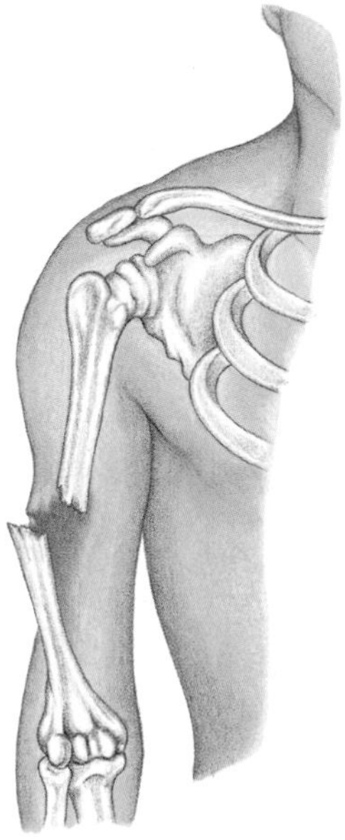

FIGURE 1B
Open fracture.

FIGURE 2
Open tibia-fibula fracture.

LEARNING OBJECTIVES

After reading this chapter, you should be able to

1. Describe the common signs and symptoms of bone, joint, and muscle injuries

2. Describe the first aid for a fracture, dislocation, sprain, strain, contusion, and cramps

3. Identify the reasons for splinting fractures and dislocations

4. Describe the various types of splints

5. Stabilize one or more of the following body parts: shoulder, clavicle, upper arm, forearm, fingers and hand, elbow (straight and bent), knee (straight and bent), thigh, lower leg, and ankle/foot

FRACTURES

The terms "fracture" and "broken bone" have the same meaning: a break or crack in a bone. There are two categories of fractures:

- In a *closed (simple) fracture,* the skin is intact and there are no open wounds anywhere near the fracture site (**FIGURE 1A**).

- In an *open (compound) fracture,* the overlying skin has been damaged or broken. The wound may be the result of the bone protruding through the skin or of a direct blow that cuts the skin at the time of the fracture. The bone might not always be visible in the wound (**FIGURE 1B**).

It may be difficult to tell if a bone is fractured. When in doubt, treat the injury as a fracture. Use the mnemonic "DOTS" in assessing the injury — Deformity, Open wound, Tenderness, Swelling:

- Deformity might or might not be obvious (**FIGURE 2**). Compare the injured part with the uninjured part on the other side.

- Open wound may indicate an underlying fracture.

- Tenderness and pain are commonly found only at the injury site. The victim usually will be able to point to the site of the pain. A useful procedure for detecting a fracture is to gently feel along the bone; a victim's complaint about pain or tenderness is a reliable sign of a fracture.

- Swelling caused by bleeding happens rapidly after a fracture.

Additional signs and symptoms of fractures include the following:

- Loss of use might or might not occur. Guarding occurs when motion produces pain; the victim tries to avoid using the injured part. Sometimes, however, the victim is able to move a fractured limb with little or no pain.

- A grating sensation can be felt and sometimes even heard when the ends of the broken bone rub together. Do not move the injured limb in an attempt to detect it.

- The history of the injury can lead you to suspect a fracture whenever a serious accident has happened. The victim may have heard or felt the bone snap.

Care for a Fracture

1. Check and treat the ABCDs. Fractures, even open fractures, seldom present an immediate threat to life.

2. Treat the victim for shock.

3. Determine what happened and the location of the injury.

4. Gently remove clothing covering the injured area. Cut clothing at the seams if necessary.

5. Look and feel the extremity.

   - Look at the injury site. Swelling and black-and-blue marks, which indicate escape of blood into the tissues, may come from either the bone end or associated muscular and blood vessel damage. Shortening or severe deformity (angulation) between the joints (FIGURE 3) or deformity around the joints, shortening of the extremity, and rotation of the extremity when compared with the opposite extremity indicate a bone injury. Lacerations or even small puncture wounds near the site of a bone fracture are considered open fractures.

   - Feel the injured area. If a fracture is not obvious, gently press, touch, or feel along the length of the bone for deformities, tenderness, and swelling.

6. Check blood flow and nerves. Use the mnemonic "CSM" — Circulation, Sensation, Movement:

   - Circulation. Feel for the radial pulse (located on the thumb side of the wrist) for an arm injury and the posterior tibial pulse (located between the inside ankle bone and the Achilles tendon) for a leg injury. A pulseless arm or leg is a significant emergency that requires immediate surgical care. Because the major blood vessels of an extremity run close to bone, they may be torn by bone fragments or pinched off between the ends of the broken bone. The tissues of the arms and legs cannot survive without a continuing blood supply for more than two or three hours. A lack of a pulse requires seeking immediate medical attention.

   - Sensation. Lightly touch or squeeze the victim's toes or fingers and ask the victim what he or she feels. Loss of sensation is an early sign of nerve damage or spinal damage.

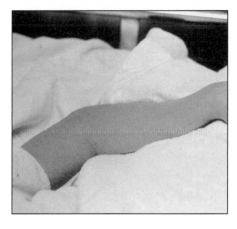

FIGURE 3A
Deformity of forearm fracture.

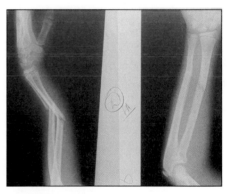

FIGURE 3B
X-rays of forearm fracture before and after setting.

B O N E
I N J U R I E S

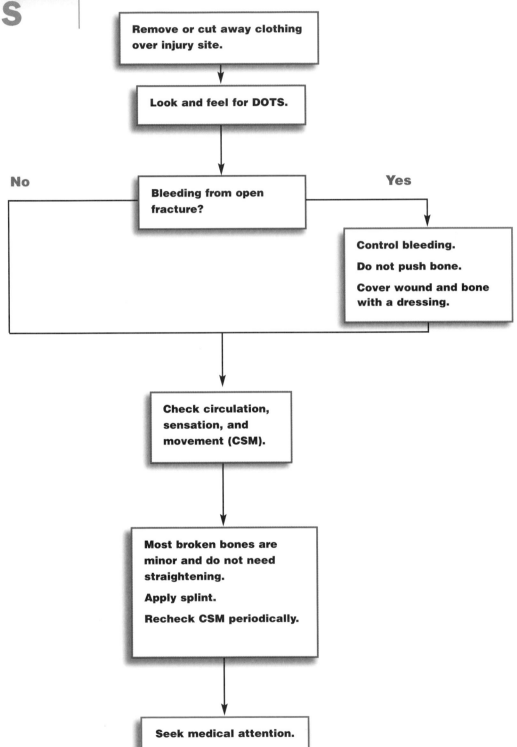

Remove or cut away clothing over injury site.

↓

Look and feel for DOTS.

↓

No ← Bleeding from open fracture? → **Yes**

Control bleeding.

Do not push bone.

Cover wound and bone with a dressing.

↓

Check circulation, sensation, and movement (CSM).

↓

Most broken bones are minor and do not need straightening.

Apply splint.

Recheck CSM periodically.

↓

Seek medical attention.

- Movement. Check for nerve damage by asking the victim to wiggle the toes or fingers, unless they are injured.

7. Use the RICE (**R**est, **I**ce, **C**ompression, **E**levation) procedures (see pages 250-254).

8. Use a splint to stabilize the fracture (see pages 254-259). Most fractures do not require rapid transportation. An exception is an arm or a leg without a pulse, indicating insufficient blood flow to that extremity. In that case, immediate medical attention is necessary.

JOINT INJURIES

Dislocations

A dislocation occurs when a joint comes apart and stays apart with the bone ends no longer in contact. The shoulders, elbows, fingers, hips, kneecaps, and ankles are the joints that are most frequently affected. Dislocations cause signs and symptoms similar to those of a fracture: deformity, severe pain, swelling, and the inability of the victim to move the injured joint. The main sign of a dislocation is deformity: Its appearance is different from an uninjured joint.

Care for Dislocations

1. Check CSM (circulation, sensation, movement). If the end of the dislocated bone is pressing on nerves or blood vessels, numbness or paralysis may exist below the dislocation. Always check the pulses. If there is no pulse in the injured extremity, transport the victim to a medical facility immediately.

2. Use the RICE procedures (see pages 250-254).

3. Use a splint to stabilize the joint in the position in which it was found.

4. Do not try to reduce the joint (put the displaced parts back into their normal positions), since nerve and blood vessel damage could result.

5. Seek medical attention for reduction of the dislocation.

Sprains

A sprain is an injury to a joint in which the ligaments and other tissues are damaged by violent stretching or twisting. Attempts to move or use the joint increase the pain. The skin around the joint may be discolored because of bleeding from torn

---

**CRITICAL CONCEPTS:
IS IT A FRACTURE?**

- It can be difficult to tell if a bone is fractured.
- Look at the injury site and check circulation, sensation, and movement if possible.
- When in doubt, treat the injury as if it is a fracture.
- Use RICE: Rest, Ice, Compression, and Elevation.

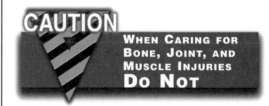

CAUTION WHEN CARING FOR BONE, JOINT, AND MUSCLE INJURIES **DO NOT**

- apply heat for at least 48 hours.

CHECKING AN EXTREMITY'S CSM

Check an upper extremity for:

1. **Circulation: radial pulse** (FIGURE 4A).
2. **Sensation: squeeze fingers** (FIGURE 4B).
3. **Movement: wiggle fingers** (FIGURE 4C).

Check a lower extremity for:

4. **Circulation: posterior tibial pulse** (FIGURE 4D).
5. **Sensation: squeeze toe** (FIGURE 4E).
6. **Movement: wiggle toes** (FIGURE 4F).

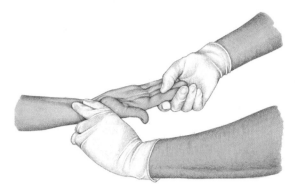

FIGURE 4A

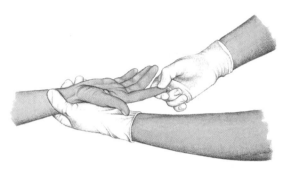

FIGURE 4B

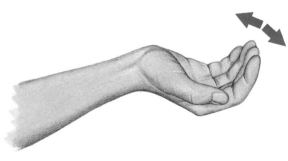

FIGURE 4C

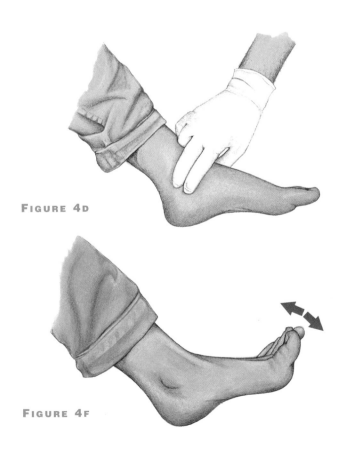

FIGURE 4D

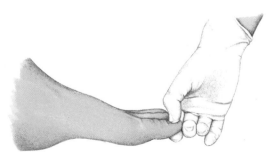

FIGURE 4E

FIGURE 4F

FLOW CHART
SPRAINS, STRAINS, CONTUSIONS, DISLOCATIONS

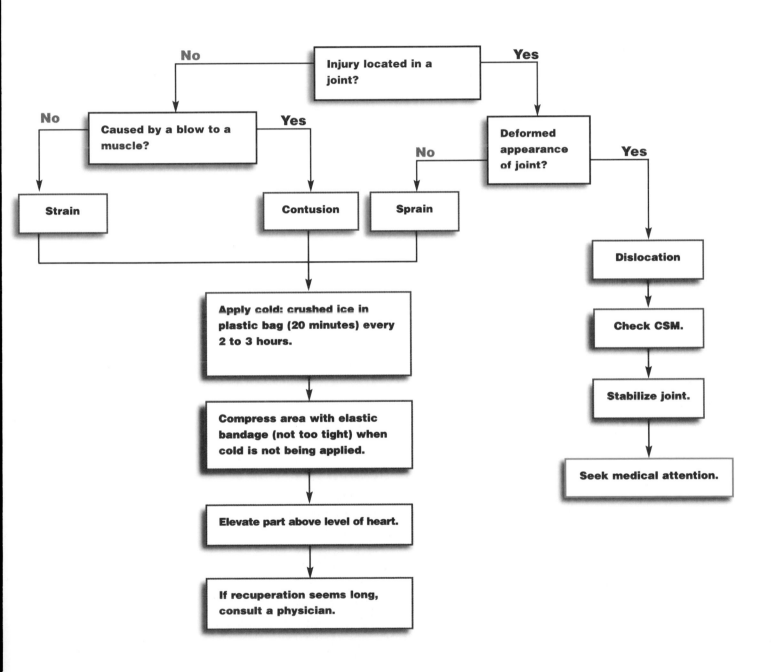

No ← **Injury located in a joint?** → **Yes**

No ← **Caused by a blow to a muscle?** → **Yes**

No ← **Deformed appearance of joint?** → **Yes**

Strain

Contusion

Sprain

Dislocation

Apply cold: crushed ice in plastic bag (20 minutes) every 2 to 3 hours.

Check CSM.

Compress area with elastic bandage (not too tight) when cold is not being applied.

Stabilize joint.

Elevate part above level of heart.

Seek medical attention.

If recuperation seems long, consult a physician.

tissues. It often is difficult to distinguish between a severe sprain and a fracture, because their signs and symptoms are similar. Give this first aid:

1. Use the RICE treatment: rest, ice, compression, and elevation. See pages 250-254 for the RICE procedure for bone, joint and muscle injuries.

2. Use cold promptly to keep swelling out of a joint, and make the swelling recede as quickly as possible with a compression (elastic) bandage.

MUSCLE INJURIES

Strains

A muscle strain, or pull, occurs when a muscle is stretched beyond its normal range of motion, resulting in the muscle's tearing. Any of the following signs and symptoms may indicate a muscle strain:

- Sharp pain
- Extreme tenderness when the area is touched
- A cavity, indentation, or bump that can be felt or seen
- Severe weakness and loss of function of the injured part
- Stiffness and pain when the victim moves the muscle

For first aid for a muscle strain, use the RICE procedures (pages 250-254).

Contusions

A muscle contusion, or bruise, results from a blow to the muscle. Any of the following signs and symptoms may occur in a muscle contusion:

- Swelling
- Pain and tenderness
- A black-and-blue mark appearing hours later

For first aid for a contusion, use the RICE procedures (pages 250-254).

Cramps

A cramp occurs when a muscle goes into an uncontrolled spasm and contraction, resulting in severe pain and restriction or loss of movement.

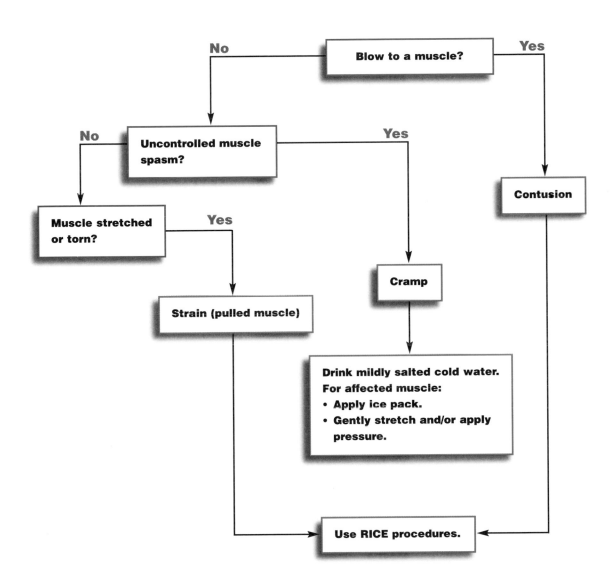

No → **Blow to a muscle?** ← Yes

Uncontrolled muscle spasm?

No

Yes

Contusion

Muscle stretched or torn?

Yes

Cramp

Strain (pulled muscle)

Drink mildly salted cold water.
For affected muscle:
• **Apply ice pack.**
• **Gently stretch and/or apply pressure.**

Use RICE procedures.

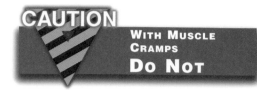

CAUTION

WITH MUSCLE CRAMPS
DO NOT

- give salt tablets to a person with muscle cramps. Salt tablets can cause stomach irritation, nausea, and vomiting.
- massage or rub the affected muscle. This only causes more pain and does not relieve the cramping.

Care for Cramps

There are many treatments for cramps. Try one or more of the following:

1. Have the victim gently stretch the affected muscle. Because a muscle cramp is an uncontrolled muscle contraction or spasm, a gradual lengthening of the muscle may help to lengthen the muscle fibers and relieve the cramp.

2. Relax the muscle by applying pressure to it.

3. Apply ice to the cramped muscle to make it relax (except in a cold environment).

4. Pinch the upper lip hard (an acupressure technique) to reduce calf muscle cramping.

5. Drink lightly salted cool water (dissolve 1/4 teaspoon salt in a quart of water) or a commercial sports drink.

RICE PROCEDURE FOR BONE, JOINT, AND MUSCLE INJURIES

RICE is the acronym for the first aid procedures Rest, Ice, Compression, Elevation for bone, joint, and muscle injuries. What is done in the first 48 to 72 hours after such an injury can do a lot to relieve, even prevent, aches and pains. Treat all extremity bone, joint, and muscle injuries with the RICE procedure described below. In addition to RICE, fractures and dislocations should be splinted to stabilize the injured area. (See pages 255-259 for splinting techniques.)

Care for Bone, Joint, and Muscle injuries

R = Rest

Injuries heal faster if they are rested. Rest means that the victim stays off the injured part. Use of a body part increases the blood circulation to that area, which can cause more swelling of an injured part. Crutches may be used to rest injuries to the leg.

I = Ice

An ice pack should be applied to the area as soon as possible after the injury for 20 to 30 minutes every 2 to 3 hours during the first 24 to 48 hours. Skin that is being treated with cold passes through four stages: cold, burning, aching, and numbness. When the skin becomes numb, usually in 20 to 30 minutes, remove the ice pack. Then compress the injured part with an elastic bandage and keep it elevated.

Cold constricts the blood vessels to and in the injured area, which helps to reduce the swelling and inflammation and at the same time dulls the pain and relieves muscle spasms. Heat has the opposite effect when applied to fresh injuries: It increases circulation to the area and greatly increases both the swelling and the pain.

Use either of the following methods to apply cold to an injury:

- Put crushed ice (or cubes) into a double plastic bag, ice bag, or hot water bottle. Place the ice pack on the skin directly over the injury and shape or mold it to the general contour of the body part. Secure it in place with an elastic bandage.
- Use a chemical cold pack, a sealed pouch that contains two chemical envelopes. Squeezing the pack mixes the chemicals, producing a chemical reaction that has a cooling effect. Although they do not cool as well as other methods, they are convenient to use when ice is not readily available. They lose their cooling power quickly, however, and can be used only once. Also, they may be impractical because of their expense and the possibility of breakage.

C = Compression

Compression of the injured area may squeeze some fluid and debris out of the injury site. Compression limits the ability of the skin and of other tissues to expand and reduces internal bleeding. Apply an elastic bandage to the injured area, especially the foot, ankle, knee, thigh, hand, or elbow. Fill the hollow areas with padding (eg, a sock or a washcloth) before applying the elastic bandage.

Elastic bandages come in various sizes, for different body areas:

- 2″ width, used for the wrist or hand
- 3″ width, used for the elbow or arm
- 4″ or 6″ width, used for the ankle, knee, or leg

Start the elastic bandage several inches below the injury and wrap in an upward, overlapping (about one-half the bandage's width) spiral, starting with even and somewhat tight pressure, then gradually wrapping more loosely above the injury.

Applying compression may be the most important step in preventing swelling. The victim should wear the elastic bandage continuously for 18 to 24 hours (except when cold is applied). At night, have the victim loosen but not remove the elastic bandage.

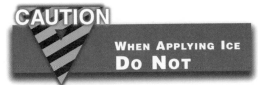

CAUTION

WHEN APPLYING ICE
DO NOT

- apply an ice pack for more than 20 to 30 minutes at a time. Frostbite or nerve damage can result.
- apply an ice pack on the back outside part of the knee. Nerve damage can occur.
- apply cold if the victim has a history of circulatory disease, Raynaud's syndrome (spasms in the arteries of the extremities that reduce circulation), abnormal sensitivity to cold, or If the injured part has been frostbitten previously.
- stop using an ice pack too soon. A common mistake is using heat too early, which will result in swelling and pain.

RICE PROCEDURES FOR AN ANKLE

1. **R = Rest**

   Stop using the injured part. Continued use could cause further injury, delay healing, increase pain, and stimulate bleeding. Get the victim into a comfortable position, either sitting or lying down. This slows blood flow to the injured area.

2. **I = Ice** (FIGURE 5A–B)

   An ice pack should be applied as soon as possible after the injury to the area for 20 to 30 minutes every 2 to 3 hours during the first 24 to 48 hours.

3. **C = Compression** (FIGURE 5C–E)

   Compression limits the ability of the skin and of other tissues to expand and reduces internal bleeding. Apply an elastic bandage to the injured area, especially the foot, ankle, knee, thigh, hand, or elbow.

4. **E = Elevation**

   Elevating the injured part is another way to decrease swelling and pain. While icing or compressing, elevate the part in whatever way is most convenient. The aim of this step is to get the injured part higher than the heart, if possible.

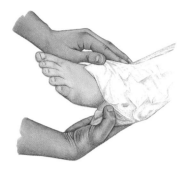

FIGURE 5A
Place ice bag on skin.

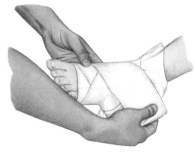

FIGURE 5B
Use elastic to hold ice pack.

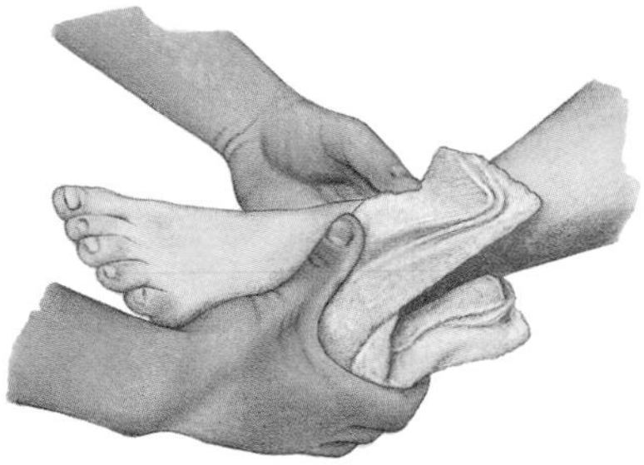

FIGURE 5C
Remove ice pack. Place "U" shaped cloth around ankle knob.

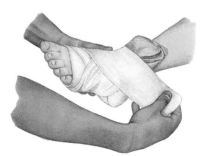

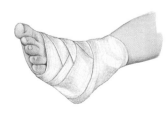

FIGURE 5D
Use elastic bandage to hold "U" shaped cloth.

FIGURE 5E
Cover heel and close to the toes.

ANKLE INJURIES

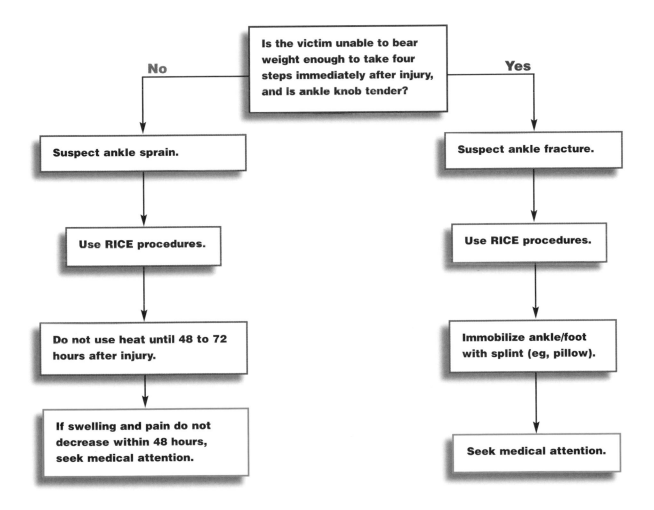

Is the victim unable to bear weight enough to take four steps immediately after injury, and is ankle knob tender?

No → Suspect ankle sprain. → Use RICE procedures. → Do not use heat until 48 to 72 hours after injury. → If swelling and pain do not decrease within 48 hours, seek medical attention.

Yes → Suspect ankle fracture. → Use RICE procedures. → Immobilize ankle/foot with splint (eg, pillow). → Seek medical attention.

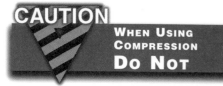

CAUTION

WHEN USING
COMPRESSION
DO NOT

- apply an elastic bandage too tightly, which will restrict circulation.

Stretch a new elastic bandage to about one-third its maximum length for adequate compression. Leave fingers and toes exposed so that possible color change can be observed. Compare the toes or fingers of the injured extremity with those of the uninjured one. Pale skin, pain, numbness, and tingling are signs that an elastic bandage is too tight. If any of these signs or symptoms appears, immediately remove the elastic bandage. Leave the elastic bandage off until all the symptoms disappear, then rewrap the area, but less tightly. Always wrap from below the injury and move toward the heart.

For an ankle injury, place a horseshoe-shaped pad around the ankle knob and under the elastic bandage. The pad will permit compression of the soft tissues rather than just the bones. Wrap the bandage most tightly nearest the toes and most loosely above the ankle. It should be tight enough to decrease swelling but not tight enough to inhibit blood flow.

For a contusion or a strain, place a pad between the injury and the elastic bandage.

E = Elevation

Gravity slows the return of blood to the heart from lower parts of the body. Accumulation of fluid leads to swelling in that part of the body. Once fluid gets to the hands or feet, the fluid has nowhere else to go, and those parts of the body swell. Elevating the injured area, in combination with ice and compression, limits circulation to that area, which in turn helps to limit internal bleeding and minimize swelling.

It is simple to prop up an injured leg or arm to limit bleeding. Whenever possible, elevate the injured part above the level of the heart for the first 24 hours after an injury. If a fracture is suspected, do not elevate an extremity until it has been stabilized with a splint. Along with RICE, fractures and dislocations should be splinted.

SPLINTING EXTREMITIES

Most extremity fractures are minor. Because medical help is usually nearby, the injury can be stabilized by splinting the extremity in the position in which it was found. To stabilize means to use any method to hold a body part still and prevent movement. All fractures should be stabilized by splinting before a victim is moved to

- Reduce pain
- Prevent damage to muscle, nerves, and blood vessels
- Prevent a closed fracture from becoming an open fracture
- Reduce bleeding and swelling

Types of Splints

A splint is any device that is used to stabilize a fracture or a dislocation. Such a device can be improvised (eg, a newspaper), or it can be one of several commercially available splints (eg, SAM Splint™ or air splint). The lack of a commercial splint should never prevent you from properly stabilizing an injured extremity. Splinting sometimes requires ingenuity or improvisation.

A rigid splint is an inflexible device that is attached to an extremity to maintain stability. It may be a padded board, a piece of heavy cardboard, or a SAM Splint™ molded to fit the extremity. Whatever its construction, a rigid splint must be long enough to be secured well above and below the fracture site. A soft splint, such as an air splint, is useful mainly for stabilizing fractures of the lower leg or the forearm.

A self splint, or anatomic splint, is almost always available. A self splint is one in which the injured body part is tied to an uninjured part. For example, an injured finger can be splinted to an adjacent finger, the legs can be splinted together, or an injured arm can be splinted to the chest.

Care for Fractures: Splinting

All fractures and dislocations should be stabilized before the victim is moved. When in doubt, apply a splint:

1. Cover all open wounds, if any, with a dry, sterile dressing before applying a splint.

2. Check CSM in the extremity. If pulses are absent and medical help is hours away, try to straighten a mid-shaft fracture or a shoulder dislocation to restore blood flow.

3. Determine what to splint by using the *Rule of Thirds*. Imagine each long bone as being divided into thirds. If the injury is located in the upper or lower third of a bone, assume that the nearest joint is injured. Therefore, the splint should extend to stabilize the bones above and below the unstable joint; for example, for a fracture of the upper third of the tibia (shinbone), the splint must extend to include the upper leg, as well as the lower leg, because the knee is unstable.

   For a fracture of the middle third of a bone, stabilize the joints above and below the fracture (eg, wrist and elbow for fractured radius or ulna; shoulder and elbow for fractured humerus; knee and ankle for fractured tibia or fibula). An upper extremity fracture, in addition to being splinted, should be placed in an arm sling and a swathe (binder).

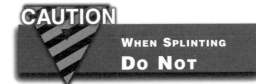

CAUTION

WHEN SPLINTING

DO NOT

- straighten dislocations or fractures of the spine, elbow, wrist, hip, or knee because of the proximity of major nerves and arteries.

4. If two first aiders are present, one should support the injury site and minimize movement of the extremity until splinting is completed.

5. When possible, place splint materials on both sides of the injured part, especially when two bones are involved (eg, radius/ulna or tibia/fibula). This "sandwich splint" prevents rotation of the injured extremity and keeps the two bones from touching. With rigid splints, use extra padding in natural body hollows and around any deformities.

6. Apply splints firmly but not so tight that blood flow into an extremity is affected. Check CSM before and periodically after the splint is applied. If the pulse disappears, loosen the splint enough so you can feel the pulse. Leave the fingers or toes exposed so that CSM can be checked easily.

7. Use RICE on the injured part. When practical, elevate the injured extremity after stabilization to promote drainage and reduce swelling. Do not apply ice packs if a pulse is absent.

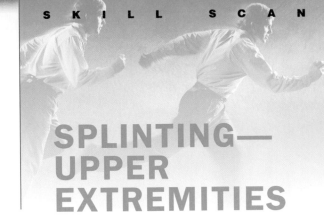

SPLINTING— UPPER EXTREMITIES

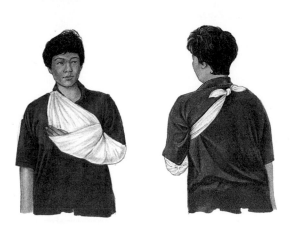

FIGURE 6A
Arm sling: shoulder and clavicle injuries.

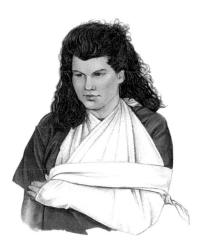

FIGURE 6B
Arm sling and swathe for upper extremity injuries.

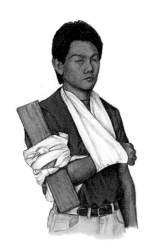

FIGURE 6C
Upper arm (humerus).

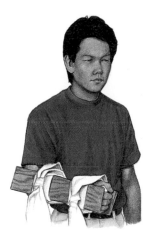

FIGURE 6D
Forearm (radius/ulna).

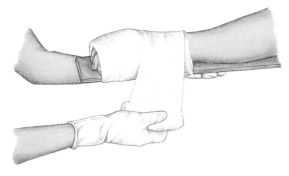

FIGURE 6E
Fingers and hand (position of function).

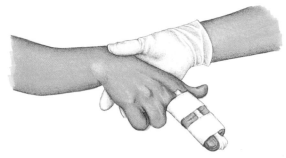

FIGURE 6F
Self-splint: fingers.

SPLINTING— ELBOW AND KNEE

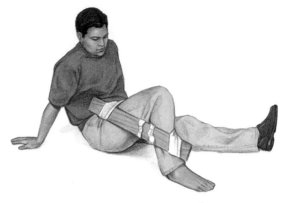

FIGURE 7C
Knee in bent position.

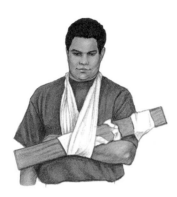

FIGURE 7A
Elbow in bent position.

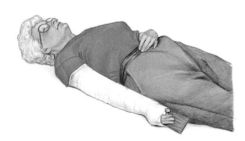

FIGURE 7B
Elbow in straight position.

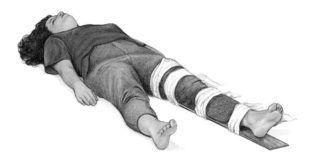

FIGURE 7D
Knee in straight position.

SPLINTING— LOWER EXTREMITIES

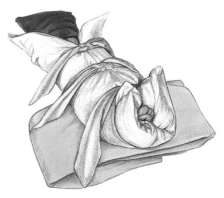

FIGURE 8A
Ankle/foot.

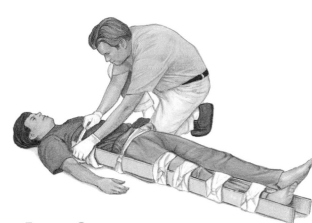

FIGURE 8C
Thigh (femur).

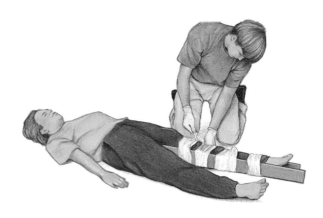

FIGURE 8B
Lower leg (tibia/fibula).

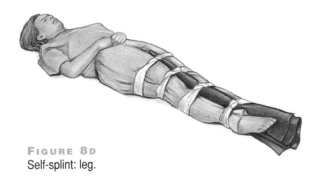

FIGURE 8D
Self-splint: leg.

SUMMARY

The RICE procedure (rest, ice, compression, elevation) is used for bone, joint, and muscle injuries. Rest and immobilize the injured area. Apply ice to the area frequently over the first 1 to 2 days. Use an elastic bandage to apply compression of the injured area, but check that circulation is not cut off. Elevate the area for the first 24 hours to help prevent swelling.

In addition, for fractures check the ABCDs and treat the victim for shock. Check for circulation, sensation, and movement (CSM). Use a splint to stabilize the fracture. For dislocations, check the CSM and splint the joint in the position found.

RICE procedures are also used for muscle contusions. For muscle cramps, use stretching, pressure, or ice.

Fractures and dislocations should be splinted to reduce pain, prevent damage, and reduce bleeding and swelling. Splints may be rigid splints, commercial splints, or anatomic splints. Splint above and below the injury. Splint both sides of an extremity. Apply splints firm enough to immobilize the area but not so tight that circulation is cut off.

REVIEW QUESTIONS

Fractures

Directions: Circle Yes if you agree with the statement, and circle No if you disagree.

Yes   **No**   1. For a suspected arm or leg fracture, check blood flow and nerves.

Yes   **No**   2. Apply cold on a suspected fracture.

Yes   **No**   3. A splint can help to stabilize (keep in place) a fracture.

Dislocations and Sprains

Yes   **No**   1. The letters RICE represent the treatment for sprains and dislocations.

Yes   **No**   2. When using ice, place it directly on the skin.

Yes   **No**   3. Applying heat to the injury too soon is a mistake.

Yes   **No**   4. An elastic bandage, if used correctly, can help to control swelling in a joint.

Muscle Injuries

Yes   **No**   1. Give salt tablets to a person who is suffering from muscle cramps.

Yes   **No**   2. Apply heat initially to a muscle injury.

Yes   **No**   3. An elastic bandage, if used correctly, can help to limit swelling.

Scenario 1. While changing a light bulb in a high ceiling lighting fixture, an electrician falls off a 10-foot ladder. He complains about pain in his left lower leg. You look at the leg and feel it. You find slight swelling, and when compared with the uninjured leg, the injured one has a slight bend in it. What should you do?

_____

_____

_____

Scenario 2. While descending a set of stairs in a warehouse, a worker misses a step, slips, and bounces her knee on the landing. Upon checking it, you find a bony prominence on the outside of the knee. It looks as though the kneecap (patella) is dislocated. What should you do?

_____

_____

_____

Scenario 3. During a company picnic's "flag football" game, one of your teammates suddenly stops and sits on the ground holding her calf muscle. It's a hot, humid summer afternoon. What should you do?

_____

_____

_____

Scenario 4. During a city league basketball game, one of the players turns his ankle. He hobbles with difficulty and pain off the court. What should you do?

_____

_____

_____

HOW DID YOU DO?

Fractures
1. Yes; **2.** Yes; **3.** Yes

Dislocations and Sprains
1. Yes; **2.** Yes; **3.** Yes; **4.** Yes

Muscle Injuries
1. No; **2.** No; **3.** Yes

SUDDEN ILLNESS

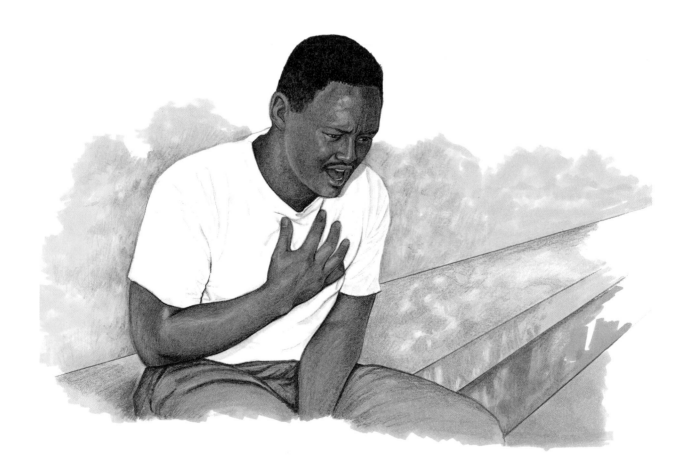

CONTENTS

17

LEARNING OBJECTIVES

After reading this chapter, you should be able to

1. Describe the signs and symptoms of asthma, hyperventilation, fainting, seizures, diabetic emergencies, vaginal bleeding, and pregnancy emergencies

2. Describe the first aid for asthma, hyperventilation, fainting, seizures, diabetic emergencies, vaginal bleeding, and pregnancy emergencies

ASTHMA

The signs and symptoms of a person having an asthma attack are

- Coughing
- Cyanosis (bluish skin color)
- Inability to speak in complete sentences without pausing for breath
- Nostrils flaring with each breath
- Difficulty breathing, including wheezing (high-pitched whistling sound during breathing)

Care for Asthma

1. Check the ABCs.

2. Keep the victim in a comfortable upright position that makes it easier to breathe.

3. Ask the victim about any **asthma medication** he or she may be using. Most asthma sufferers will have some form of asthma medication, usually administered through physician-prescribed, hand-held inhalers **(FIGURE 1).**

4. If the victim does not respond well to his or her inhaled medication or is having an extreme asthma attack (known as status asthmaticus), seek medical attention immediately.

HYPERVENTILATION

Fast, deep breathing, called hyperventilation, is common during psychological stress. The signs and symptoms are

- Dizziness or lightheadedness
- Numbness
- Tingling of the hands and feet
- Shortness of breath
- Breathing rates faster than 40 per minute

CAUTION

WITH AN ASTHMA VICTIM DO NOT

- delay getting medical help for the victim of a severe asthma attack.

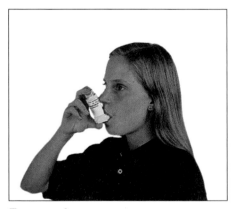

FIGURE 1

Care for Hyperventilation

1. Calm and reassure the person.

2. Encourage the person to breathe slowly, using the abdominal muscles: Inhale through the nose, hold the full inhalation for several seconds, then exhale slowly through pursed lips.

FAINTING

Most fainting is caused by decreased blood flow to the brain, which may result from a medical condition or from fright, anxiety, drugs, or fatigue. Sitting or standing for a long time without moving, especially in a hot environment, can also cause a person to faint. Someone who is about to faint usually will have one or more of the following signs and symptoms:

- Dizziness
- Weakness
- Seeing spots
- Visual blurring
- Nausea
- Pale skin
- Sweating

Most fainting episodes are not serious, and the victim regains consciousness quickly. However, seek medical attention if the victim

- Has had repeated attacks of unconsciousness
- Does not quickly regain consciousness
- Loses consciousness while sitting or lying down
- Faints for no apparent reason

Care for Fainting

1. Prevent the person from falling.

2. Help the person to lie down and raise his or her legs 8″ to 12″. This position increases venous blood flow back to the heart, which in turn pumps more blood to the brain.

3. Loosen tight clothing and belts.

4. If the victim has fallen, check for any sign of injury. If no injury is suspected, have the victim slowly regain an upright posture.

5. Fresh air and a cool, wet cloth for the face usually aid recovery.

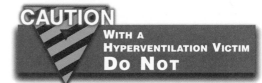

CAUTION

WITH A HYPERVENTILATION VICTIM DO NOT

- have the person breathe into a paper bag.

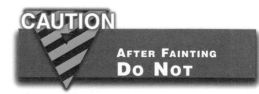

CAUTION

AFTER FAINTING DO NOT

- splash or pour water on the victim's face.
- use smelling salts or ammonia inhalants.
- slap the victim's face in an attempt to revive him or her.
- give the victim anything to drink until he or she has fully recovered and can swallow.

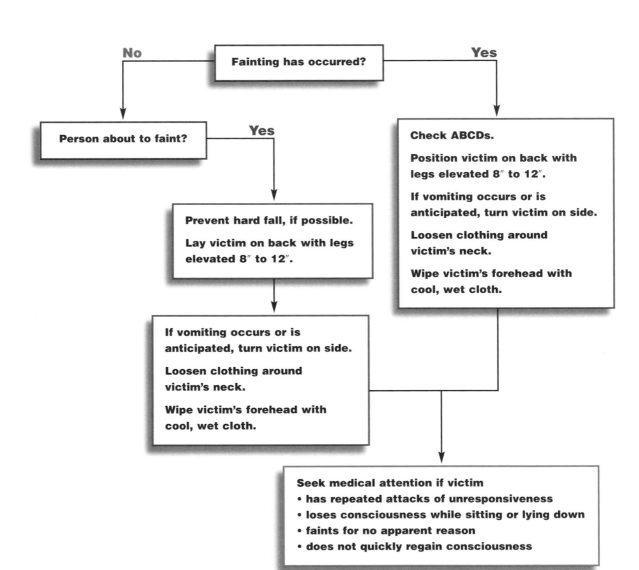

No ← **Fainting has occurred?** → **Yes**

Person about to faint? → **Yes**

Check ABCDs.

Position victim on back with legs elevated 8″ to 12″.

If vomiting occurs or is anticipated, turn victim on side.

Loosen clothing around victim's neck.

Wipe victim's forehead with cool, wet cloth.

Prevent hard fall, if possible.

Lay victim on back with legs elevated 8″ to 12″.

If vomiting occurs or is anticipated, turn victim on side.

Loosen clothing around victim's neck.

Wipe victim's forehead with cool, wet cloth.

Seek medical attention if victim
- **has repeated attacks of unresponsiveness**
- **loses consciousness while sitting or lying down**
- **faints for no apparent reason**
- **does not quickly regain consciousness**

SEIZURES

A seizure is the result of an abnormal stimulation of the brain's cells. It can be mild, whereby the victim looks as if he or she is daydreaming, or severe, involving convulsions of the entire body. A variety of medical conditions increase the instability or irritability of the brain and can lead to seizures, including the following:

- Epilepsy
- Heatstroke
- Poisoning
- Electric shock
- Hypoglycemia
- High fever in children
- Brain injury, tumor, or stroke
- Alcohol withdrawal, drug abuse/overdose

Epilepsy is not a mental illness, and it is not a sign of low intelligence. It also is not contagious. Between seizures, a person with epilepsy can function as normally as a nonepileptic.

Care for Seizures

The Epilepsy Foundation lists the following first aid procedures for seizures:

1. Cushion the victim's head; **remove items that could cause injury** if the victim bumped into them.

2. Loosen any tight neckwear.

3. Turn the victim onto his or her left side.

4. **Look for a medical-alert identification tag** (bracelet or necklace).

5. As the seizure ends, offer your help. Most seizures in people with epilepsy are not medical emergencies. They end after a minute or two without harm and usually do not require medical attention.

6. **Call EMS if any of the following exists:**

   - A seizure happens to someone who is not known to have a seizure disorder. It could be a sign of serious illness.

   - A seizure lasts more than 5 minutes.

   - The victim is slow to recover, has a second seizure, or has difficulty breathing afterward.

   - The victim is pregnant or has another medical condition.

   - There are any signs of injury or illnesses.

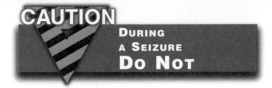

CAUTION

DURING A SEIZURE DO NOT

- give the victim anything to eat or drink.
- hold the victim down.
- put anything between the victim's teeth.
- throw any liquid on the victim's face or pour liquid into the victim's mouth.
- move the victim to another location, unless needed for safety.

SEIZURES

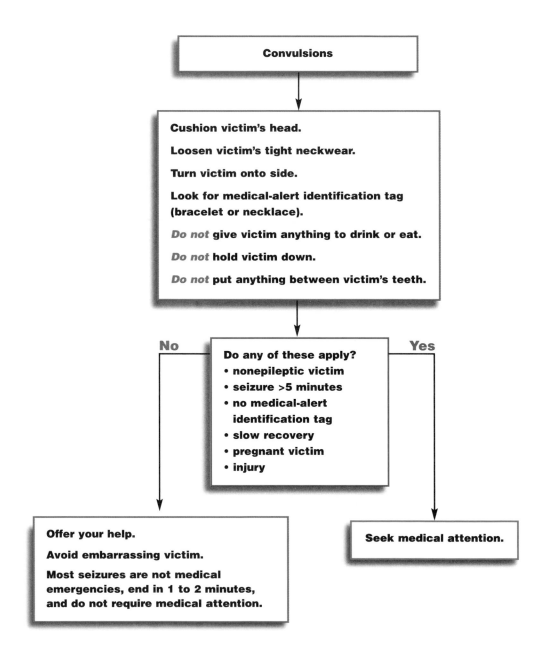

Convulsions

Cushion victim's head.

Loosen victim's tight neckwear.

Turn victim onto side.

Look for medical-alert identification tag (bracelet or necklace).

Do not give victim anything to drink or eat.

Do not hold victim down.

Do not put anything between victim's teeth.

No   **Yes**

Do any of these apply?
- nonepileptic victim
- seizure >5 minutes
- no medical-alert identification tag
- slow recovery
- pregnant victim
- injury

Offer your help.

Avoid embarrassing victim.

Most seizures are not medical emergencies, end in 1 to 2 minutes, and do not require medical attention.

Seek medical attention.

DIABETIC EMERGENCIES

Diabetes is a condition in which insulin, a hormone produced by the pancreas that helps the body to use the energy in food, is either lacking or ineffective. Insulin is needed to take sugar from the blood and carry it into body cells. When insulin levels are low, diabetes results. There are two types of diabetes:

- *Type I: juvenile-onset or insulin-dependent diabetes.* Type I diabetics require external (not made by the body) insulin to allow sugar to pass from the blood into cells. When deprived of external insulin, the diabetic becomes quite ill.

- *Type II: adult-onset or noninsulin-dependent diabetes.* Type II diabetics tend to be overweight. They may not be dependent on external insulin. If their insulin level is low, problems result, including dehydration.

The body is continuously balancing sugar and insulin (**FIGURE 2**). Too much insulin and not enough sugar lead to low blood sugar, possibly insulin shock. Too much sugar and not enough insulin lead to high blood sugar, possibly diabetic coma.

Low Blood Sugar

Very low blood sugar, called hypoglycemia, is sometimes referred to as an "insulin reaction." This condition can be caused by too much insulin, too little or delayed food intake, exercise, alcohol, or any combination of these factors.

The American Diabetes Association lists the following signs and symptoms of insulin reaction and hypoglycemia as diabetic emergencies requiring first aid:

- Sudden onset
- Staggering, poor coordination
- Anger, bad temper
- Pale color
- Confusion, disorientation
- Sudden hunger
- Excessive sweating
- Trembling
- Eventual unconsciousness

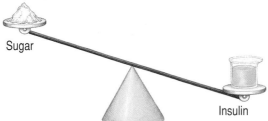

FIGURE 2A
Excess insulin is the cause of insulin shock.

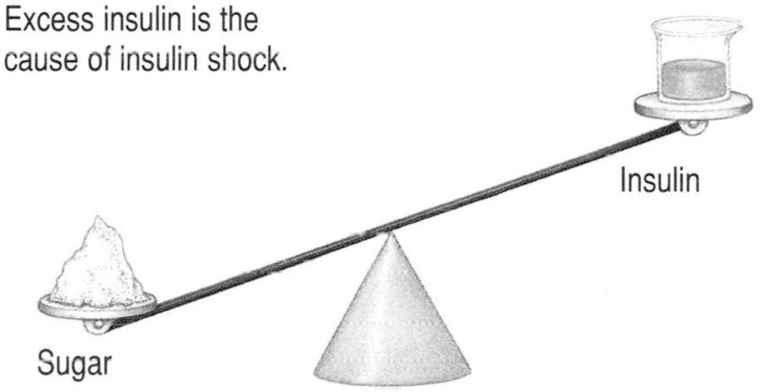

FIGURE 2B
Insufficient insulin is the cause of diabetic coma.

**CRITICAL CONCEPTS:
IS IT A DIABETIC COMA
OR INSULIN SHOCK?**

If you are uncertain whether a
conscious victim is in a diabetic
coma or insulin shock, give sugar.

Care for Low Blood Sugar

Give sugar if all three conditions are present:

- The victim is a known diabetic, and
- The victim's mental status is altered, and
- The victim is awake enough to swallow.

1. Give the victim a sugar-containing food, such as soda, candy, milk, or fruit juice. Do not use diet drinks because they do not contain sugar.

2. If improvement is not seen in 15 minutes, take the victim to a hospital.

High Blood Sugar

Hyperglycemia is the opposite of hypoglycemia. Hyperglycemia occurs when the body has too much sugar in the blood. This condition may be caused by insufficient insulin, overeating, inactivity, illness, stress, or a combination of these factors.

The American Diabetes Association lists the following signs and symptoms of diabetic coma and hyperglycemia as diabetic emergencies requiring first aid:

- Gradual onset
- Drowsiness
- Extreme thirst
- Very frequent urination
- Flushed skin
- Vomiting
- Fruity breath odor
- Heavy breathing
- Eventual unconsciousness

Care for High or Low Blood Sugar

1. If you are uncertain whether the victim has a high or low blood-sugar level, give the person a sugar-containing food or drink.

2. If improvement is not seen in 15 minutes, get the victim to the hospital.

DIABETIC EMERGENCIES

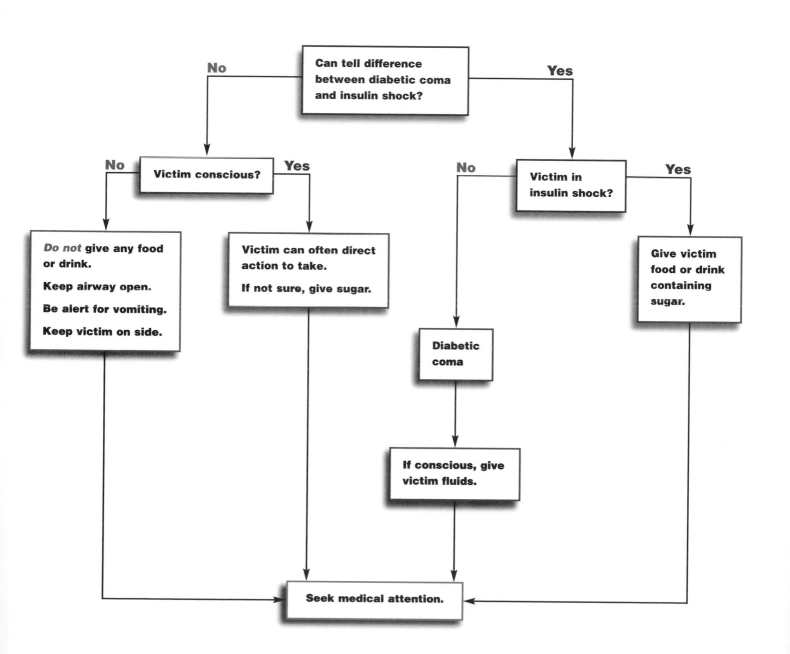

Can tell difference between diabetic coma and insulin shock?

No → **Yes**

Victim conscious?

No **Yes**

Victim in insulin shock?

No **Yes**

Do not give any food or drink.

Keep airway open.

Be alert for vomiting.

Keep victim on side.

Victim can often direct action to take.

If not sure, give sugar.

Give victim food or drink containing sugar.

Diabetic coma

If conscious, give victim fluids.

Seek medical attention.

A miscarriage

is a premature

delivery of a

nonviable fetus.

VAGINAL BLEEDING AND PREGNANCY EMERGENCIES

Miscarriage

Miscarriages usually occur during the first 3 months (first trimester) of pregnancy. The signs and symptoms of a threatened miscarriage include vaginal bleeding and pain that resembles menstrual cramps. Signs of an inevitable miscarriage include heavy vaginal bleeding and uterine contractions.

Care for Miscarriage

1. Have the victim place a sanitary pad over the outside of the vagina.

2. Seek medical attention.

Vaginal Bleeding in Late Pregnancy

If a woman has vaginal bleeding late in her pregnancy (third trimester), she should be asked how long she has been bleeding and how many sanitary pads she has used so that this can be reported to medical personnel. An increase in pulse rate of more than 20 beats per minute when the victim goes from a lying-down to a sitting position suggests blood loss greater than 1 pint.

Care for Vaginal Bleeding in Late Pregnancy

1. **Place the victim on her left side** to help prevent vomiting, to prevent aspiration of vomitus should it occur, and to relieve pressure the fetus places on the mother's circulatory system.

2. Seek medical attention.

Care for Injury-related Vaginal Bleeding

1. Use direct pressure to control bleeding.

2. Apply an ice pack to reduce swelling and pain.

3. Apply a diaper-type bandage to hold dressings in place. Never place or pack dressings into the vagina.

4. Seek medical attention.

Care for Noninjury-related Vaginal Bleeding

Noninjury-related vaginal bleeding can result from various causes, but treatment is similar.

1. Have the victim place a sanitary pad over the vaginal opening.

2. Seek medical attention.

A sudden illness

is a medical

condition that

occurs without

warning, for

which the victim

needs first aid.

SUMMARY

A sudden illness is a medical condition that occurs without warning, for which the victim needs first aid. In all cases, check or monitor the victim's ABCDs and be prepared to call 911 when necessary.

An asthma attack may be indicated by coughing and wheezing and an inability to speak without pausing for breath. Monitor the ABCs, help the victim into a position that is comfortable for breathing, and ask the victim about his or her asthma medication. Call 911 immediately if the victim does not have medication available or is having an extreme attack.

A person who is hyperventilating because of stress is breathing very fast and may experience dizziness or lightheadedness and shortness of breath. Calm the person and encourage him or her to breathe slowly and deeply.

Fainting may result from medical conditions, fear or anxiety, or simply standing or sitting too long in a hot environment. Fainting may be prevented by lying down with the legs raised. After fainting, check for injury and help the person to recover. If the fainting occurs for no apparent reason, is persistent or recurrent, the victim should seek medical attention.

Seizures occur in people suffering from epilepsy but may also be caused by other medical conditions. Give supportive care and prevent injury during the seizure. Call the EMS if the victim is not known to have epilepsy, if the victim is pregnant or has another medical condition, or if the victim is injured.

Diabetic emergencies can occur whenever insulin and blood sugar become unbalanced in a diabetic person; this may result from various factors. The signs and symptoms of *low* blood sugar include poor coordination, pale color, confusion or disorientation, sweating, and sudden hunger. If the victim is known to be a diabetic and demonstrates altered mental status, give him or her a sugar-containing food. Seek medical attention if there is no improvement in 15 minutes. The signs and symptoms of *high* blood sugar include drowsiness, thirst, flushed skin, and a fruity breath odor — but these symptoms may be confused with those of low blood sugar. The victim needs immediate medical attention. If you are unsure whether the victim has high or low blood sugar, give food or drink containing sugar but be prepared to get the person to a hospital if there is no improvement in 15 minutes.

Vaginal bleeding early in a pregnancy may be a sign of miscarriage, and the victim should place sanitary pads over the outside of the vagina and seek medical attention. In late pregnancy, if bleeding is accompanied by an increased pulse upon sitting up, place the victim on her left side and seek medical attention. For nonpregnancy vaginal bleeding, have the victim put a sanitary pad or dressing over the vagina, and seek medical attention.

REVIEW QUESTIONS

Sudden Illness

Directions: Circle Yes if you agree with the statement and circle No if you disagree.

Yes No 1. Most asthma victims usually have a doctor-prescribed inhaler.

Yes No 2. A victim who is breathing fast (hyper-ventilation) should be encouraged to breathe slowly by holding inhaled air for several seconds, then exhaling slowly.

Fainting

Yes No 1. Splash or sprinkle water on a person who has fainted.

Yes No 2. Have a fainting victim inhale smelling salts or ammonia inhalants.

Scenario 1. During a first aid training video showing a bloodied injured victim, a young man suddenly falls from his chair to the floor. He is breathing and has a pulse but is unresponsive. No other injuries from the fall are detected. A person sitting behind him reports that he didn't hit his head on the floor. What should you do?

_____

_____

_____

Scenario 2. An Army private on guard duty has been at her post for about 3 hours standing rigidly at attention with her knees locked. She suddenly but slowly collapses to the ground. What should you do?

_____

_____

_____

Seizures

Yes No 1. Place a strong stick or similar object between a seizure victim's teeth.

Yes No 2. A person who is having seizures always requires medical attention.

Scenario 3. You see some of your coworkers holding down another employee on the floor. They are trying to force a couple of pencils between her teeth. The person is unresponsive and is having severe muscle jerks. What should you do?

_____

_____

_____

Scenario 4. A coworker slumps over in his chair and then onto the floor. He is having a seizure; his eyes are rolled back, his body is rigid, and he is shaking from head to foot. His head is pounding on the concrete floor. What should you do?

_____

_____

_____

Diabetic Emergencies

Yes   **No**   **1.** If in doubt about whether a victim has an insulin reaction or is in a diabetic coma, give sugar to a responsive victim who can swallow.

Yes   **No**   **2.** During a diabetic emergency, if improvement is not seen in 15 minutes, seek medical attention for the victim.

Scenario 5. In your carpool after work, the driver is driving fast, has been weaving, and almost crossed some traffic lanes. When he stops to let the first rider out, he just sits in the car, staring at the car's steering wheel. He then slumps over onto the steering wheel. His skin is cold and sweaty. You are aware that the driver is diabetic. What should you do?

_____

_____

_____

Scenario 6. A coworker yells for your help and says that someone has passed out in the company's lunchroom. You find a middle-aged worker collapsed on the floor but responsive to questions. In one hand, she is holding a wrapped candy bar. You find a medical-alert identification indicating that she has diabetes and takes insulin daily. When asked, she says that she is having an insulin reaction. What should you do?

_____

_____

_____

HOW DID YOU DO?

Sudden Illness
1. Yes; 2. Yes
Fainting
1. No; 2. No
Seizures
1. No; 2. No
Diabetic Emergencies
1. Yes; 2. Yes

POISONING

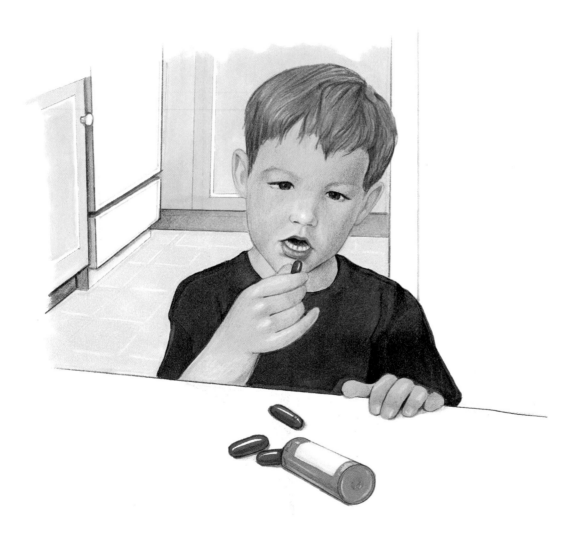

CONTENTS

18

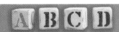

LEARNING OBJECTIVES

After reading this chapter, you should be able to

1. Identify the signs and symptoms of poisoning

2. Describe the appropriate first aid for ingested, inhaled, and absorbed poisoning

3. Describe the appropriate first aid care for alcohol and other drug-related emergencies

INGESTED (SWALLOWED) POISON

Fortunately, most poisonings involve weak toxic poisons or small amounts. Severe poisonings do occur, however.

The signs and symptoms of ingested poison include

- Abdominal pain and cramping
- Nausea or vomiting
- Diarrhea
- Burns, odor, stains around and in mouth
- Drowsiness or unconsciousness
- Poison containers nearby

Care for Ingested Poison

1. Determine critical information:
   - Age and size of the victim
   - What was swallowed
   - How much was swallowed (eg, a "taste," half a bottle, a dozen tablets)
   - When it was swallowed

2. For a responsive victim, call a poison control center immediately. Some poisons do not cause harm until hours later; others cause damage immediately. Most poisonings can be treated with instructions over the telephone from a poison control center. The center also will advise you if medical attention is needed. Poison control centers routinely follow up calls to check whether additional symptoms or unexpected effects occur. The inside front covers or first pages of many telephone directories list the poison control center's number.

3. If chemicals or household products were swallowed, dilute them by having the victim drink water or milk. (Cold milk or water tends to absorb heat better than room-temperature or warmer liquids do.)

4. For an unresponsive victim, or if the poison control center number is unknown, call 911 or the local emergency number. Monitor the ABCs often.

5. Place the victim on his or her left side to position the end of the stomach where it enters the small intestine (pylorus) straight up. Gravity can delay the movement of the poison into the small intestine up to 2 hours (**FIGURE 1**). The side position also helps to prevent aspiration (inhalation) into the lungs if vomiting begins.

6. **Induce vomiting only if a poison control center or a physician advises it.** Inducing vomiting must be done within 30 minutes of swallowing the poison. If you are instructed by a poison control center or a physician to induce vomiting, use syrup of ipecac. It can be purchased without a prescription and is easily given. Follow the directions carefully. Ipecac will not work unless sufficient water also is given.

7. Give activated charcoal if a poison control center advises. In prehospital settings it is the single most effective agent for most swallowed poisons.

8. Save poison containers, plants, and the victim's vomit to help medical personnel identify the poison.

ALCOHOL AND OTHER DRUG EMERGENCIES

Alcohol Intoxication

Helping an intoxicated person is often difficult because the person may be belligerent and combative, or may be unpleasant to be near because of poor personal hygiene. However, it is important that alcohol abusers be helped, and not just labeled as "drunks." Their condition may be quite serious, even life-threatening.

Following are signs of alcohol intoxication (some of these may also indicate an illness or injury other than alcohol abuse, such as diabetes or heat injury):

- The odor of alcohol on a person's breath or clothing
- Unsteady, staggering walking
- Slurred speech and the inability to carry on a conversation
- Nausea and vomiting
- Flushed face

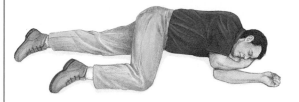

FIGURE 1
Put a victim who has ingested poison on his or her left side.

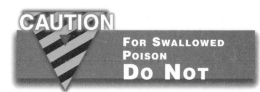

CAUTION

FOR SWALLOWED POISON
DO NOT

- give water or milk to dilute poisons other than chemicals or household products unless instructed to do so by a poison control center. Fluids may dissolve a dry poison (eg, tablets or capsules) more rapidly and fill up the stomach, forcing stomach contents (ie, the poison) into the small intestine, where poisons are absorbed more quickly.

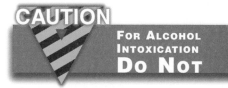

CAUTION

FOR ALCOHOL INTOXICATION
DO NOT

- let an intoxicated person sleep on his or her back.
- leave an intoxicated person alone.
- try to handle a hostile drunk by yourself. Find a safe place, then call the police for help.

SWALLOWED POISON

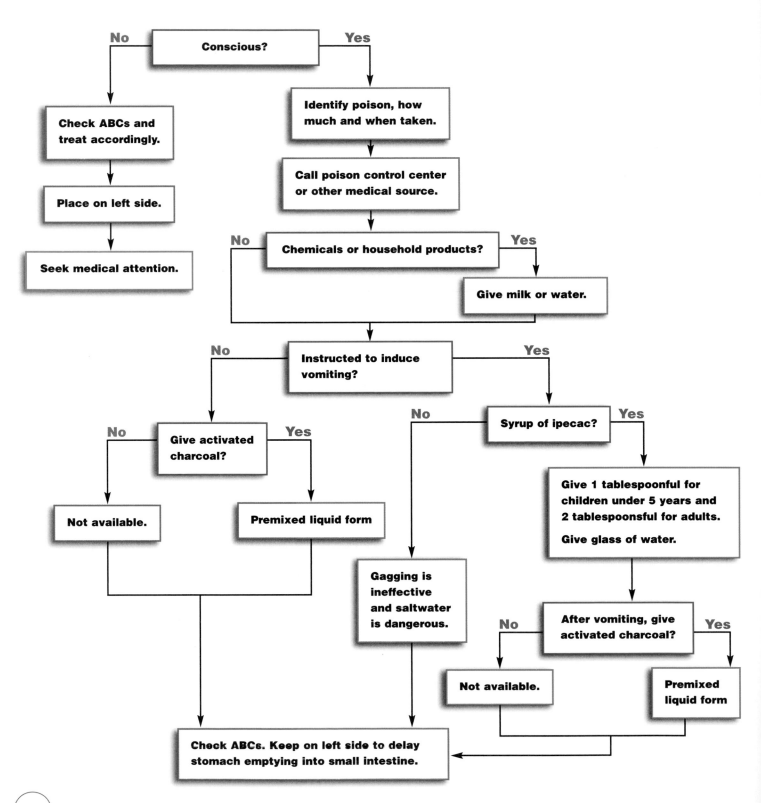

Conscious?

No → **Check ABCs and treat accordingly.** → **Place on left side.** → **Seek medical attention.**

Yes → **Identify poison, how much and when taken.** → **Call poison control center or other medical source.** → **Chemicals or household products?**

Chemicals or household products? Yes → **Give milk or water.**

No / Yes → **Instructed to induce vomiting?**

Instructed to induce vomiting? No → **Give activated charcoal?**

Give activated charcoal? No → **Not available.**
Give activated charcoal? Yes → **Premixed liquid form**

Instructed to induce vomiting? Yes → **Syrup of ipecac?**

Syrup of ipecac? No → **Gagging is ineffective and saltwater is dangerous.**

Syrup of ipecac? Yes → **Give 1 tablespoonful for children under 5 years and 2 tablespoonsful for adults. Give glass of water.** → **After vomiting, give activated charcoal?**

After vomiting, give activated charcoal? No → **Not available.**
After vomiting, give activated charcoal? Yes → **Premixed liquid form**

Check ABCs. Keep on left side to delay stomach emptying into small intestine.

Drugs

A person who is on drugs may experience a medical emergency. Some drugs that may cause an emergency are marijuana, barbiturates, amphetamines, and narcotics.

Care for Alcohol and Drug Emergencies

Alcohol Intoxication

1. **Look for any injuries.** Alcohol can mask pain.

2. **Check the ABCDs** and treat accordingly.

3. If the intoxicated person is lying down, place him or her in the recovery (left side) position to reduce the likelihood of vomiting and aspiration of vomit and to delay absorption. Be sure to check that the victim is breathing and does not have a spinal injury before you move him or her. The recovery position can be used for both responsive and unresponsive victims.

4. Call the poison control center for advice or the local emergency number for help. It may be best to let EMS personnel decide whether the police should be alerted.

5. **If the victim becomes violent, leave the scene** and find a safe place until police arrive.

6. Provide emotional support.

7. Assume that an injured or unresponsive victim has a spinal injury and needs to be stabilized against movement. Because of decreased pain perception, an intoxicated victim cannot be assessed reliably. If you suspect a spinal injury, wait for EMS personnel to arrive. They have the proper equipment and training to stabilize and move a victim.

8. Intoxicated individuals often are exposed to the environment, so on a cold day, suspect hypothermia and move the person to a warm place. Remove wet clothing and cover the individual with warm blankets. Handle a hypothermic victim gently, since rough handling could induce a heart attack.

Drugs

1. **Check the ABCDs.**

2. **Call the poison control center for advice, or EMS for help.**

3. Check for injuries.

4. Keep the person on the left side to reduce the likelihood of vomiting and aspiration of vomit and to delay absorption.

5. Provide reassurance and emotional support.

6. If the person becomes violent, **seek safety** until the police arrive. Let law enforcement officers handle dangerous situations.

7. Seek medical attention.

Because of decreased pain perception, an intoxicated victim cannot be assessed reliably.

It is difficult to

tell if a person is

a CO victim.

Sometimes, a

complaint of the

"flu" is really a

symptom of CO

poisoning.

INHALED POISONS

Carbon Monoxide

Victims of carbon monoxide (CO) often are unaware of its presence. The gas is invisible, tasteless, odorless, and nonirritating. It is produced by the incomplete burning of organic material such as gasoline, wood, paper, charcoal, coal, and natural gas.

It is difficult to tell whether a person is a CO victim. Sometimes, a complaint of the "flu" is really a symptom of CO poisoning. Although many symptoms of CO poisoning resemble those of the flu, there are differences. For example, CO poisoning does not cause low-grade fever or generalized aching and does not involve the lymph nodes.

The following conditions are signs of possible CO poisoning:

- The symptoms come and go
- The symptoms worsen or improve in certain places or at certain times of the day
- People around the victim have similar symptoms
- Pets seem ill

The signs and symptoms of CO poisoning are as follows:

- Headache
- Ringing in the ears (tinnitus)
- Chest pain (angina)
- Muscle weakness
- Nausea and vomiting
- Dizziness and visual changes (blurred or double vision)
- Unconsciousness
- Respiratory and cardiac arrest

Care for Carbon Monoxide Poisoning

1. Remove the victim from the toxic environment and into fresh air immediately.
2. Call EMS, which will be able to give the victim 100% oxygen, improving oxygenation and disassociating the linkage between the CO and the hemoglobin.
3. Monitor the ABCs.
4. Place an unresponsive victim on one side.
5. Seek medical attention. All suspected CO victims should obtain a blood test to determine the level of CO in their system.

ABSORBED POISONS

Poison Ivy, Oak, and Sumac

Most people cannot identify poison ivy, poison oak, and poison sumac (**FIGURES 2–4**). A helpful method of identifying them is the "black-spot test." When the sap is exposed to the air, it turns brown in a matter of minutes and is black by the next day.

The primary signs and symptoms are itching and rash.

Care for Poison Ivy, Oak, and Sumac

1. For those who know that they have contacted a poisonous plant, decontaminate the skin as soon as possible (within 5 minutes for sensitive people, up to 1 hour for moderately sensitive individuals). (Most victims do not know about their contact until several hours or days later, when the itching and rash begin.) Use soap and cold water to clean the skin of the oily resin or apply rubbing (isopropyl) alcohol liberally (not in swab-type dabs). If too little isopropyl alcohol is used, the oil will actually be spread to another site and will enlarge the injury. Other solvents (eg, paint thinner, gasoline) can be used, but they are hard on the skin. Rinse with water to remove the solubilized material. Water removes urushiol (plant resin) from the skin, oxidizes and inactivates it, and does not penetrate the skin as do solvents. This might prevent the rash (**FIGURE 5**).

2. For the mild stage, have the victim soak in a lukewarm bath sprinkled with 1 to 2 cups of colloidal oatmeal (eg, Aveeno™) (colloidal oatmeal makes a tub slick, so take appropriate precautions) or apply any of the following:

   - Wet compresses soaked with Burow's solution (aluminum acetate) for 20 to 30 minutes three or four times a day

   - Calamine lotion (calamine ointment if the skin becomes dry and cracked) or zinc oxide

   - Baking soda paste: 1 teaspoon of water mixed with 3 teaspoons of baking soda

3. For the mild to moderate stage, care for the skin as you would for the mild stage, and use a physician-prescribed corticosteroid ointment.

4. For the severe stage, care for the skin as you would for the mild and moderate stages, and use a physician-prescribed oral corticosteroid (eg, prednisone). Apply a topical corticosteroid ointment or cream, cover it with a transparent plastic wrap, and lightly bind the area with an elastic or self-adhering bandage.

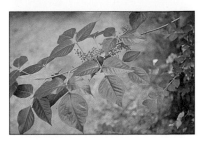

FIGURE 2
Poison ivy.

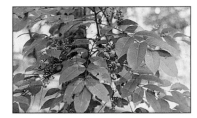

FIGURE 3
Poison sumac.

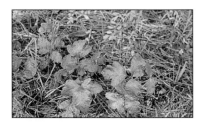

FIGURE 4
Poison oak.

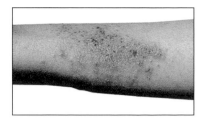

FIGURE 5
Poison ivy rash.

POISON IVY, OAK, AND SUMAC

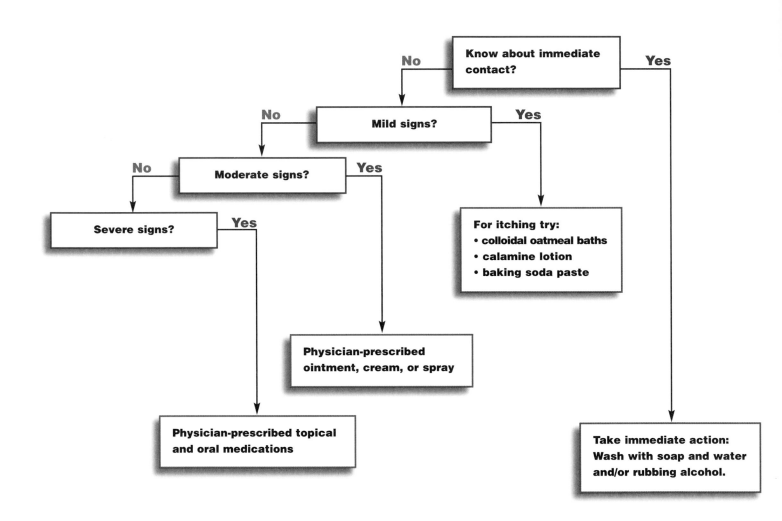

Know about immediate contact?

No

Yes

Mild signs?

No

Yes

Moderate signs?

No

Yes

Severe signs?

Yes

For itching try:
- colloidal oatmeal baths
- calamine lotion
- baking soda paste

Physician-prescribed ointment, cream, or spray

Physician-prescribed topical and oral medications

Take immediate action: Wash with soap and water and/or rubbing alcohol.

SUMMARY

Poisons may enter the body by being ingested, inhaled, or through contact with the skin. A poisoning may result in a range of health problems from a mild rash to life-threatening emergencies.

Ingested poisons may cause gastrointestinal effects and drowsiness or unconsciousness. Try to determine what was swallowed. For a responsive victim, call a poison control center immediately and follow their instructions. If the victim is unconscious, call 911. Monitor the ABCs and place the victim in the recovery position to delay the advancement of poison into the small intestine.

Alcohol intoxication and other drug emergencies are special types of poisoning. Check the ABCDs and call 911 or the poison control center if necessary. Maintain your own safety if the person becomes violent. If the victim becomes unresponsive, place the victim in the recovery position to delay the advancement of poison into the small intestine.

Carbon monoxide poisoning is the most common poisoning caused by inhalation. Move the victim to fresh air immediately and call 911. Monitor the ABCs and place an unresponsive victim on one side.

The effects of poison ivy, oak, and sumac can be mild to severe. Care may include colloidal oatmeal baths, compresses soaked with Burow's lotion, or calamine lotion, and possibly physician-prescribed corticosteroids.

Poisons may enter the body by being ingested, inhaled, or through contact with the skin.

REVIEW QUESTIONS

Directions: Circle Yes if you agree with the statement, and circle No if you disagree.

Yes   No   1. If chemicals or household products were swallowed, dilute them by having the victim drink water or milk.

Yes   No   2. For a poisoned victim, call a poison control center immediately.

Yes   No   3. Induce vomiting with ipecac syrup only if so advised by a poison control center or a doctor.

Yes   No   4. Place a swallowed poison victim on his or her left side to delay the poison reaching the small intestine.

Yes   No   5. Do NOT let an intoxicated person sleep on his or her back.

Yes   No   6. If an intoxicated or drugged person becomes violent, leave the scene and let law enforcement officers handle the situation.

Yes   No   7. Seek medical attention for all carbon monoxide victims.

Yes   No   8. Calamine lotion can help to relieve itching caused by poison ivy, oak, or sumac.

Yes   No   9. Some cases of poison ivy, oak, or sumac require medical attention.

Scenario 1. You find your two-year-old son, Scott, vomiting. You notice that the top of a nearby medicine bottle is off. The label on the bottle reveals that the medicine inside belongs to your visiting mother. You realize that Scott must have swallowed some of the highly potent medicine. What should you do?

_____

_____

_____

Scenario 2. You are at a party and, while walking to the bathroom, see someone you know lying in the hallway unconscious. Right next to her is a bottle for medicine prescribed to another person at the party for migraine headaches. The bottle is empty. What should you do?

_____

_____

_____

Scenario 3. While weeding around a vacant lot, you pull up a batch of weeds with shiny leaves in clusters of three. You finish the job about an hour later. The next morning, your arms are itching, and you notice a rash beginning to appear. What should you do?

_____

_____

_____

Scenario 4. Your friend complains of a rash on his arms and legs. He has no known allergies and has never had a similar rash. He cannot associate it with any new medications, soaps, foods, or colognes. However, he did just return from a two-day camping trip. The rash is red, with mild swelling, itching, and blisters. What should you do?

_____

_____

_____

HOW DID YOU DO?
1. Yes; 2. Yes; 3. Yes; 4. Yes; 5. Yes; 6. Yes;
7. Yes; 8. Yes; 9. Yes

BITES AND STINGS

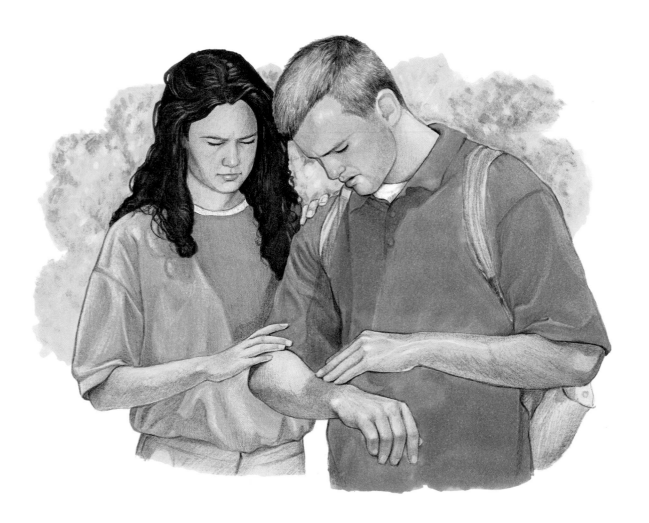

CONTENTS

19

Rattlesnakes only

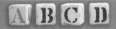

FIGURE 1
Dog bite.

FOUNDATION FACTS: RABIES

A virus that is found in warm-blooded animals causes rabies and spreads from one animal to another in the saliva, usually through a bite or by licking.

Consider an animal possibly rabid if any of these are true:

- The animal attacked unprovoked.

- The animal acted strangely or out of character (eg, a usually friendly dog is aggressive, or a wild fox seems docile and "friendly").

- The animal was of a high-risk species (skunk, raccoon, or bat).

A B C D

LEARNING OBJECTIVES

After reading this chapter you should be able to

1. Describe what to do for an animal bite

2. Describe what to do for a human bite

3. Describe the first aid for

   - Snakebite

   - Insect sting

   - Spider bite

   - Scorpion sting

   - Mosquito bite

4. Describe how best to remove an embedded tick

ANIMAL BITES

It is estimated that one of every two Americans will be bitten at some time by an animal* or by another person. Dogs are responsible for about 80% of all animal-bite injuries (**FIGURE 1**).

Handling the Animal

If the victim was bitten in the United States (except for the area along the border with Mexico) by a healthy domestic dog or cat, the animal should be confined and observed for 10 days for any illness. If the offending animal is a stray or unwanted dog or cat, it should be killed immediately and its head should be submitted for rabies examination. If feasible, only a veterinarian should kill the animal (domesticated or wild) and decapitate it for sending the head to a laboratory. If the animal is dead, transport the entire body; do not attempt decapitation. Precautions must be taken to prevent exposure to potentially infected tissues and saliva.

Report animal bites to the police or animal control officers, who should capture the animal for observation. If the dog or cat escapes and is not suspected to be rabid, consult local public health officials.

If the victim was bitten in the United States by a skunk, raccoon, bat, fox, or other mammal, it should be considered a rabies exposure and treatment should be started immediately. The only exception is when the bite occurred in a part of the continental United States that is known to be free of rabies. If the wild animal is captured, it should be killed and its head should be shipped to a qualified laboratory immediately.

Care for Animal Bites

1. Clean the wound with a soap solution, rinse it with water under pressure.

---

*The term "animal bite" refers to a bite by a mammal, not by an insect or reptile.

2. Stop the bleeding and give wound care.

3. **Seek medical attention for further wound cleaning and a possible tetanus shot.** The physician will determine whether sutures are needed to close the wound. If needed, a vaccination against rabies will be started.

HUMAN BITES

Because the human mouth contains a wide range of bacteria, the risk of infection is greater from a human bite than from bites of other warm-blooded animals.

Care for Human Bites

1. If the wound is not bleeding heavily, wash it with soap and water (under the pressure from a faucet) for 5 to 10 minutes. Avoid scrubbing, which can traumatize tissues.

2. Rinse the wound thoroughly with running water under pressure.

3. Control bleeding with direct pressure.

4. Cover the wound with a sterile dressing. Do not close the wound with tape or butterfly bandages. That traps bacteria in the wound, increasing the chance of infection.

5. Seek medical attention for possible further wound cleaning, a tetanus shot, and sutures applied to close the wound.

SNAKEBITES

Only four snake species in the United States (FIGURE 2) are venomous: rattlesnakes (which account for about 65% of all venomous snakebites and nearly all the snakebite deaths in the United States), copperheads, water moccasins (also known as cottonmouths), and coral snakes. The first three are pit vipers (FIGURES 3–5). The coral snake is small and colorful, with a series of bright red, yellow, and black bands around its body (every other band is yellow). It also has a black snout (FIGURE 6).

Pit Viper Bites

In about 25% of poisonous snakebites, there is no venom injection, only fang and tooth wounds (known as a "dry" bite).

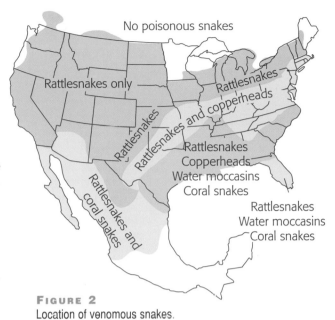

FIGURE 2
Location of venomous snakes.

No poisonous snakes

Rattlesnakes only

Rattlesnakes

Rattlesnakes and copperheads

Rattlesnakes
Copperheads
Water moccasins
Coral snakes

Rattlesnakes
Water moccasins
Coral snakes

Rattlesnakes and coral snakes

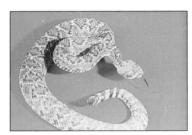

FIGURE 3
Rattlesnake.

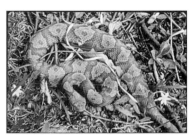

FIGURE 4
Copperhead.

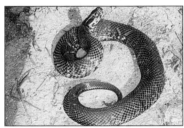

FIGURE 5
Water moccasin (cottonmouth).

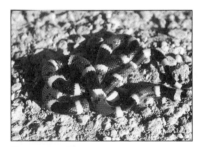

FIGURE 6
Coral snake.

ANIMAL BITES

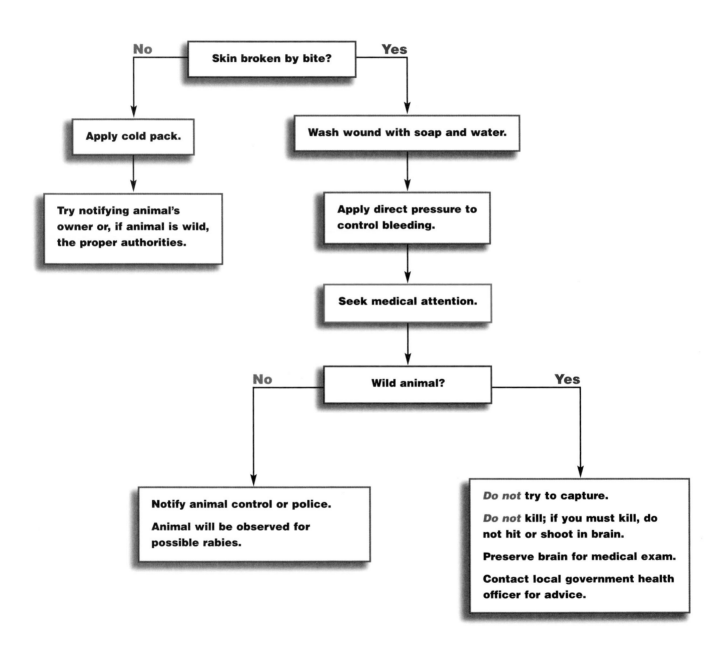

Skin broken by bite?

No → Apply cold pack. → Try notifying animal's owner or, if animal is wild, the proper authorities.

Yes → Wash wound with soap and water. → Apply direct pressure to control bleeding. → Seek medical attention. → **Wild animal?**

Wild animal?

No → Notify animal control or police.

Animal will be observed for possible rabies.

Yes → *Do not* try to capture.

Do not kill; if you must kill, do not hit or shoot in brain.

Preserve brain for medical exam.

Contact local government health officer for advice.

The signs and symptoms of pit viper bites include the following:

- Severe burning pain at the bite site
- Two small puncture wounds about ½ inch apart (some cases may have only one fang mark) **(FIGURE 7)**
- Swelling developing within 5 minutes; can involve an entire extremity
- Discoloration and blood-filled blisters possibly developing in 6 to 10 hours **(FIGURE 8)**
- In severe cases, nausea, vomiting, sweating, and weakness

Coral Snake Bites

The coral snake is the most venomous snake in the United States, but it rarely bites people. The coral snake has short fangs and tends to hang on and "chew" its venom into the victim rather than to strike and release, like a pit viper.

Nonpoisonous Snakebites

A nonpoisonous snake leaves a horseshoe shape of toothmarks on the victim's skin. If you are not positive about a snake, assume that it was venomous. Some so-called nonpoisonous North American snakes (eg, hognose and garter snakes) have venom that can cause painful local reactions but no systemic (whole-body) symptoms.

Care for Snakebites

Nonpoisonous snakebites

1. Gently clean the bite site with soap and water.
2. Care for the bite as you would a minor wound.
3. Seek medical advice.

Pit Vipers Identifying the type of pit viper is of minimal importance, since the same antivenin is used with bites from all North American pit vipers. The Wilderness Medical Society lists the following guidelines for dealing with bites by pit vipers:

1. Get the victim and bystanders away from the snake. Snakes have been known to bite more than once. Pit vipers can strike about one-half their body length. Be careful around a decapitated snake head, because head reactions can persist for 20 minutes or longer.
2. Keep the victim quiet. If possible, carry the victim or have the victim walk very slowly to help.
3. Gently wash the bitten area with soap and water.
4. If you are more than 1 hour from a medical facility with antivenin, or if the snake was large and the victim's skin is

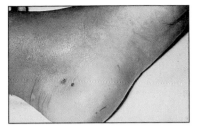

FIGURE 7
Rattlesnake bite.

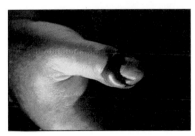

FIGURE 8
Copperhead bite hours later.

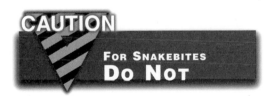

CAUTION

FOR SNAKEBITES
DO NOT

- apply cold or ice to a snakebite. It does not inactivate the venom, and it poses a danger of frostbite.
- use the "cut-and-suck" procedure. You could damage underlying structures (eg, blood vessels, nerves).
- apply mouth suction. Your mouth is filled with bacteria increasing the likelihood of wound infection.
- apply electric shock.

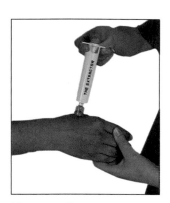

FIGURE 9
Use of Extractor™.

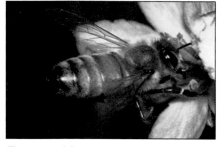

FIGURE 10
Honeybee.

swelling rapidly, immediately apply suction with the Extractor™ (from Sawyer Products). It does not require cutting **(FIGURE 9)**.

5. Seek medical attention immediately. This is the most important thing to do for the victim.

Coral Snakes

1. Keep the victim calm.

2. Gently clean the bite site with soap and water.

3. Apply mild pressure by wrapping several elastic bandages (eg, Ace™ bandages) over the bite site and the entire arm or leg. Applying such pressure is recommended only for bites from elapid (eg, coral) snakes, not pit vipers. Do not cut the victim's skin or use an Extractor™.

4. **Seek medical attention for antivenin.**

INSECT STINGS

Severe allergic reactions to insect stings are reported by about 0.5% of the population in the United States **(FIGURE 10)**. Fortunately, localized pain, itching, and swelling, the most common consequences of an insect bite, can be treated with first aid. Generally, the sooner the symptoms develop after a sting, the more serious the reaction will be.

Care for Insect Stings

Most people who have been stung can be treated on site, but everyone should know what to do if a **life-threatening allergic reaction (anaphylaxis)** occurs. In particular, those who have had a severe reaction to an insect sting should be instructed on what they can do to protect themselves. They also should be advised to wear a medical-alert identification tag identifying them as allergic to insects.

1. Look at the sting site for a stinger embedded in the skin. Bees are the only stinging insects that leave their stingers behind. If the stinger is still embedded, remove it or it will continue to inject poison for 2 to 3 minutes. Scrape the stinger and venom sac away with a hard object such as a long fingernail, credit card, scissor edge, or knife blade. If applied in the first 3 minutes, a Sawyer Extractor™ can remove a portion of the venom.

2. Wash the sting site with soap and water to prevent infection.

3. Apply an ice pack over the sting site to slow absorption of the venom and relieve pain. Because bee venom is acidic, a paste made of baking soda and water can help. Sodium bicarbonate is an alkalinizing agent that draws out fluid and reduces

itching and swelling. Wasp venom, by contrast, is alkaline, so apply vinegar or lemon juice instead.

4. To further relieve pain and itching, use aspirin (adults only), acetaminophen, or ibuprofen. A topical steroid cream, such as hydrocortisone, can help to combat local swelling and itching. An antihistamine may prevent some local symptoms if it is given early, but it works too slowly to counteract a life-threatening allergic reaction.

5. Observe the victim for at least 30 minutes for signs of an allergic reaction. **For a person who is having a severe allergic reaction, a dose of epinephrine is the only effective treatment.** A person with a known allergy to insect stings should have a physician-prescribed emergency kit that includes prefilled syringes of epinephrine. Because epinephrine is short-acting, watch the victim closely for signs of returning anaphylaxis. Inject another dose of epinephrine as often as every 15 minutes, if needed.

SPIDER BITES

Most spiders are venomous, but lack the long fangs and strong jaws that are needed to bite a human. Death occurs rarely and only from bites by brown recluse and black widow spiders.

A spider bite is difficult to diagnose, especially if the spider was not seen or recovered, because the bites typically cause little pain initially.

Black Widow Spiders

Black widow spiders have round abdomens that are gray or brown or black, depending on the species. The female black widow's abdomen is shiny black with a red or yellow spot (often in the shape of an hourglass) or white spots or bands **(FIGURE 11)**. Black widow spiders are found throughout the world.

It is difficult to determine whether a person has been bitten by a black widow spider (or any spider). Following are signs and symptoms:

- The victim might feel a sharp pinprick when the spider bites, although some victims are not even aware of the bite. Within 15 minutes, a dull, numbing pain develops in the bite area.

- Two small fang marks might be seen as tiny red spots.

- Within 15 minutes to 4 hours, muscle stiffness and cramps occur, usually affecting the abdomen when the bite is on a lower part of the body and the shoulders, back, or chest when the bite is on an upper part. Victims often describe the pain as the most severe they have ever experienced.

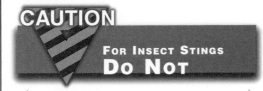

FOR INSECT STINGS
DO NOT

- pull the stinger with tweezers or your fingers because you may squeeze more venom into the victim from the venom sac.

- use epinephrine unless the victim has their own, prescribed by a physician, and is having a severe allergic reaction.

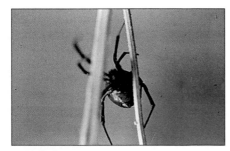

FIGURE 11
Black widow spider.

SNAKE BITES

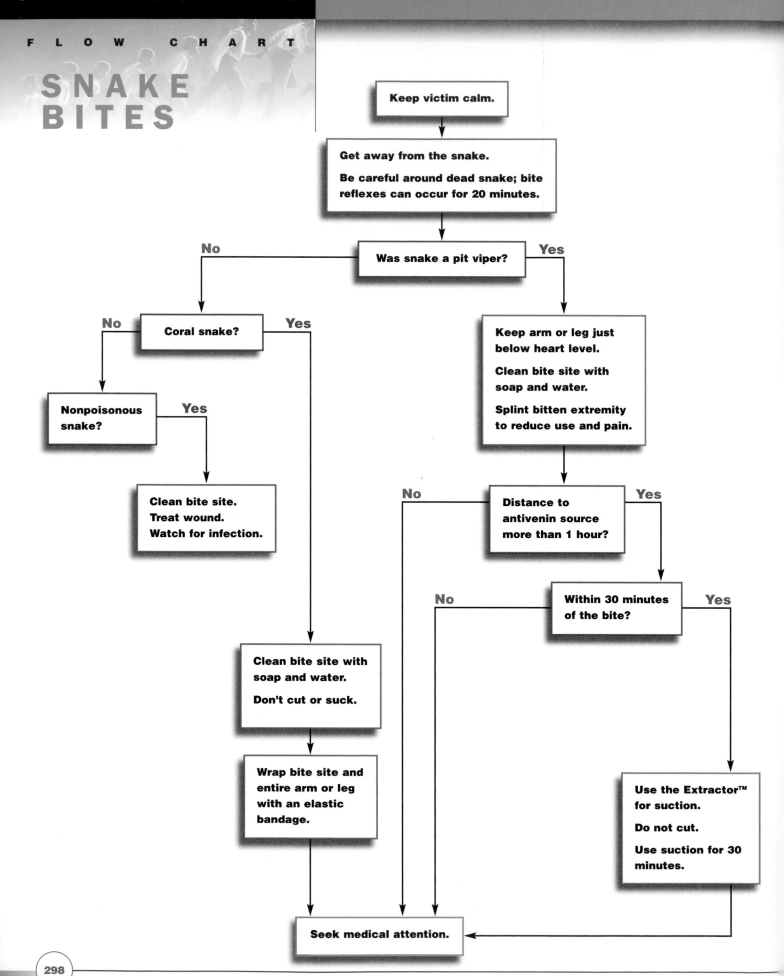

Keep victim calm.

Get away from the snake.

Be careful around dead snake; bite reflexes can occur for 20 minutes.

Was snake a pit viper?

No — Yes

Coral snake?

No — Yes

Nonpoisonous snake? — Yes

Clean bite site.
Treat wound.
Watch for infection.

Keep arm or leg just below heart level.

Clean bite site with soap and water.

Splint bitten extremity to reduce use and pain.

Distance to antivenin source more than 1 hour?

No — Yes

Within 30 minutes of the bite?

No — Yes

Clean bite site with soap and water.

Don't cut or suck.

Wrap bite site and entire arm or leg with an elastic bandage.

Use the Extractor™ for suction.

Do not cut.

Use suction for 30 minutes.

Seek medical attention.

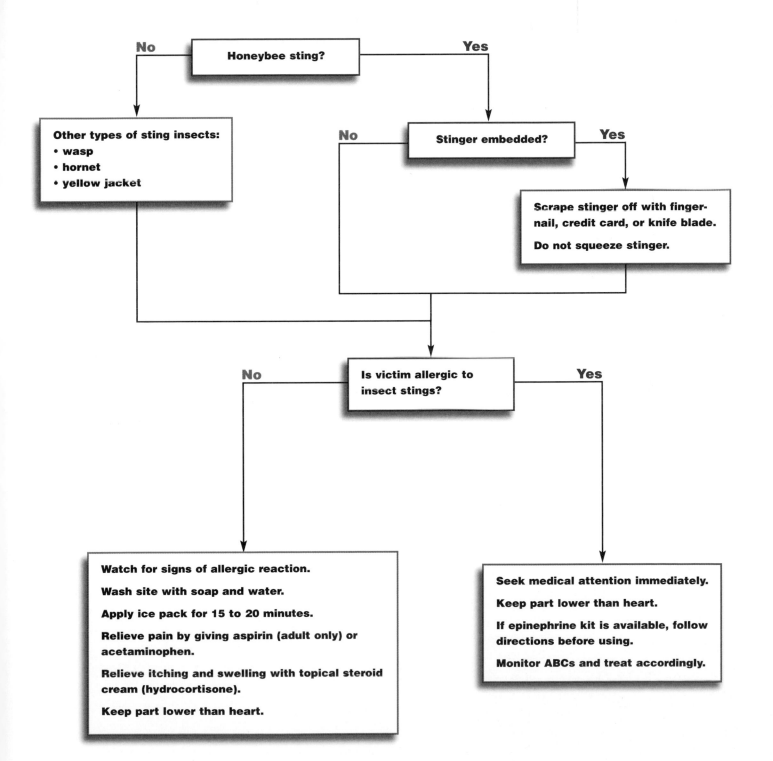

No ← **Honeybee sting?** → **Yes**

Other types of sting insects:
- wasp
- hornet
- yellow jacket

No ← **Stinger embedded?** → **Yes**

Scrape stinger off with finger-nail, credit card, or knife blade.

Do not squeeze stinger.

No ← **Is victim allergic to insect stings?** → **Yes**

Watch for signs of allergic reaction.

Wash site with soap and water.

Apply ice pack for 15 to 20 minutes.

Relieve pain by giving aspirin (adult only) or acetaminophen.

Relieve itching and swelling with topical steroid cream (hydrocortisone).

Keep part lower than heart.

Seek medical attention immediately.

Keep part lower than heart.

If epinephrine kit is available, follow directions before using.

Monitor ABCs and treat accordingly.

• Headache, chills, fever, heavy sweating, dizziness, nausea, and vomiting appear next. Severe pain around the bite site peaks in 2 to 3 hours and can last 12 to 48 hours.

Brown Recluse Spiders

Brown recluse spiders are also known in North America as fiddle-back, violin, and brown spiders. They have a violin-shaped figure on their backs (several other spider species have a similar configuration on their backs). Color varies from fawn to dark brown, with darker legs (FIGURE 12).

Brown recluse spiders are found primarily in the Southern and Midwestern states; other, less toxic, related spiders are found throughout the rest of the country. They are not found in the Pacific Northwest.

Following are signs and symptoms of a brown recluse spider bite:

• A local reaction usually occurs within 2 to 8 hours, with mild to severe pain at the bite site and the development of redness, swelling, and local itching.

• In 48 to 72 hours, a blister develops at the bite site, becomes red, and bursts. During the early stages, the affected area often takes on a bullseye appearance, with a central white area surrounded by a reddened area, ringed by a whitish or blue border (FIGURE 13). A small red crater remains, over which a scab forms. When that scab falls away in a few days, a still larger crater remains. That too scabs over and falls off, leaving yet a larger crater. The craters are known as volcano lesions. This process of slow tissue destruction can continue for weeks or even months. The ulcer sometimes requires skin grafting.

• Fever, weakness, vomiting, joint pain, and a rash may occur.

• Stomach cramps, nausea, and vomiting may occur.

Tarantulas

Tarantulas bite only when they are vigorously provoked or roughly handled (FIGURE 14). The bite varies from almost painless to a deep throbbing pain lasting up to 1 hour. When upset, the tarantula will roughly scratch the lower surface of its abdomen with its legs and flick hairs onto a person's skin nearby. The hairs cause itching and hives that can last several weeks. Treatment is cortisone cream and antihistamines.

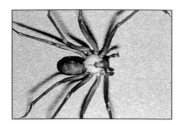

FIGURE 12
Brown recluse spider.

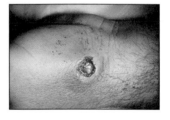

FIGURE 13
Brown recluse spider bite.

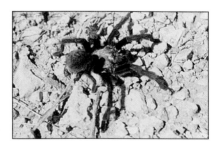

FIGURE 14
Tarantula.

Care for All Spider Bites

1. If possible, catch the spider to confirm its identity. Even if the body has been crushed, save it for identification. The species helps to determine the treatment, so if the dead spider is found, it should be taken with the victim to the hospital.

2. Clean the bite area with soap and water or rubbing alcohol.

3. Place an ice pack over the bite to relieve pain and to delay the effects of the venom.

4. **Monitor the ABCs.**

5. **Seek medical attention immediately.** For black widow spider bites, there is an antivenin. It is usually reserved for children (under age 6), older adults (over age 60 and with high blood pressure), pregnant women, and victims with severe reactions. The antivenin will give relief in 1 to 3 hours. Antivenin for brown recluse and other spider bites is not currently available.

SCORPION STINGS

Scorpions look like miniature lobsters, with lobsterlike pincers and a long upcurved "tail" with a poisonous stinger (FIGURE 15). Several species of scorpions inhabit the Southwestern United States, but only the bark scorpion poses a threat to humans.

The most frequent symptom of a scorpion sting, especially in an adult victim, is local, immediate pain and burning around the sting site. Later, numbness or tingling occurs.

Care for Scorpion Stings

1. **Monitor the ABCs.**

2. Gently clean the sting site with soap and water or rubbing alcohol.

3. Apply an ice pack over the sting site.

4. **Seek medical attention.** Small children are prime candidates for receiving antivenin, which is available only in Arizona.

MOSQUITO BITES

Mosquitoes not only are a nuisance, but also may carry disease. In developing countries, mosquitoes transmit malaria, yellow fever, and dengue fever. In the United States, mosquitoes may carry encephalitis. There is no evidence that mosquitoes transmit HIV, the virus that causes AIDS.

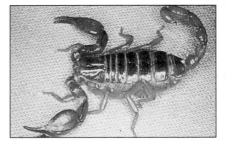

FIGURE 15
Scorpion.

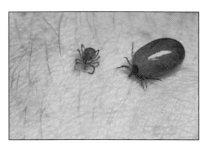

FIGURE 16
Deer ticks not engorged and blood-engorged.

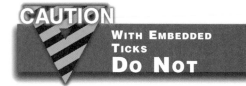

CAUTION

WITH EMBEDDED TICKS
DO NOT

- use the following popular methods of tick removal, which have been proved useless:
  - petroleum jelly
  - fingernail polish
  - rubbing alcohol
  - a hot match
  - a petroleum product, such as gasoline
- grab a tick at the rear of its body. The internal gut may rupture and the contents be squeezed out, causing infection.
- twist or jerk the tick, which may result in incomplete removal.

Care for Mosquito Bites

1. Wash the bitten area with soap and water.

2. Apply an ice pack.

3. Apply calamine lotion to decrease redness and itching.

4. For a victim who is suffering a number of bites or a delayed allergic reaction, an antihistamine (Benadryl™) every 6 hours or a physician-prescribed cortisone may prove useful.

EMBEDDED TICKS

Remove ticks as soon as possible **(FIGURE 16).** If a tick is carrying a disease, the longer it stays embedded, the greater the chance of the disease being transmitted.

Because its bite is painless, a tick can remain embedded for days without the victim realizing it. Most tick bites are harmless, although ticks can carry serious diseases.

Care for Embedded Ticks

1. To pull a tick off, use tweezers or one of the specialized tick-removal tools. Grasp the tick as close to the skin as possible and lift it with enough force to "tent" the skin surface. Hold until the tick lets go. This may take several seconds.

2. Wash the bite site with soap and water. Apply rubbing alcohol to further disinfect the area.

3. Apply an ice pack to reduce pain.

4. Apply calamine lotion to relieve any itching. Keep the area clean.

5. Continue to watch the bite site for 1 month for a rash. If a rash appears, see a doctor. **Watch for other signs such as fever, muscle aches, sensitivity to bright light, and paralysis that begins with leg weakness.**

TICK REMOVAL

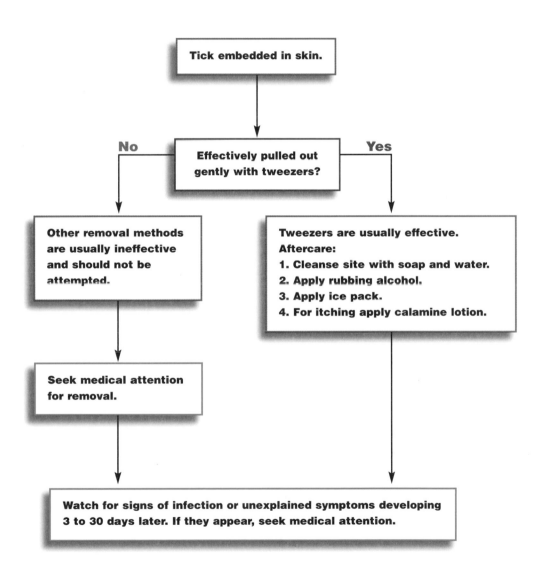

Tick embedded in skin.

No ← Effectively pulled out gently with tweezers? → **Yes**

Other removal methods are usually ineffective and should not be attempted.

Tweezers are usually effective.
Aftercare:
1. Cleanse site with soap and water.
2. Apply rubbing alcohol.
3. Apply ice pack.
4. For itching apply calamine lotion.

Seek medical attention for removal.

Watch for signs of infection or unexplained symptoms developing 3 to 30 days later. If they appear, seek medical attention.

Bites from

dogs, other

mammals, snakes,

and insects

are common

first aid

situations.

SUMMARY

Bites from dogs, other mammals, snakes, and insects are common first aid situations. Because the skin is broken and there is a potential for infection, the wound should be washed with soap and water. If the bite or sting may have been from a venomous snake, seek medical attention immediately. Other specific care depends on the animal or insect.

The bites of dogs and other mammals can be serious because of the risk of rabies or tetanus. Seek medical care immediately, and report the animal to police or animal control officers, who will take appropriate steps if rabies is suspected. Human bites, too, should receive medical attention.

The bites of pit vipers and coral snakes are poisonous and can be very serious. Seek medical attention immediately. Keep the victim calm and clean the bite site. Do not apply ice or cold or attempt to cut the wound open and suck out the venom.

The bites of black widow spiders and brown recluse spiders and the sting of scorpions are poisonous. Try to catch the spider and save it for identification. Seek medical attention immediately.

Ticks that are embedded in the skin can transmit disease and should be removed as soon as possible. Do not cover the tick with any substance or try to burn it off. Use tweezers to grasp the tick and pull it from the skin with steady pressure. Then wash the site with soap and water and disinfectant.

REVIEW QUESTIONS

Animal Bites

Directions: Circle Yes if you agree with the statement, and circle No if you disagree.

Yes   No   1. Report animal bites to the police or animal control officers.

Scenario 1. A mail carrier is heard crying for help while being attacked by a neighbor's large dog. The dog's owner calls off the dog and takes it inside the house. You run up the street and help the victim over to a nearby yard. You find several severe bite marks on the mail carrier's legs and arms. What should you do?

_____

_____

_____

Scenario 2. Your 18-month-old son wants to pet a mother dog and a litter of pups. He crawls over to her and her pups, he startles her, and, in reaction, she bites his forearm. What should you do?

_____

_____

_____

Snake and Insect Bites and Stings

Yes   No   1. Apply cold or ice over a snakebite.

Yes   No   2. Use the "cut-and-suck" method for a snakebite.

Yes   No   3. In remote settings, suction pit viper snake venom out with an Extractor™.

Yes   No   4. Apply a cold or ice pack over an insect sting or a suspected spider bite.

Yes   No   5. A baking soda paste can help to reduce itching and swelling caused by an insect sting.

Yes   No   6. A victim's doctor-prescribed epinephrine may have to be given if the victim has a life-threatening reaction to an insect sting.

Yes   No   7. Spider bite antivenin is available only for black widow spider bites, and not all victims need it.

Yes   No   8. An antihistamine or cortisone can be useful for mosquito bites.

Scenario 3. You rush to a vacant lot to help a young woman who is calling for help. She is sitting upright and says that some type of snake bit her on the leg. You see two puncture wounds (fang marks) on her leg. What should you do?

_____

_____

_____

Scenario 4. Tom screams as the large eastern diamondback rattlesnake buries its fangs in his leg just above his boot. You are hiking with him on a forest trail but are some 50 yards behind him. After hearing him, you run to help and find him on the ground in agony, clutching his painful leg. What should you do?

_____

_____

_____

Scenario 5. A garden shop employee complains about her face swelling and a feeling of tightness across her chest. She is having some breathing difficulty. She says that a bee stung her. She has a medical-alert identification tag around her neck indicating an allergy to insects. She tells you that she has medication for such an emergency. There is an ice machine nearby. What should you do?

_____

_____

_____

Scenario 6. While conducting a bird survey, a wildlife biologist is stung by a honeybee. You look at the site and find the bee's stinger still embedded. You ask him about allergies to bees, and he says that he has never reacted before. What should you do?

_____

_____

_____

Scenario 7. While resting during lunch on your company's office patio, you feel a sharp pinprick on your arm. About 15 minutes later, a dull, numbing pain develops in your back. You look at your arm and see two tiny red spots. Abdominal cramping starts about an hour later and steadily gets worse. What should you do?

_____

_____

Scenario 8. Your four-year-old daughter runs into the house crying and holding her arm. She complains about having a black bug with lots of legs on her that made her arm hurt. You look at her arm and find a slight redness and swelling around what appears to be a bite. What should you do?

_____

_____

_____

_____

Ticks

Yes   **No**   1.   Apply a blown-out, glowing match head or heated needle to cause an embedded tick to back out of a victim's skin.

Yes   **No**   2.   Cover an embedded tick with heavy oil or grease to cause a tick to back out because of lack of oxygen.

Scenario 9. On a Monday morning, one of your coworkers returns from a weekend camping trip. When he rubs the back of his head, he feels a bump and asks you to look at it. You see a tick embedded in his scalp. What should you do?

_____

_____

_____

How did you do?

Animal Bites
1. Yes
Snake and Insect Bites and Stings
1. No; 2. No; 3. Yes; 4. Yes;
5. Yes; 6. Yes; 7. Yes; 8. Yes
Ticks
1. No; 2. No

COLD- AND HEAT-RELATED EMERGENCIES

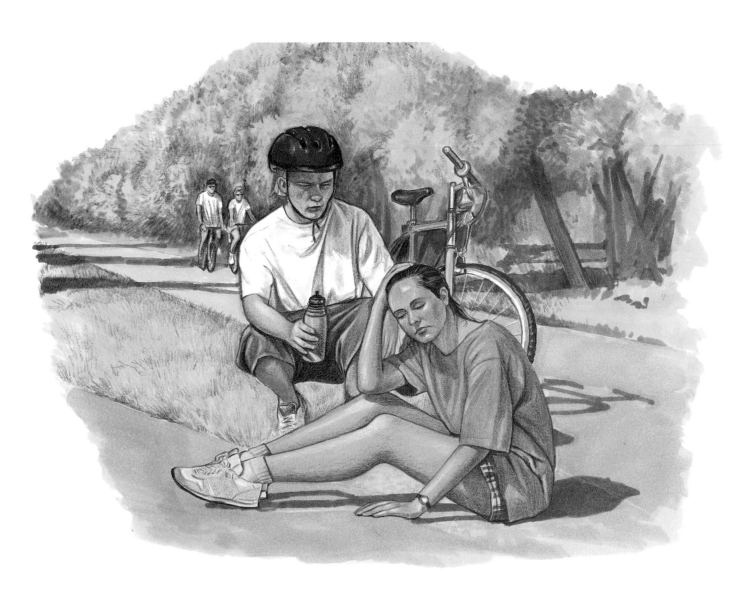

CONTENTS

Frostnip

should be taken

seriously, since

it may be the

first sign of

impending

frostbite.

LEARNING OBJECTIVES

After reading this chapter, you should be able to

1. Describe frostnip and frostbite
2. Describe how to determine the wind-chill factor
3. Describe the first aid for frostnip and frostbite
4. Describe hypothermia
5. Describe the first aid for hypothermia
6. Describe several heat illnesses:
   - Heat cramps
   - Heat exhaustion
   - Heatstroke
7. Describe what to do for:
   - Heat cramps
   - Heat exhaustion
   - Heatstroke
8. Describe other less serious heat illnesses and their care:
   - Heat syncope
   - Heat edema
   - Prickly heat
9. Describe how to determine the apparent temperature

COLD-RELATED EMERGENCIES

Freezing Cold Injuries

Freezing cold injuries can occur whenever the air temperature is below freezing (32°F/0°C). Freezing that is limited to the skin surface is called frostnip. Freezing that extends deeper through the skin and into the flesh is frostbite.

Frostnip involves the freezing of water on the skin surface. The skin becomes reddened and possibly swollen. Although it is painful, there usually is no further damage after rewarming. Repeated frostnip in the same spot can dry the skin, causing it to crack and become sensitive. It is difficult to tell the difference between frostnip and frostbite. Frostnip should be taken seriously, since it may be the first sign of impending frostbite.

Care for Frostnip

1. Gently warm the affected area by placing it against a warm body part (eg, bare hands, armpit, stomach) or by blowing warm air on the area. After rewarming, the affected area may be red and tingling.
2. Do not rub the area.

Frostbite occurs when temperatures drop below freezing. Frostbite affects mainly the feet, hands, ears, and nose. Those areas do not contain large heat-producing muscles and are some distance from the body's heat-generation sources. The most severe consequences of frostbite are gangrene and amputation.

The severity and extent of frostbite are difficult to judge until hours after thawing. The signs and symptoms of superficial frostbite are as follows:

- Skin color is white, waxy, or grayish-yellow
- The affected part is cold and numb
- There might be tingling, stinging, or an aching sensation
- The skin surface feels stiff or crusty, and the underlying tissue feels soft when depressed gently and firmly

Deep frostbite is indicated by the following signs and symptoms:

- The affected part feels cold, hard, and solid, and cannot be depressed
- The affected part is pale, and skin may appear waxy
- A painfully cold part suddenly stops hurting
- Blisters may appear after rewarming **(FIGURES 1–3)**

After a part has thawed, frostbite can be categorized by degrees, similar to the classification of burns.

Care for Frostbite

All frostbite injuries require the same first aid treatment:

1. Get the victim to a warm place.
2. Remove any clothing or constricting items that could impair blood circulation (eg, rings).
3. Seek immediate medical attention.
4. If the affected part is partially thawed, or the victim is in a remote or wilderness situation (more than 1 hour from a medical facility), use the following wet, rapid rewarming method.

   Place the frostbitten part in warm (102°F to 105°F; 39°C to 40.5°C) water. If you do not have a thermometer, pour some of the water over the inside of your arm, or put your elbow into it to test that it is warm, not hot. Maintain water temperature by adding warm water. Rewarming usually takes 20 to 40 minutes, or until the tissues are soft. To help control the severe pain during rewarming, give the victim aspirin (adults only) or ibuprofen. For ear or facial injuries, apply warm moist cloths, changing them frequently.

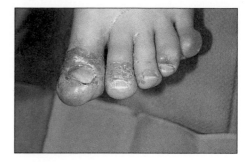

FIGURE 1
Second degree frostbite.

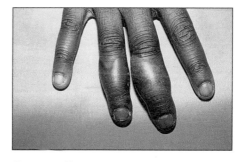

FIGURE 2
Frostbitten fingers 6 hours after rewarming.

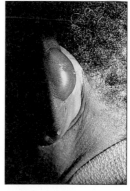

FIGURE 3
Frostbitten ear 8 hours after rewarming.

FROSTBITE

Remove victim from cold exposure if possible.

Remove constricting garments or jewelry from affected part(s).

No ← **Near medical facility?** → Yes

No ← **Any chance of refreezing if thawed?** → Yes

Transport to medical facility.

No ← **Warm water available?** → Yes

Place part(s) next to victim's or someone's body.

Put part(s) in warm water (about 104°F/40°C).

Stop rewarming when part(s) become soft.

Do not rub.

Put dry, clean gauze or cloth between fingers and toes, and over broken blisters.

Seek medical attention.

HYPOTHERMIA

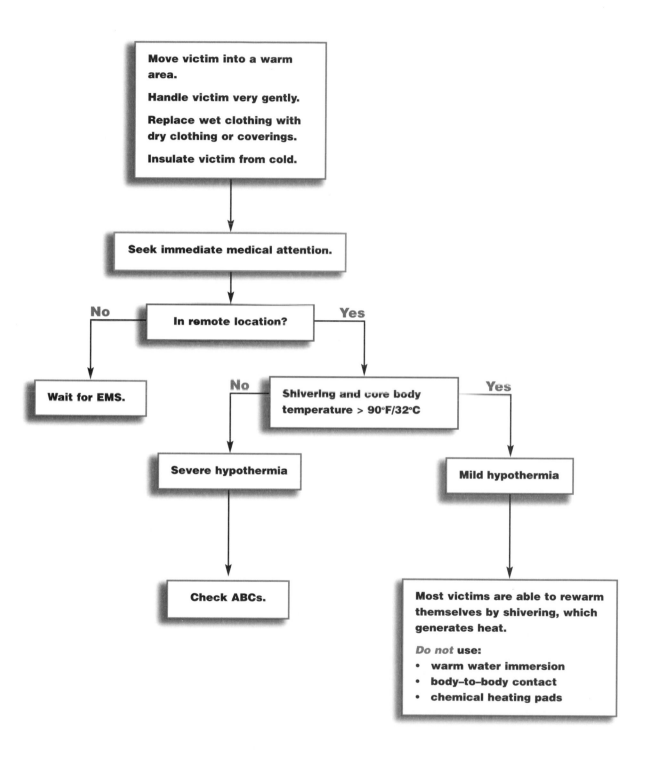

Move victim into a warm area.

Handle victim very gently.

Replace wet clothing with dry clothing or coverings.

Insulate victim from cold.

↓

Seek immediate medical attention.

↓

No ← In remote location? → **Yes**

Wait for EMS.

No ← Shivering and core body temperature > 90°F/32°C → **Yes**

Severe hypothermia

Mild hypothermia

Check ABCs.

Most victims are able to rewarm themselves by shivering, which generates heat.

Do not use:
- warm water immersion
- body–to–body contact
- chemical heating pads

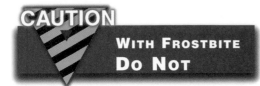

CAUTION

WITH FROSTBITE
DO NOT

- **rub or massage the part. Ice crystals can be pushed into body cells, rupturing them.**

- **rewarm the part with a heating pad, hot-water bottle, stove, sunlamp, radiator, or exhaust pipe or over a fire. Excessive temperatures cannot be controlled, resulting in burns.**

- **allow the victim to drink alcoholic beverages. Alcohol dilates blood vessels and causes a loss of body heat.**

- **allow the victim to smoke. Smoking constricts blood vessels, thus impairing circulation.**

- **rewarm if there is any possibility of refreezing.**

- **allow the thawed part to refreeze. Ice crystals that are formed will be larger and more damaging. If refreezing is likely or even possible, it is better to leave the part frozen.**

- **use the "dry" rewarming technique (putting the victim's hands in your armpits). That takes three to four times longer than the wet, rapid method to thaw frozen tissue. Slow rewarming results in greater tissue damage than rapid rewarming.**

5. After thawing
   - If a person's lower extremities are affected, they will be unable to walk
   - Protect the affected area from contact with clothing and bedding
   - Place dry, sterile gauze between the toes and the fingers to absorb moisture and to keep them from sticking together
   - Slightly elevate the affected part to reduce pain and swelling
   - Apply aloe vera gel to promote skin healing
   - Give the victim aspirin (adults only) or ibuprofen to limit pain and inflammation

Hypothermia

Body temperature falls when the body cannot produce heat as fast as it is being lost. Hypothermia is a life-threatening condition when the body's core temperature falls below 95°F (35°C). It can happen indoors, in the Southern states, and even on a summer day. It does not require subfreezing temperatures.

Following are the signs and symptoms of hypothermia:

- Change in responsiveness or mental status. This is one of the first symptoms of developing hypothermia. Examples are disorientation, apathy, and changes in personality, such as unusual aggressiveness.

- Shivering. This is the first and most important body defense against a falling body temperature. Shivering starts when the body temperature drops 1°F (0.55°C). Shivering can produce more heat than many rewarming methods. As the core temperature continues to fall, shivering usually stops at about 90°F (32°C). Shivering also stops as body temperature rises. If shivering stops while responsiveness is decreasing, assume that the core temperature is falling. On the other hand, if shivering stops while the victim is becoming more coordinated and feeling better, assume that the core temperature is rising.

- Cool abdomen. Place the back of your hand between the clothing and the victim's abdomen to assess the victim's temperature. When the victim's abdominal skin under clothing is cooler than your hand, consider the victim hypothermic until proved otherwise.

- Low core body temperature. The best indicator of hypothermia is a thermometer reading of the core body temperature. Normal thermometers do not register below 94°F (34.5°C) and therefore cannot indicate whether the hypothermia is mild or severe. Because first aid for mild hypothermia is different from that for severe hypothermia, it would be helpful to use a rectal thermometer that registers below 90°F (32°C). However, measuring rectal temperatures is seldom practical because low-reading rectal thermometers usually are not readily available. Also, taking a rectal temperature can be difficult, inconvenient, and embarrassing to victim and rescuer. If done outdoors, such a procedure can expose the already cold victim.

Types of Hypothermia The difference between mild and severe hypothermia is based on the core body temperature. The other most significant difference is that with severe hypothermia, the victim becomes so cold that shivering stops. That means that the victim's body cannot rewarm itself internally, and requires external heat for recovery.

A mild hypothermia victim has a core body temperature above 90°F (32°C). Symptoms are shivering, slurred speech, memory lapses, and fumbling hands. Victims frequently stumble and stagger, but they are usually responsive and can talk. Although many people suffer cold hands and feet, a victim of mild hypothermia experiences a cold abdomen.

Victims of severe hypothermia have a core body temperature below 90°F (32°C). Shivering has stopped. Muscles may be stiff and rigid, similar to rigor mortis. The victim's skin is ice cold and has a blue appearance. Pulse and breathing slow down, and the pupils dilate. The victim may appear to be dead.

Care for Hypothermia

1. For all hypothermia victims, stop further heat loss:
   - Get the victim out of the cold.
   - Handle the victim gently. Rough handling can cause a cardiac arrest.
   - Replace wet clothing with dry clothing.
   - Add insulation (eg, blankets, towels, pillows, newspapers) beneath and around the victim. Cover the victim's head (50% to 80% of the body's heat loss is through the head).
   - Keep the victim in a horizontal (flat) position.

2. Call EMS for immediate medical transportation. Remember that hypothermia is more common in urban settings than in victims found in the wilderness.

3. For mild hypothermia in a remote or wilderness location, the goal is to prevent further heat loss. If protected from further heat loss, most mildly hypothermic victims are able to rewarm themselves by shivering, which generates heat.

FOUNDATION FACTS: THE DANGER OF REWARMING A HYPOTHERMIA VICTIM

Adding heat to a hypothermia victim is extremely difficult. The longer the victim has been exposed to the cold, the longer it will take to raise the core temperature to normal. Trying to rewarm a hypothermic victim may cause a cardiac arrest.

Although surface rewarming suppresses shivering, it may be the only option when the victim is far from medical care. In that case, the victim must be warmed by any available external heat source.

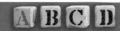

The AHA recognizes 3 types of hypothermia:

Mild (34°–36°C), moderate (30°–34°C), and severe (less than 30°C).

4. For severe hypothermia in a remote or wilderness situation

- Check the victim's ABCs (airway, breathing, circulation).
- If possible, evacuate the victim by helicopter. Rewarming in a remote location is difficult and rarely effective.

Table 20-1: How Cold Is It?

In addition to coldness, two other factors account for body heat loss: moisture and wind. Moisture—whether from rain, snow, or perspiration—speeds the conduction of heat away from the body.

Windchill Factor

Wind causes sizable amounts of body-heat loss. If the thermometer reads 20°F and the wind speed is 20 mph, the exposure is comparable to −10°F. This is called the windchill factor. Use the following rough measures of wind speed: If you feel the wind on your face, the speed is about 10 mph; if small branches move or dust or snow is raised, 20 mph; if large branches are moving, 30 mph; and if a whole tree bends, about 40 mph.

To determine the windchill factor:

1. Estimate the wind speed by checking for the signs described above.

2. Look at a thermometer reading (in Fahrenheit degrees) outdoors.

3. Match the estimated wind speed with the actual thermometer reading in the table below.

Estimated Wind Speed (mph)	Actual Thermometer Reading (°F)											
	50	40	30	20	10	0	−10	−20	−30	−40	−50	−60
	Equivalent Temperature (°F)											
Calm	50	40	30	20	10	0	−10	−20	−30	−40	−50	−60
5	48	37	27	16	6	−5	−15	−26	−36	−47	−57	−68
10	40	28	16	3	−9	−21	−33	−46	−58	−70	−83	−95
15	36	22	9	−5	−18	−32	−45	−58	−72	−85	−99	−112
20	32	18	4	−10	−25	−39	−53	−67	−82	−96	−110	−124
25	30	15	0	−15	−29	−44	−59	−74	−89	−104	−118	−133
30	25	13	−2	−18	−33	−48	−63	−79	−94	−109	−125	−140
35	27	11	−4	−20	−35	−51	−67	−82	−98	−113	−129	−145
40	26	10	−6	−21	−37	−53	−69	−85	−101	−117	−132	−148

(Wind speeds greater than 40 mph have little additional effect.)	**Little danger.** (In less than 5 hours with dry skin. Greatest hazard from false sense of security.)	**Increasing danger.** (Exposed flesh may freeze within 1 minute.)	**Great danger.** (Flesh may freeze within 30 seconds.)

HEAT-RELATED EMERGENCIES

Heat illnesses include a range of disorders. Some of them are common, but only heatstroke is life threatening. Untreated heatstroke victims always die.

Heat Cramps

Heat cramps are painful muscular spasms that happen suddenly. They usually involve the muscles in the back of the leg (calf and hamstring muscles) or the abdominal muscles. They tend to occur during or after exertion.

Heat Exhaustion

Heat exhaustion is characterized by heavy perspiration with normal or slightly above normal body temperatures. It is caused by water depletion, salt depletion, or both. Heat exhaustion affects workers and athletes who do not drink enough fluids while working or exercising in hot environments. Symptoms include severe thirst, fatigue, headache, nausea, vomiting, and sometimes diarrhea. The affected person often mistakenly believes that he or she has the flu. Uncontrolled heat exhaustion can evolve into heatstroke.

Heatstroke

Two types of heatstroke exist: classic and exertional. Classic heatstroke, also known as the "slow cooker," may take days to develop. It is often seen during summer heat waves, and typically affects poor, elderly, chronically ill, alcoholic, or obese persons. (Classic heatstroke victims are not sweating.) Because the elderly are frequently afflicted, this type of heatstroke has a 50% death rate even with medical care. It results from a combination of a hot environment and dehydration. Exertional heatstroke is also more common in the summer. It is frequently seen in athletes, laborers, and military personnel. This type of heatstroke is known as the "fast cooker." It affects healthy, active individuals who are working or playing strenuously in a warm environment. Because its rapid onset does not allow enough time for severe dehydration to occur, 50% of exertional heatstroke victims usually are sweating.

There are several ways to tell the difference between heat exhaustion and heatstroke:

- If the victim's body feels extremely hot when touched, suspect heatstroke.

- Altered mental status (behavior) occurs with heatstroke, ranging from slight confusion and disorientation to coma. Between those extreme conditions, victims usually become irrational, agitated, or even aggressive, and may have seizures.

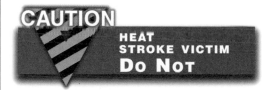

CAUTION

HEAT STROKE VICTIM
DO NOT

- delay initiating cooling while waiting for an ambulance. The longer the delay, the greater the risk of tissue damage and prolonged hospitalization.

- continue cooling after the victim's mental status has improved. Unnecessary cooling could lead to hypothermia.

- use rubbing alcohol to cool the skin. It can be absorbed into the blood and cause alcohol poisoning. Also, the vapors are a potential fire hazard.

....

Less serious

heat illnesses

include heat

syncope (fainting),

heat edema

(swelling),

and prickly

heat (itching).

....

- In severe heatstroke, the victim can go into a coma in less than an hour. The longer a coma lasts, the lower the chance for survival.
- Rectal temperature can also distinguish heatstroke from heat exhaustion, although obtaining this is usually not practical. A responsive heatstroke victim might not cooperate, taking a rectal temperature can be embarrassing to both victim and rescuer, and rectal thermometers are seldom available.

Other Heat Illnesses

Less serious heat illnesses include heat syncope (fainting), heat edema (swelling), and prickly heat (itching).

- Heat syncope, in which a person becomes dizzy or faints after exposure to high temperatures, is a self-resolving condition. Victims should lie down in a cool place and, if not nauseated, drink water.
- Heat edema, which is also a self-resolving condition, causes the ankles and feet to swell from heat exposure. It is more common in women who are unacclimatized to a hot climate. It is related to salt and water retention, and tends to disappear after acclimatization. Wearing support stockings and elevating the legs may help to reduce the swelling.
- Prickly heat, also known as a heat rash, is an itchy rash that develops because of unevaporated moisture on skin wet from sweating. Treat by drying and cooling the skin.

Care for Heat Illnesses

Heat Cramps To relieve heat cramps (it may take several hours), follow these steps:

1. Rest in a cool place.
2. Drink lightly salted cool water (dissolve 1/4 teaspoon salt in a quart of water) or a commercial sports drink.
3. Stretch the cramped calf muscle. Also, try an acupressure method: pinch the upper lip just below the nose.

Heat Exhaustion To relieve heat exhaustion, follow these steps:

1. Move the victim immediately out of the heat to a cool place.
2. Give cool liquids, adding electrolytes (lightly salted water or a commercial sports drink) if plain water does not improve

HEAT-RELATED EMERGENCIES

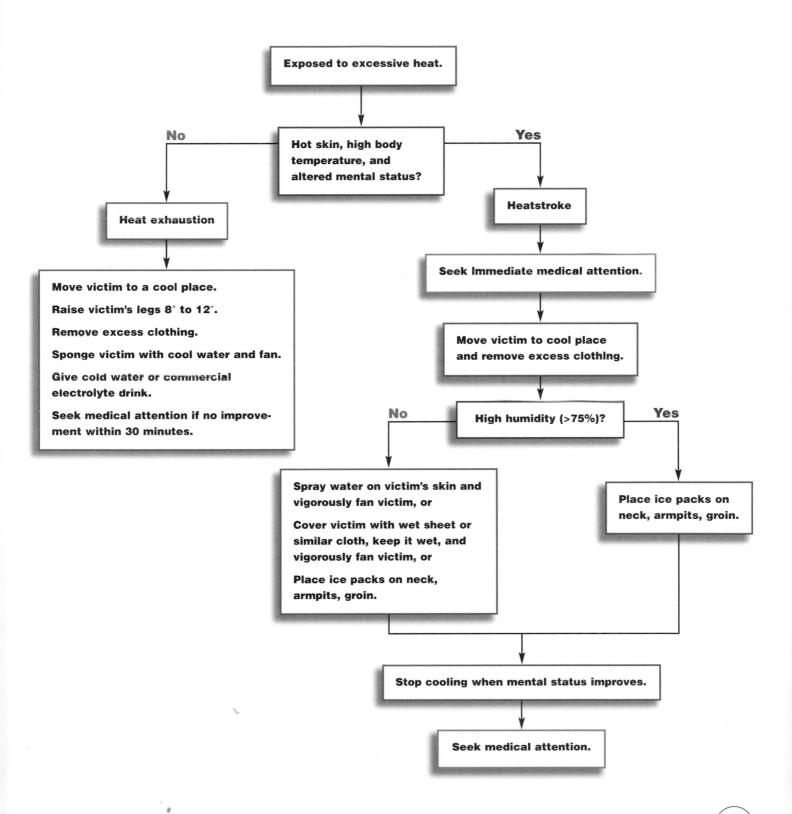

Exposed to excessive heat.

No ← Hot skin, high body temperature, and altered mental status? → **Yes**

Heat exhaustion

Move victim to a cool place.

Raise victim's legs 8″ to 12″.

Remove excess clothing.

Sponge victim with cool water and fan.

Give cold water or commercial electrolyte drink.

Seek medical attention if no improvement within 30 minutes.

Heatstroke

Seek immediate medical attention.

Move victim to cool place and remove excess clothing.

No ← High humidity (>75%)? → **Yes**

Spray water on victim's skin and vigorously fan victim, or

Cover victim with wet sheet or similar cloth, keep it wet, and vigorously fan victim, or

Place ice packs on neck, armpits, groin.

Place ice packs on neck, armpits, groin.

Stop cooling when mental status improves.

Seek medical attention.

Heatstroke

is a medical

emergency

and must be

treated rapidly!

the victim's condition in 20 minutes. Do not give salt tablets; they can irritate the stomach and cause nausea and vomiting.

3. Raise the victim's legs 8″ to 12″ (keep the legs straight).

4. Remove excess clothing.

5. Sponge with cool water and fan the victim.

6. If no improvement is seen within 30 minutes, seek medical attention.

Heatstroke Heatstroke is a medical emergency and must be treated rapidly! Every minute of delay increases the likelihood of serious complications or death.

1. Seek immediate medical attention, even if the victim seems to be recovering.

2. Move the victim immediately out of the heat to a cool place.

3. Remove clothing down to the victim's underwear.

4. Keep the victim's head and shoulders slightly elevated.

5. The only way to prevent damage to the body is to cool the victim quickly by any means possible. Cooling methods include the following:

   • Spraying the victim with water and then fanning. The water droplets act as artificial sweat and cool through evaporation. This method is effective in low-humidity (less than 75%) conditions.

   • Ice bags placed against the large veins in the groin, armpits, and sides of the neck cool the body regardless of humidity.

HOW HOT IT FEELS

Under normal conditions, temperature and humidity are the most important elements influencing body comfort. The Heat Index compiled by the National Weather Service lists apparent temperatures—how hot it feels at various combinations of temperature and humidity.

Relative Humidity, %	Air Temperature, °F										
	70	75	80	85	90	95	100	105	110	115	120
	Apparent Temperature, °F										
0	64	69	73	78	83	87	91	95	99	103	107
10	65	70	75	80	85	90	95	100	105	111	116
20	66	72	77	82	87	93	99	105	112	120	130
30	67	73	78	84	90	96	104	113	123	135	148
40	68	74	79	86	93	101	110	123	137	151	
50	69	75	81	88	96	107	120	135	150		
60	70	76	82	90	100	114	132	149			
70	70	77	85	93	106	124	144				
80	71	78	86	97	113	136					
90	71	79	88	102	122						
100	72	80	91	108							

Above 130°F = heatstroke imminent
105°–130°F = heat exhaustion and heat cramps likely; heatstroke with long exposure and activity
90°–105°F = heat exhaustion and heat cramps with long exposure and activity
80°–90°F = fatigue during exposure and activity

Source: National Weather Service.

fyi

Environmental

extremes can

result in cold-

and heat-related

emergencies

if precautions

are not taken to

maintain normal

skin and body

temperatures.

SUMMARY

Environmental extremes can result in cold- and heat-related emergencies if precautions are not taken to maintain normal skin and body temperatures. Remember that wind increases the effects of cold and humidity increases the effects of heat.

Frostbite is the freezing of skin and possibly the flesh beneath. Deep frostbite can be serious and result in the loss of a body part. Medical attention should be sought immediately. If medical attention will be delayed, the frostbitten part can be rewarmed in warm water and then protected from contact.

Hypothermia is a life-threatening condition that results when the body's core temperature falls below 95°F (35°C). Bring the victim in from the cold, remove wet clothing, and cover the victim with blankets. Call the EMS immediately, and monitor the ABCs.

Heat illnesses include heat cramps, heat exhaustion, and heatstroke. For heat cramps, rest in a cool place, drink lightly salted water, and stretch the muscle. For heat exhaustion, move the victim to a cool place, remove excess clothing, give cool liquid, and sponge the victim with cool water and a fan. For heatstroke, which is a medical emergency requiring immediate action, move the victim to a cool place, remove clothing while maintaining modesty, elevate the head and shoulders, and cool the victim by any means available. For heatstroke, call EMS immediately.

REVIEW QUESTIONS

Frostbite

Directions: Circle Yes if you agree with the statement, and circle No if you disagree.

Yes   No   1. Rub or massage to rewarm a frostbitten part.

Yes   No   2. Frostbite damage becomes more severe if the affected area is thawed and then refrozen.

Yes   No   3. It's best to rewarm a frostbitten part by using warm water.

Yes   No   4. Placing frostbitten hands in another person's armpits is the best rewarming method.

Yes   No   5. When near a hospital, it's best to let medical personnel thaw the frostbitten part.

Scenario 1. In subfreezing temperatures during a snowstorm, you find a stalled truck on a little-used road. Inside the truck is an elderly man. He tells you that his truck is out of gasoline and that when he tried to refill the truck's gas tank, he dropped the gas can and some of the gasoline spilled on his hands. He has been stranded for over 3 hours. The man complains of numb fingers and cold feet. He did not know about a cabin about a quarter of mile away. What should you do?

_____

_____

_____

Scenario 2. An 18-year-old has been in the woods in below freezing temperatures for most of the afternoon. She complains that her toes are numb. You find that they look grayish-blue and feel hard and frozen. What should you do?

_____

_____

_____

Hypothermia

Yes   No   1. Add insulation (blankets) around and under the victim.

Yes   No   2. Replace wet clothing with dry clothing.

Yes   No   3. Shivering is sufficient to rewarm a victim of mild hypothermia.

Yes   No   4. For mild hypothermia, applying chemical heat packs or using a rescuer's body heat are preferred methods of rewarming a victim.

Yes No 5. Victims of severe hypothermia should be transported to a hospital for rewarming.

Yes No 6. Check a severe hypothermic victim's pulse for at least 30 to 45 seconds.

Scenario 3. It is a cold winter day, and you feel the need to check on your 80-year-old grandfather, who lives alone. As you enter his home, you notice that it is not much warmer inside the house than it is outside. You find your grandfather wrapped in a blanket lying on top of his bed. You speak to him, but you get only mumbling. He is shivering severely. What should you do?

_____

_____

_____

Scenario 4. A 50-year-old woman has fallen through the ice of a local pond during her attempt to rescue a dog. Several bystanders have formed a human chain and have pulled her to safety. She is awake and has cold, pale skin. She has intense, uncontrollable shivering. What should you do?

_____

_____

_____

Heat-Related Emergencies

Yes No 1. For heat cramps, stretch a cramped leg muscle.

Yes No 2. Salt tablets should be given to victims suffering from heat illnesses.

Yes No 3. Move heat illness victims out of the heat to a cool place.

Yes No 4. Heat exhaustion victims need immediate medical attention because it's a life-threatening condition.

Yes No 5. Heatstroke victims need immediate cooling by any means possible.

Yes No 6. Apply rubbing alcohol on a heatstroke victim's skin for cooling.

Yes No 7. In high-humidity conditions, wet down or spray and fan the heatstroke victim.

Yes No 8. In low-humidity conditions, only cold or ice packs applied to the neck, armpits, and groin will work well to cool a heatstroke victim.

Scenario 5. On your vacation, you spend a day at a large amusement park. It is an extremely hot and humid day. During the afternoon, you decide to rest and watch one of the special shows. Soon after you have been seated, an elderly man in front of you suddenly falls forward out of his seat. When you reach him, his wife reports that they have been walking around the park practically all day without stopping. His skin feels very hot and dry, and he is unresponsive. What should you do?

_____

_____

_____

Scenario 6. A college student's summer job is landscaping and involves mowing lawns for various companies in an industrial park. She is sweating heavily on a very hot, humid day. She complains about being very thirsty and nauseated and says that she has a headache. What should you do?

_____

_____

_____

How did you do?

Frostbite

1. No; 2. Yes; 3. Yes; 4. No; 5. Yes

Hypothermia

1. Yes; 2. Yes; 3. Yes; 4. No; 5. Yes; 6. Yes

Heat-Related Emergencies

1. Yes; 2. No; 3. Yes; 4. No;
5. Yes; 6. No; 7. No; 8. No

FIRST AID LEARNING RESOURCES

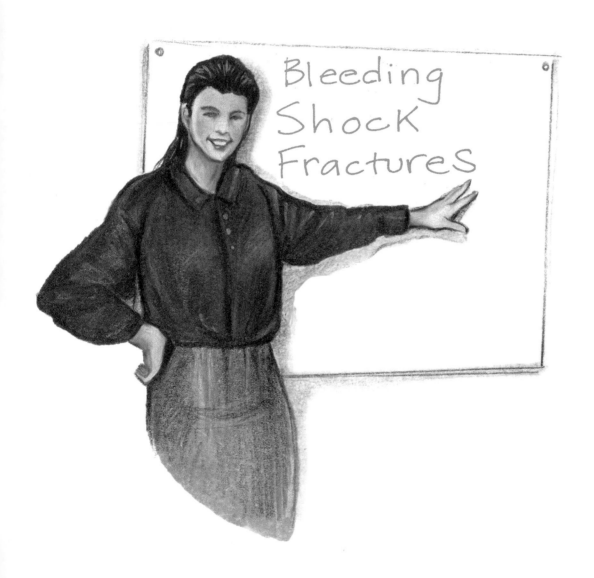

Bleeding
Shock
Fractures

CONTENTS

FREQUENTLY ASKED QUESTIONS ABOUT FIRST AID

Fractures

1. **How can you tell whether an ankle is broken or sprained?**

   An accurate test consists of having the victim try to take four steps, after which the first aider feels for bone tenderness on the victim's ankle bones (knobs). The inability to take four steps and pain when the ankle knob bone is felt indicate a broken ankle.

2. **What is important about how to wrap an injured ankle?**

   A horseshoe-shaped pad is needed around the ankle knob under the elastic bandage. Swelling must be kept out of the joint, since synovial fluid will immobilize a joint and later require extensive therapy for full recovery.

3. **Can an ice bag be applied directly on the skin in treating musculoskeletal injuries?**

   Frostbite can occur when ice is applied directly on the skin for a long period of time. As a precaution, some people suggest placing a dry cloth or towel between the ice pack and the skin to prevent frostbite. However, this method insulates against the cold and reduces the therapeutic effect. Using a wet cloth or towel over the skin to allow more cold through has also been recommended, but the cloth still insulates and is therefore less effective. Therefore, when applying an ice pack, place it directly on the skin for about 30 minutes; this prevents frostbite, and the victim receives the full benefit of the cold on the injury.

Wounds

4. **Are over-the-counter medications effective in treating wounds?**

   A shallow or small wound that does not require sutures can be covered by an antibiotic ointment. Among the recommended ones are polysporin and neosporin. Over-the-counter medications that can prolong healing time and therefore should not be used include Merthiolate (thimerosal), hydrogen peroxide, and tincture of iodine.

5. **How can the pain be relieved from a smashed fingernail with blood accumulating under the nail?**

There are several methods of relieving pain from blood collecting under a nail. The fastest one is melting a hot paper clip through the nail; this procedure is painless.

6. **How much water pressure is needed for effective wound cleaning?**

Irrigating wounds with pressurized water is highly recommended. A minimum water pressure of 5 to 8 pounds per square inch (psi) is needed to effectively clean a wound. Such force occurs with water faucets or in using an irrigation syringe in remote locations. Bulb syringes, pouring, and soaking do not have sufficient force.

7. **When should wounds be stitched (sutured) by a physician?**

Generally, stitches are needed to close a wound when the edges of skin do not fall together and/or when the wound is more than an inch long and is deep. Stitches speed the healing process, lessen the risk of infection, and improve the look of scars.

8. **What is the single most important thing I can do to prevent wound infection?**

Irrigate, irrigate, irrigate. Irrigation with forceful water (minimum of 5 to 8 psi), which can be obtained under a forceful household faucet or with an irrigation syringe, has proven to be the single most important method for lowering the risk of infection in open wounds.

Bites and Stings

9. **How can pit viper snake venom be removed without cutting the victim's skin?**

If you are near a medical facility with antivenin, transport the victim. However, if you are more than 1 hour from a source of antivenin, or for immediate and extensive swelling, a device known as the Extractor™ can remove up to 30% of the venom if it is applied within the first 3 minutes of the bite. It does not require cutting the victim's skin. Not only does cutting the skin expose the first aider to possible bloodborne exposure, but wound infections and increased injuries often result.

10. What is the first aid for stinging nettle?

Whereas about 50% of people in North America are sensitive to poison ivy, oak, and sumac, everyone can be affected by the stinging nettle. First aid includes washing the exposed area with soap and water; applying a cold, wet pack, calamine lotion, or hydrocortisone cream (1%); and taking an over-the-counter antihistamine.

11. What is the best method for removing an embedded tick?

Use tweezers and avoid useless methods such as petroleum jelly, rubbing alcohol, a hot match, and fingernail polish. Grasp the tick as close to the skin as possible and lift the tick up until it pulls the skin up. Hold it in this position for about 30 seconds, when the tick will usually release itself. Don't jerk or twist the tick.

12. How should a bee's stinger be removed?

Care should be taken not to squeeze the stinger, because if the venom sac is still attached, this maneuver may inject more venom. Rather, the stinger should be scraped off the victim as soon as possible to minimize the amount of venom that is injected.

13. What should be done when someone is bitten by a dog?

Dog bites are very common in the United States; an estimated 4.5 million people are bitten annually. Cleanse bite wounds with lots of soap and water for at least 15 minutes. Afterward, flush the wound with forceful water from a faucet. Apply pressure with a sterile dressing to control bleeding. Report the incident to the proper authority in your community (eg, police, animal control officer). Seek medical advice about wound care involving stitches. If rabies may be involved, promptly seek the advice of a physician, the Department of Health, or the local animal control officer.

Fainting

14. Should smelling salts or ammonia inhalant capsules be used on a person who has fainted?

No, and neither should you splash water on the person's face or slap the victim. Inhalants can adversely affect the victim by causing an asthma attack or other complications.

Poisoning

15. Why should a poisoned victim be kept on his or her left side?

Placing the victim on his or her left side positions the end of the stomach where it enters the small intestine (pylorus) straight up. Gravity will delay (by as much as 2 hours) the advancement of the poison into the small intestine, where absorption into the victim's circulatory system is faster and therefore more dangerous.

16. What is the role of syrup of ipecac in treating ingested poisoning?

Although syrup of ipecac induces vomiting within 20 to 30 minutes in most people, very little poison is removed. Use of syrup of ipecac also prevents other treatments from being used. Many toxicologists haven't used ipecac in years. Although ipecac is becoming less popular, activated charcoal should be considered for prehospital situations but is seldom found. Always call the Poison Control Center for advice on what to do before treating poisoning victims.

Heat and Cold Emergencies

17. What are the best ways to cool a heatstroke victim?

One method of cooling a victim suffering from heatstroke, is the "wetting and fanning" method. This method uses evaporation to cool the victim, and works best in low humidity circumstances (under 75%).

18. Why are the traditional methods of rewarming wrong for treating mild hypothermia?

For a victim of mild hypothermia, shivering is the best method of rewarming. Warm water immersion, body-to-body contact, and chemical heating pads all have problems, but primarily they warm the skin, signaling the victim's brain to stop the shivering. Since shivering is the best way of rewarming a mildly hypothermic person, avoid measures that stop it by adding heat to the skin.

19. Why should I know about hypothermia?

Because most places in the United States become cold, wet, or both, hypothermia can occur anywhere. Also, the injured, the sick, the young, and the old are especially susceptible to cold.

20. What is the difference between fever and hyperthermia?

They are caused by different things. Fevers are associated with disease; hyperthermia is related to environmental heat exposure. Fever changes our body's "set point," and we seek a warmer environment (eg, under blankets). Attempts at cooling will cause shivering and discomfort. Hyperthermia is caused by an inability to cool the body, and we seek cooler environments (eg, in shade).

Burn Injuries

21. Why does it take several days to determine how deep a burn injury goes?

Because of blisters, having clothing melted into the skin, or being covered with dirt, it can take several days of wound cleaning before proper assessment can be done.

22. Does it matter whether first aiders estimate the extent of a burn?

Estimating the extent of a burn is necessary for determining proper care. Several methods can be used to determine the extent of a burn, including the "Rule of Nines" and the "Rule of the Palm."

23. What is the "Rule of the Palm"?

This is most useful on small burned areas. The victim's palm represents about 1% of the victim's body surface area. For extensive burns, you can use this method to measure the unburned area and then subtract it from 100%.

24. Can home remedies or ointments be used on burns?

Home remedies on burns have included anything from butter to toothpaste. Unfortunately, these home remedies usually just contaminate the wound, make it impossible to assess the depth of injury, and interfere with appropriate care. The best procedure is to initially cool superficial burns and small (less than 20% of body surface area) partial-thickness burns with cool water until the pain subsides. Afterwards (hours later and over the ensuing days), aloe vera gel can be applied on superficial burns and bacitracin ointment on partial-thickness burns. Ibuprofen can help to relieve the pain and swelling. You need to cover only large partial-thickness and full-thickness burns with a sterile dressing.

25. **Are wet dressings or dry dressings better for major burns?**

    Generally, it is recommended that dry sterile dressings be applied over large burns to prevent further contamination and hypothermia. Cool, moist sterile dressings will stop the burning process, help to hydrate the tissues, and lessen pain. However, the risk of hypothermia is very high, and a damp wound offers a breeding ground for bacteria. Therefore, moist dressings are usually not recommended.

Bleeding

26. **Are tourniquets ever needed to control severe bleeding?**

    A tourniquet is rarely needed to control life-threatening bleeding that cannot be stopped by any other means. A tourniquet can damage nerves and blood vessels and can result in the loss of an arm or leg.

Legal

27. **Am I required to give first aid to anyone I encounter who needs it?**

    Only people who have a "duty to act" are legally required to give first aid either because of employment (eg, paramedic, lifeguard, worksite-designated first aider) or a preexisting relationship (parent to child, driver to passenger). In many cases, a lay first aider might not be legally required to give first aid, but most people believe that, morally, he or she should give it.

28. **How can I avoid a lawsuit resulting from giving first aid?**

    Before giving first aid, get the victim's consent or permission. Then provide good care, be nice to the victim, have witnesses, and afterward, write down what you did and who took over the victim's care.

General

29. **Isn't 911 the universal number for calling the Emergency Medical Service for help?**

    Not necessarily, though 911 is used in most major population centers nationwide, and the vast majority of the population can access the EMS by calling 911. However, in some large geographical areas, predominately rural ones, 911 service is still not available. In these locations, the EMS system is called with a seven-digit telephone number.

30. **What should I do when faced with several people who are injured or ill at the same time?**

When this happens, the first aider must decide which victims should be treated first. Triage is the process of prioritizing victim care on the basis of severity of injury or illness. The intent is to select the victims who are in greatest need of immediate care. You can enlist bystanders to help perform various functions, such as calling the EMS and directing their care of others.

31. **What is the purpose of a physical exam?**

The goal of doing a hands-on physical exam is to identify a victim's injuries. It is done after the initial assessment, which checks for life-threatening conditions. The physical exam is performed by looking and feeling primarily for deformities, open wounds, tenderness, and swelling. You cannot properly care for a victim until you determine what is wrong.

32. **What does "altered mental status" mean?**

This phrase describes the state of awareness between two extremes: normal consciousness and coma. There are a variety of causes, such as alcohol, drugs, epilepsy, insulin reactions, brain trauma, heatstroke, severe hypothermia, poisons, stroke, and many more.

33. **How do I remember all of the first aid skills?**

Remembering skills is impossible without periodically reviewing first aid procedures. Try to set aside time periodically to reread your book. Also, when you hear or read about an injury on television or radio or in the newspaper and you aren't sure what first aid should have been given to the victim, review the procedures in your book. Take another first aid course well before two years are up, since new procedures are constantly being developed and it's a good way to review what you learned previously.

34. Do I have to perform a complete victim assessment for every injured or suddenly ill victim?

No. Check every victim's ABCs (airway, breathing, and circulation) and acquire as much of each victim's SAMPLE history as you can. Performing a complete victim assessment, which includes a head-to-toe physical exam, is crucial for the unresponsive ill and significantly injured victim. However, for the responsive ill person and the nonsignificantly injured victim, the physical exam focuses primarily on the victim's complaint. This is obvious for the majority of injuries, such as sunburns and small cuts.

Glossary of Terms

abandonment The termination of a helping relationship by a first aider without the victim's consent and without replacement care to the victim by qualified medical personnel.

ABCs Airway, Breathing, and Circulation; the first three steps in the examination of any victim; basic life support.

abdomen The large body cavity below the diaphragm and above the pelvis.

abdominal thrusts A method of dislodging food or other material from the throat of a choking victim. Also known as the *Heimlich maneuver.*

abrasion Loss of or damage to the superficial layer of skin after a body part rubs or scrapes across a rough or hard surface.

activated charcoal Powdered charcoal that has been treated to increase its powers of absorption for an ingested poison.

algorithm 1. A visual learning aid that teaches how to make decisions in emergencies. Using a branching, tree-like format, algorithms display conditions, treatment options, and points where decisions must be made. **2.** The process that computer chips in AEDs follow as they analyze the heart rhythm for presence or absence of a shockable rhythm (ventricular fibrillation or pulseless ventricular tachycardia).

allergic reaction A local or general reaction to an allergen, usually characterized by hives or tissue swelling or difficulty in breathing.

amputation Complete removal of an appendage.

anaphylactic shock A rapidly occurring state of collapse caused by hypersensitivity to drugs or other foreign materials (insect venom, certain foods, inhaled allergens); symptoms may include hives, wheezing, tissue edema, bronchospasm, and vascular collapse.

anaphylaxis An exaggerated allergic reaction, usually caused by foreign proteins.

angina A condition in which the heart muscle receives an insufficient blood supply, causing temporary pain in the chest and often in the left arm and shoulder, usually during physical activity or when the patient is emotionally upset.

antivenin An antiserum containing antibodies against reptile or insect venom.

artery A blood vessel that carries blood away from the heart to the various parts of the body.

asthma A condition marked by recurrent attacks of breathing difficulty with wheezing, due to spasmodic constriction of the bronchi, often as a response to allergens or to mucous plugs in the bronchioles.

automated external defibrillator (AED) A restricted medical device that can assess the cardiac rhythm and determine if a shockable rhythm is present. When powered ON, the AED analyzes the rhythm and "advises" the operator to press the SHOCK control if a shockable rhythm is detected.

avulsion An injury that leaves a piece of skin or other tissue either partially or completely torn away from the body.

bandage A material used to hold a dressing in place.

barrier devices Plastic devices that allow a rescuer to provide rescue breathing without touching the victim's mouth or nose. There are two types: *face shields,* which are flexible and mold closely to the face, and *face masks,* which are rigid plastic and increase the distance between the victim and the rescuer.

basic life support Maintenance of the ABCs (Airway, Breathing, and Circulation) without adjunctive equipment.

blood pressure The force or pressure exerted by the heart in pumping blood; the pressure of blood in the arteries.

bloodborne pathogen Virus or other disease organism carried by blood or blood-tinged bodily fluids.

body substance isolation (BSI) An infection control concept and practice that assumes all body fluids are potentially infectious.

brachial artery The main artery of the upper arm; used to check the pulse of an infant.

brain The soft, large mass of nerve tissue that is contained in the skull.

burn An injury caused by heat, electrical current, or a chemical of extreme acidity or alkalinity.

carbon monoxide (CO) A colorless, odorless, and dangerous gas formed by incomplete combustion of carbon; associated especially with the burning of fuels such as wood, kerosene, gasoline, and natural gas.

cardiopulmonary resuscitation (CPR) A series of actions that include assessment of breathing, rescue breathing, assessment of a pulse, and chest compressions. These actions keep oxygen-rich blood flowing to the brain until defibrillation and advanced life support can be started.

cardiovascular Pertaining to the heart and blood vessels, including the major blood vessels that supply blood to the brain.

carotid artery The principal artery found on either side of the neck; used to check the pulse of persons greater than 1 year in age.

circulatory system The heart and blood vessels (arteries, veins, and capillaries).

closed fracture A fracture that does not cause a break in the skin; a simple fracture.

compound fracture A fracture in which the bone ends pierce the skin; an open fracture.

confidentiality Maintaining a victim's privacy by not revealing personal information about the victim, except to medical or other prehospital personnel directly involved in caring for the victim.

consent An agreement by a patient or victim to accept treatment offered as explained by medical personnel or first aiders.

contusion A bruise; an injury that causes a hemorrhage in or beneath the skin but does not break the skin.

coronary arteries Arteries arising from the aorta, circling the surface of the heart, and conducting blood to the heart muscle.

Coronary Care Unit (CCU) An in-hospital specialized facility or emergency mobile unit equipped with monitoring devices, staffed with trained personnel, and designed to treat coronary patients.

coronary occlusion An obstruction or narrowing of one of the coronary arteries that hinders or completely blocks blood flow to part of the heart muscle. See heart attack.

coronary thrombosis Formation of a clot in one of the arteries that conduct blood to the heart muscle. Also known as *coronary occlusion*.

cyanosis A blueness of the skin due to insufficient oxygen in the blood.

defibrillator A restricted medical device that supplies an electric current to the heart to treat ventricular fibrillation. The current is delivered through either adhesive electrode pads that attach to the chest or hand-held metal paddles. Defibrillators can be either automated or manual.

dehydration Loss of water and electrolytes; excessive loss of body water.

depressed fracture A skull fracture in which there is obvious inward deformation of the fragmented bone.

diabetes mellitus A disease marked by a relative lack of insulin production resulting in an unusually high level of glucose in the blood.

dislocation A joint injury resulting in misalignment of the bone ends so that they are no longer in contact.

DOTS The acronym or mnemonic used to remember the signs of injury; Deformity, Open wounds, Tenderness, and Swelling.

dressing A protective covering for a wound; used to stop bleeding and to prevent contamination of the wound.

edema A condition in which fluid escapes from vessels and moves into nearby body tissues causing local or generalized swelling.

electrocution Death caused by the passage of an electrical current through the body.

EMS Emergency medical service.

EMT Emergency medical technician.

fainting A momentary loss of consciousness caused by insufficient blood supply to the brain; also known as *syncope*.

femur The bone that extends from the pelvis to the knee; the longest and largest bone of the body; the thigh bone.

first-degree burn A burn causing only reddening of the outer layer of skin; sunburn is usually a first-degree burn.

fracture A break or rupture in a bone.

frostbite Damage to tissues as a result of prolonged exposure to extreme cold.

glucose Blood sugar.

Good Samaritan laws Laws that protect an individual who voluntarily helps an injured or suddenly ill person from legal liability for any error of omission in rendering good faith emergency medical care.

heart attack A nonspecific term usually referring to complete blockage of a diseased coronary artery by a blood clot, resulting in the death of the heart muscle supplied by that artery. Also known more specifically as *myocardial infarction.*

hemorrhage Abnormally large amount of bleeding.

high blood pressure (hypertension) Persistent elevation of blood pressure above the normal range.

hyperglycemia An abnormally increased concentration of sugar in the blood.

hyperthermia An abnormally increased body temperature.

hypoglycemia An abnormally diminished concentration of sugar in the blood; insulin shock.

hypothermia Decreased body temperature.

hypoxia A low oxygen content in the blood; lack of oxygen in inspired air.

implied consent An assumed consent given by an unconscious adult when emergency lifesaving treatment is required.

infectious disease A communicable disease.

informed consent Consent given by a mentally competent adult who understands what the treatment will involve; it can also be given by the parent or guardian of a child, as defined by the state, or for a mentally incompetent adult.

insulin A hormone secreted by the pancreas; essential for maintaining a normal level of blood sugar.

laceration A wound made by tearing or cutting of body tissues.

log roll A method for placing a person on a carrying device, usually a long spineboard or a flat litter; the person is rolled onto his or her side, then back onto the litter.

mouth-to-mask ventilation Rescue breathing through a device that eliminates direct mouth-to-mouth contact between rescuer and victim.

mouth-to-mouth ventilation The preferred emergency method of artificial ventilation when adjuncts are not available.

myocardial infarction See heart attack.

myocardium Heart muscle.

nervous system The brain, spinal cord, and all nerves of the body.

nitroglycerin Drug that causes dilation of blood vessels; often used in the treatment of angina.

occluded artery One in which blood flow has been impaired by a blockage.

open fracture A fracture in which the skin is open; a compound fracture.

oxygen A colorless, odorless, tasteless gas that is essential to life and that makes up 21% of the atmosphere; chemical formula O_2.

palpation The act of palpating; the act of feeling with the hands for the purpose of determining the consistency of the part beneath, or using your fingers to feel for a pulse.

palpitation A sensation felt under the left breast when the heart skips a beat.

personal protective equipment (PPE) Specialized clothing or equipment worn for protection against potentially infectious blood- or air-borne hazards.

poison Substance whose chemical action could damage structures or impair functions when introduced into the body in a relatively small amount.

pulmonary Pertaining to the lungs.

pupil The small opening in the center of the iris of the eye.

rabies An acute viral infection of the central nervous system, transmitted by the bite of a rabid animal.

radial artery One of the major arteries of the forearm; the pulse in that artery can be felt in the wrist at the base of the thumb.

recovery position Position used to help maintain a clear airway in a victim with a decreased level of consciousness who has not had traumatic injuries and is breathing on his or her own.

respiration The act of breathing; the exchange of oxygen and carbon dioxide in the tissues and lungs.

respiratory system The system of organs that controls the inspiration of oxygen and the expiration of carbon dioxide.

resuscitation The act of reviving an unconscious victim.

RICE The acronym for the first aid procedures of Rest, Ice, Compression, and Elevation for bone, joint, and muscle injuries.

second-degree burn A burn extending through the outer layer of skin, causing blisters and edema; a scald is usually a second-degree burn.

seizure A sudden attack or recurrence of a disease; a convulsion; an attack of epilepsy.

shock A state of inadequate tissue perfusion that may be a result of heart failure (cardiogenic shock), blood loss or internal bleeding (hypovolemic shock), reflexive widening of the blood vessels (neurogenic shock), or any combination of these.

sign Any objective evidence or physical manifestation of a disease.

simple fracture A fracture in which the skin is not broken; a closed fracture.

skeleton The hard, bony structure that forms the main support of the body.

skin The outer covering of the body, consisting of an inner layer (the dermis) and an outer layer (the epidermis); the largest organ of the body, it contains various sensory and regulatory mechanisms.

splint Any support used to immobilize a fracture or to restrict movement of a part.

sprain Trauma to a joint that injures the ligaments.

strain An injury to a muscle caused by a violent contraction or an excessive, forcible stretching.

stroke A sudden onset of weakness or paralysis on one side of the body (such as the hand, arm, or leg) caused by an insufficient supply of blood to part of the brain. A stroke can also affect balance, coordination, speech, or vision. Older terms for stroke are apoplexy, cerebrovascular accident, and cerebral vascular accident.

symptom A subjective sensation or awareness of a disturbance in one's bodily functions.

syncope Fainting; a brief period of unconsciousness.

tetanus An infectious disease caused by the bacterium *Clostridium tetani* that is usually introduced through a wound, characterized by extreme body rigidity and spasms of voluntary body muscles.

third-degree burn A burn extending through all layers of skin, at times through muscle or connective tissue, having a white, leathery look and lacking sensation; grafting is more often necessary with a third-degree burn; a flame burn is usually third-degree.

tourniquet A constrictive device used on the extremities to impede venous blood return to the heart or to obstruct arterial blood flow to the extremities.

unconscious Without awareness; comatose.

vagina The canal in the female extending from the uterus to the vulva; the birth canal.

vascular Pertaining to the blood vessels.

vein Any one of a series of vessels of the cardiovascular system that carry blood from various parts of the body back to the heart.

venom A poison, usually derived from reptiles or insects.

ventricular fibrillation (VF) A chaotic, uncoordinated quivering of the cardiac muscle that prevents effective cardiac contractions. VF causes cardiac arrest; biological death follows within minutes if VF is not defibrillated. VF can be removed only by "stunning" the heart with a strong electric shock (defibrillation).

ventricular tachycardia (VT or V-Tach) An abnormal heart rhythm causing the heart to beat too fast to pump blood effectively. Depending on the severity, a pulse may or may not be felt.

wound A soft tissue injury, generally non–life-threatening, that can range from a minor bruise to a major amputation.